COMPETENCY MANUAL
TO ACCOMPANY DELMAR'S

COMPREHENSIVE MEDICAL ASSISTING

Administrative and Clinical Competencies

Fifth Edition

Barbara M. Dahl, CMA (AAMA), CPC
Program Director, Retired
Whatcom Community College
Bellingham, WA

Julie A. Morris, RN, BSN, CBCS, CCMA, CMAA
Director of Career Services
Medtech College
Atlanta, GA

Angela P. Rein, RMA (AMT), AS, BSHM, CPC, MAHS, CPC-H
Medical Program Director
Vatterott College–Online Division
St. Louis, MO

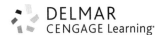

DELMAR
CENGAGE Learning

Australia • Brazil • Japan • Korea • Mexico • Singapore • Spain • United Kingdom • United States

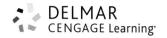

Competency Manual to Accompany Delmar's Comprehensive Medical Assisting: Administrative and Clinical Competencies, Fifth Edition
Barbara M. Dahl, Julie A. Morris, Angela P. Rein

Vice President, Careers & Computing: Dave Garza

Publisher: Stephen Helba

Executive Editor: Rhonda Dearborn

Director, Development–Career and Computing: Marah Bellegarde

Product Development Manager: Juliet Steiner

Product Manager: Lauren Whalen

Editorial Assistant: Courtney Cozzy

Executive Brand Manager: Wendy Mapstone

Senior Market Development Manager: Nancy Bradshaw

Senior Production Director: Wendy Troeger

Production Manager: Andrew Crouth

Content Project Manager: Brooke Greenhouse

Senior Art Director: Jack Pendleton

Technology Project Manager: Brian Davis

Media Editor: William Overocker

Cover image(s): www.Shutterstock.com

For product information and technology assistance, contact us at
Cengage Learning Customer & Sales Support, 1-800-354-9706
For permission to use material from this text or product,
submit all requests online at **www.cengage.com/permissions.**
Further permissions questions can be e-mailed to
permissionrequest@cengage.com

Library of Congress Control Number: 2013933619

ISBN-13: 978-1-133-60322-1

Delmar
5 Maxwell Drive
Clifton Park, NY 12065-2919
USA

Cengage Learning is a leading provider of customized learning solutions with office locations around the globe, including Singapore, the United Kingdom, Australia, Mexico, Brazil, and Japan. Locate your local office at: **www.cengage.com/global**

Cengage Learning products are represented in Canada by Nelson Education, Ltd.

To learn more about Cengage Learning, visit **www.cengage.com**

Purchase any of our products at your local college store or at our preferred online store **www.cengagebrain.com**

Notice to the Reader

Printed in the United States of America
1 2 3 4 5 6 7 16 15 14 13

CONTENTS

The Competency Assessment Checklists are designed to set criteria or standards that should be observed while a specific procedure is being performed. The procedural steps are listed in the textbook, and the Competency Assessment Checklist scoring reflects the major milestones, or outcomes, of following the specific procedural steps. As you perform each procedure, the evaluation section of this checklist can be used to judge your performance. The instructor will use this checklist to evaluate your competency in performing this skill. Your instructor may combine some Competencies and adjust others to suit individual program schedules. These checklists are provided for guidance.

A master Competency Assessment Tracking Sheet is also provided for you prior to this section of the workbook to use as an overview of all Competency Assessment Checklists. This tracking sheet can serve as a table of contents for all checklists, as well as a guide to easily view your performance on the assessment checklists.

The format of the Competency Assessment Checklists is designed to provide specific conditions, standards, milestone steps, and evaluation and documentation sections for essential skills necessary for an entry-level medical assistant. Many of the checklists include Competency Assessment information that provides specific details needed in order to complete a particular procedure. The Competency Assessment Checklists associated with the Medical Office Simulation Software (MOSS) 2.0 procedures also include step-by-step case studies with screen shots that allow you to check your work.

Forms are included in this Competency Manual and are also provided on the Premium Website for use with the Competency Assessment Checklists as you complete the procedures in your textbook. To access the Premium Website, use the instructions on the tear-out Access Card in your book to create your account and log in.

Competency Assessment Tracking Sheet

Student Name: _____

Procedure Number and Title	Date Assessment Completed and Competency Achieved			
	Date/Initials	Date/Initials	Date/Initials	Date/Initials
EXAMPLE: 22-1 Medical Asepsis Hand Wash (Hand Hygiene)	**2/23/XX DF**	**3/15/XX SL**	**4/20/XX SP**	**5/1/XX JP**
5-1 Identifying Community Resources				
9-1 Control of Bleeding				
9-2 Applying an Arm Splint				
10-1 Develop a Personal and/or Employee Safety Plan in Case of a Disaster				
10-2 Demonstrate Proper Use of a Fire Extinguisher				
11-1 Perform Routine Maintenance of Office Computers and Ancillary Equipment with Documentation				
11-2 Software Installation				
11-3 Hardware Installation				
12-1 Answering and Screening Incoming Calls				
12-2 Taking a Telephone Message				
12-3 Calling a Pharmacy to Refill an Authorized Prescription				
12-4 Handling Problem Calls				
12-5 Preparing, Sending, and Receiving a Fax				
13-1 Establishing the Appointment Matrix in a Paper System				
13-2 Establishing the Appointment Matrix Using Medical Office Simulation Software (MOSS)				
13-3 Making an Appointment Using Paper Scheduling				
13-4 Making an Appointment Using Medical Office Simulation Software (MOSS)				
13-5 Checking in Patients in a Paper System				
13-6 Checking in Patients Using Medical Office Simulation Software (MOSS)				

Procedure Number and Title	Date Assessment Completed and Competency Achieved			
	Date/Initials	Date/Initials	Date/Initials	Date/Initials
13-7 Cancelling and Rescheduling Procedures Using Paper Scheduling				
13-8 Cancelling a Patient Appointment Using MOSS				
13-9 Rescheduling a Patient Appointment Using Medical Office Simulation Software (MOSS)				
13-10 Scheduling Inpatient and Outpatient Admissions and Procedures				
14-1 Establishing a Paper Medical Chart for a New Patient				
14-2 Registering a New Patient Using Medical Office Simulation Software (MOSS)				
14-3 Correcting a Paper Medical Record				
14-4 Updating Patient Registration Information Using Medical Office Simulation Software (MOSS)				
14-5 Steps for Manual Filing with an Alphabetic System				
14-6 Steps for Manual Filing with a Numeric System				
14-7 Steps for Manual Filing with a Subject Filing System				
15-1 Preparing and Composing Business Correspondence Using All Components (Computerized Approach)				
15-2 Addressing Envelopes According to United States Postal Service Regulations				
15-3 Folding Letters for Standard Envelopes				
15-4 Creating a Mass Mailing Using Mail Merge				
15-5 Preparing Outgoing Mail According to United States Postal Service Regulations				
16-1 Transcribe Medical Referral Letters Using Medical Office Simulation Software (MOSS)				

Procedure Number and Title	Date Assessment Completed and Competency Achieved			
	Date/Initials	Date/Initials	Date/Initials	Date/Initials
17-1 Applying Managed Care Policies and Procedures				
17-2 Screening for Insurance				
17-3 Verify Insurance Eligibility Using Medical Office Simulation Software (MOSS)				
17-4 Obtaining Referrals and Authorizations				
17-5 Computing the Medicare Fee Schedule				
18-1 Current Procedural Terminology Coding				
18-2 International Classification of Diseases, 9th Revision, Clinical Modification Coding				
18-3 Applying Third-Party Guidelines				
18-4 Completing a Medicare CMS-1500 (08-05) Claim Form				
19-1 Recording/Posting Charges, Payments, and Adjustments in a Manual System				
19-2 Balancing Day Sheets in a Manual System				
19-3 Posting Procedure Charges and Payments Using Medical Office Simulation Software (MOSS)				
19-4 Insurance Billing Using Medical Office Simulation Software (MOSS)				
19-5 Posting Insurance Payments and Adjustments Using Medical Office Simulation Software (MOSS)				
19-6 Processing Credit Balances and Refunds Using Medical Office Simulation Software (MOSS)				
19-7 Preparing a Deposit				
19-8 Recording a Nonsufficient Funds Check in a Manual System				
19-9 Writing a Check				
19-10 Reconciling a Bank Statement				
19-11 Establishing and Maintaining a Petty Cash Fund				

Procedure Number and Title	Date Assessment Completed and Competency Achieved			
	Date/Initials	Date/Initials	Date/Initials	Date/Initials
20-1 Explaining Fees in the First Telephone Interview				
20-2 Prepare Itemized Patient Accounts for Billing in a Manual System				
20-3 Identifying Accounts Receivable Using Medical Office Simulation Software (MOSS)				
20-4 Preparing Itemized Patient Statements Using Medical Office Simulation Software (MOSS)				
20-5 Preparing Collection Letters Using Medical Office Simulation Software (MOSS)				
20-6 Posting Non-Sufficient Fund (NSF) Checks Using Medical Office Simulation Software (MOSS)				
20-7 Post/Record Collection Agency Adjustments in a Manual System				
20-8 Post/Record Collection Agency Adjustments Using Medical Office Simulation Software (MOSS)				
21-1 Preparing Accounts Receivable Trial Balance in a Manual System				
21-2 Preparing Accounts Receivable Trial Balance Using Medical Office Simulation Software (MOSS)				
22-1 Medical Asepsis Hand Wash (Hand Hygiene)				
22-2 Correct Use of Alcohol-Based Hand Rubs (ABHR)				
22-3 Removing Contaminated Gloves				
22-4 Transmission-Based Precautions: Donning a Gown, Mask, Gloves, and Cap (Isolation Technique)				
22-5 Sanitization of Instruments				
23-1 Taking a Medical History for a Paper Medical Record				
24-1 Measuring an Oral Temperature Using an Electronic Thermometer				
24-2 Measuring an Aural Temperature Using a Tympanic Thermometer				

Procedure Number and Title	Date Assessment Completed and Competency Achieved			
	Date/Initials	Date/Initials	Date/Initials	Date/Initials
24-3 Measuring a Temperature Using a Temporal Artery (TA) Thermometer				
24-4 Measuring a Rectal Temperature Using a Digital Thermometer				
24-5 Measuring an Axillary Temperature				
24-6 Measuring an Oral Temperature Using a Disposable Oral Strip Thermometer				
24-7 Measuring a Radial Pulse				
24-8 Taking an Apical Pulse				
24-9 Measuring the Respiration Rate				
24-10 Measuring Blood Pressure				
24-11 Measuring Height				
24-12 Measuring Adult Weight				
25-1 Assisting with a Complete Physical Examination				
26-1 Assisting with Routine Prenatal Visits				
26-2 Assisting with Pelvic Examination and Pap Test (Conventional and ThinPrep® Methods)				
26-3 Assisting with Insertion of an Intrauterine Device (IUD)				
26-4 Assisting with Insertion of a Hormonal Contraceptive (Implanon®)				
26-5 Wet Prep/Wet Mount and Potassium Hydroxide (KOH) Prep				
26-6 Amplified DNA ProbeTec Test for Chlamydia and Gonorrhea				
27-1 Administration of a Vaccine				
27-2 Maintaining Immunization Records				
27-3 Measuring the Infant: Weight, Length, and Head and Chest Circumference				
27-4 Taking an Infant's Rectal Temperature with a Digital Thermometer				

Procedure Number and Title	Date Assessment Completed and Competency Achieved			
	Date/Initials	Date/Initials	Date/Initials	Date/Initials
27-5 Taking an Apical Pulse on an Infant				
27-6 Measuring Infant's Respiratory Rate				
27-7 Obtaining a Urine Specimen from an Infant or Young Child				
28-1 Instructing Patient in Testicular Self-Examination				
30-1 Assisting the Physician during a Lumbar Puncture or Cerebrospinal Fluid Aspiration				
30-2 Assisting the Provider with a Neurologic Screening Examination				
30-3 Performing Visual Acuity Testing Using a Snellen Chart				
30-4 Measuring Near Visual Acuity				
30-5 Testing Color Vision Using the Ishihara Plates				
30-6 Performing Eye Instillation				
30-7 Performing Eye Patch Dressing Application				
30-8 Performing Eye Irrigation				
30-9 Performing Ear Irrigation				
30-10 Assisting with Audiometry				
30-11 Performing Ear Instillation				
30-12 Assisting with Nasal Examination				
30-13 Cautery Treatment of Epistaxis				
30-14 Performing Nasal Instillation				
30-15 Administer Oxygen by Nasal Cannula for Minor Respiratory Distress				
30-16 Instructing Patient in Use of Metered Dose Inhaler				
30-17 Spirometry				
30-18 Pulse Oximetry				
30-19 Assisting with Plaster Cast Application				
30-20 Assisting with Cast Removal				

Procedure Number and Title	Date Assessment Completed and Competency Achieved			
	Date/Initials	Date/Initials	Date/Initials	Date/Initials
30-21 Fecal Occult Blood Test				
30-22 Urinary Catheterization of a Male Patient				
30-23 Urinary Catheterization of a Female Patient				
31-1 Applying Sterile Gloves				
31-2 Chemical "Cold" Sterilization of Endoscopes				
31-3 Preparing Instruments for Sterilization in an Autoclave				
31-4 Sterilization of Instruments (Autoclave)				
31-5 Setting Up and Covering a Sterile Field				
31-6 Opening Sterile Packages of Instruments and Supplies and Applying Them to a Sterile Field				
31-7 Pouring a Sterile Solution into a Cup on a Sterile Field				
31-8 Assisting with Office/Ambulatory Surgery				
31-9 Dressing Change				
31-10 Wound Irrigation				
31-11 Preparation of Patient's Skin before Surgery				
31-12 Suturing of Laceration or Incision Repair				
31-13 Sebaceous Cyst Excision				
31-14 Incision and Drainage of Localized Infection				
31-15 Aspiration of Joint Fluid				
31-16 Hemorrhoid Thrombectomy				
31-17 Suture/Staple Removal				
31-18 Application of Sterile Adhesive Skin Closure Strips				
33-1 Transferring Patient from Wheelchair to Examination Table				
33-2 Transferring Patient from Examination Table to Wheelchair				

Procedure Number and Title	Date Assessment Completed and Competency Achieved			
	Date/Initials	Date/Initials	Date/Initials	Date/Initials
33-3 Assisting the Patient to Stand and Walk				
33-4 Care of the Falling Patient				
33-5 Assisting a Patient to Ambulate with a Walker				
33-6 Teaching the Patient to Ambulate with Crutches				
33-7 Assisting a Patient to Ambulate with a Cane				
34-1 Provide Instruction for Health Maintenance and Disease Prevention				
35-1 Proper Disposal of Expired Medications				
36-1 Administration of Oral Medications				
36-2 Withdrawing Medication from a Vial				
36-3 Withdrawing Medication from an Ampule				
36-4 Administration of Subcutaneous, Intramuscular, and Intradermal Injections				
36-5 Administering a Subcutaneous Injection				
36-6 Administering an Intramuscular Injection				
36-7 Administering an Intradermal Injection of Purified Protein Derivative (PPD)				
36-8 Reconstituting a Powder Medication for Administration				
36-9 Z-Track Intramuscular Injection Technique				
37-1 Perform Single-Channel or Multichannel Electrocardiogram (ECG)				
37-2 Holter Monitor Application (Cassette and Digital)				
39-1 Using the Microscope				
40-1 Palpating a Vein and Preparing a Patient for Venipuncture				

Procedure Number and Title	Date Assessment Completed and Competency Achieved			
	Date/Initials	Date/Initials	Date/Initials	Date/Initials
40-2 Venipuncture by Syringe				
40-3 Venipuncture by Vacuum Tube System				
40-4 Venipuncture by Butterfly Needle System				
40-5 Capillary Puncture				
40-6 Obtaining a Capillary Specimen for Transport Using a Microtainer Transport Unit				
40-7 Obtaining Blood for Blood Culture				
41-1 Hemoglobin Determination Using a CLIA Waived Hemoglobin Analyzer				
41-2 Microhematocrit Determination				
41-3 Erythrocyte Sedimentation Rate				
41-4 Prothrombin Time (Using a CLIA Waived ProTime Analyzer)				
42-1 Assessing Urine Volume, Color, and Clarity (Physical Urinalysis)				
42-2 Using the Refractometer to Measure Specific Gravity (Physical Urinalysis, Continued)				
42-3 Performing a Chemical Urinalysis				
42-4 Preparing Slide for Microscopic Examination of Urine Sediment				
42-5 Performing a Complete Urinalysis				
42-6 Utilizing a Urine Transport System for C&S				
42-7 Instructing a Patient in the Collection of a Clean-Catch, Midstream Urine Specimen				
43-1 Procedure for Obtaining a Throat Specimen for Culture				
43-2 Wet Mount and Hanging Drop Slide Preparations				
43-3 Performing Strep Throat Testing				
43-4 Instructing a Patient on Obtaining a Fecal Specimen				
44-1 Pregnancy Test				

Procedure Number and Title	Date Assessment Completed and Competency Achieved			
	Date/Initials	Date/Initials	Date/Initials	Date/Initials
44-2 Performing Infectious Mononucleosis Test				
44-3 Obtaining Blood Specimen for Phenylketonuria (PKU) Test				
44-4 Measurement of Blood Glucose Using an Automated Analyzer				
44-5 Cholesterol Testing				
45-1 Completing a Medical Incident Report				
45-2 Preparing a Meeting Agenda				
45-3 Supervising a Student Practicum				
45-4 Developing and Maintaining a Procedure Manual				
45-5 Making Travel Arrangements with a Travel Agent				
45-6 Making Travel Arrangements via the Internet				
45-7 Processing Employee Payroll				
45-8 Perform an Inventory of Equipment and Supplies				
45-9 Perform Routine Maintenance and Calibration of Clinical Equipment				
46-1 Develop and Maintain a Policy Manual				
46-2 Prepare a Job Description				
46-3 Conduct Interviews				
46-4 Orient Personnel				

Name_____ **Date**_____ **Score**_____

⬤ **COMPETENCY ASSESSMENT**

Procedure 5-1:   Identifying Community Resources

Task: To have a list of community resources readily available for referral to patients.

Conditions: • Competency Assessment Information
                • Computer and printer
                • Multiple resources from a variety of community services

Standards: Perform the Task within 30 minutes with a minimum score of ___ points, as determined by your instructor.

Competency Assessment Information

The following is a list of information sources to consider when beginning to put together a Community Resources Manual.

• Local public health department
• Internet
• Community service numbers in the local telephone directory
• State/federal agencies
• Visiting nurses
• Counselors/social workers at local hospitals
• Nursing home associations
• Local charities

⬤ **Time began:** _____   **Time ended:** _____   **Total time:** _____

No.	Step	Points	Check #1	Check #2	Check #3
1	With your provider, determine the types of community resources your patients may need.				
2	Create a listing of each resource including the full name, address, telephone number, and services offered by each agency.				
3	*Show initiative* by contacting each agency on the list and requesting the name of a contact person, referral instructions, and a brochure describing the facility.				
4	*Pay attention to detail.* Compile the information from steps 2 and 3 to create a Community Resources Manual.				
Student's Total Points					
Points Possible					
Final Score (Student's Total Points/Possible Points)					

Instructor's/Evaluator's Comments and Suggestions:

CHECK #1	
Evaluator's Signature:	Date:

CHECK #2	
Evaluator's Signature:	Date:

CHECK #3	
Evaluator's Signature:	Date:

ABHES Competency: MA.A.1.8.e Locate resources and information for patients and employers

CAAHEP Competencies: IV.P.12 Develop and maintain a current list of community resources related to patients' healthcare needs; XI.P.12 Maintain a current list of community resources for emergency preparedness.

Name_____   **Date**_____   **Score**_____

● **COMPETENCY ASSESSMENT**

Procedure 9-1:   Control of Bleeding

Task: To control bleeding from an open wound.

Conditions: • Sterile dressings
               • Sterile gloves
               • Mask and eye protection
               • Gown
               • Biohazard waste container

Standards: Perform the Task within 15 minutes with a minimum score of ____ points, as determined by your instructor.

Competency Assessment Information

Use the following information to demonstrate the control of bleeding in the scenarios below, and complete Progress Note (Work Documentation) accordingly.

1. Lydia Tumlin presents with a severe cut on her left index finger that she sustained while cutting vegetables.
2. Mark Harned stumbled on the stairs at his home and has a 5-cm laceration on his right shin.
3. Gwen Carr was locked out of her home and broke a small window in order to unlock the door. She received a severe laceration on her right forearm.

● **Time began:** _____   **Time ended:** _____   **Total time:** _____

No.	Step	Points	Check #1	Check #2	Check #3
1	Wash hands.				
2	Assemble equipment and supplies.				
3	Apply eye and mask protection and gown if splashing is likely to occur.				
4	Put on gloves.				
5	Apply dressing and press firmly. Did you *explain the procedure and ally patient's fears?*				
6	If bleeding continues, elevate arm above heart level.				
7	*Display sound judgment.* If bleeding continues, press adjacent artery against bone. Notify the provider if bleeding cannot be controlled. *Remain calm in a crisis.*				
8	Apply pressure bandage over the dressing.				
9	Dispose of waste in biohazard container.				

No.	Step	Points	Check #1	Check #2	Check #3
10	Remove gloves and dispose in biohazard container.				
11	Wash hands.				
12	Document procedure in patient's chart or electronic medical record.				
Student's Total Points					
Points Possible					
Final Score (Student's Total Points/Possible Points)					

Instructor's/Evaluator's Comments and Suggestions:

_____

_____

_____

_____

_____

_____

_____

CHECK #1 Evaluator's Signature:	Date:

CHECK #2 Evaluator's Signature:	Date:

CHECK #3 Evaluator's Signature:	Date:

Work Documentation Form(s)

*Progress Note Template can be downloaded from the Premium Website

ABHES Competencies: MA.A.1.9.b Apply principles of aseptic techniques and infection control; MA.A.1.9.d Recognize and understand various treatment protocols; MA.A.1.9.i Use standard precautions

CAAHEP Competencies: I.P.10 Assist the physician with patient care; III.P.2 Practice standard precautions; IX.P.7 Document accurately in the patient record; XI.P.10 Perform first aid procedures

Name _____ **Date** _____ **Score** _____

● COMPETENCY ASSESSMENT

Procedure 9-2:   Applying an Arm Splint

Task: To immobilize the area above and below the injured part of the arm in order to reduce pain, immobilize the injured part, and prevent further injury.

Conditions: • Thin piece of rigid board or commercially available splint; cardboard, wood, or rigid plastic can be used if necessary
   • Gauze roller bandage

Standards: Perform the Task within 5 minutes with a minimum score of ___ points, as determined by your instructor.

Competency Assessment Information

Use the following information to demonstrate the appropriate application of a splint in the scenario below, and complete Progress Note (Work Documentation) accordingly.

Five-year-old Addi Mountjoy fell from her swing set and sustained a greenstick fracture of her right forearm.

Time began: _____   **Time ended:** _____   **Total time:** _____

No.	Step	Points	Check #1	Check #2	Check #3
1	Wash hands.				
2	*After introducing yourself,* place the padded splint under the injured area.				
3	*While displaying a calm and professional manner,* hold the splint in place with gauze roller bandage. Pad gaps between arm and board (wrist) with gauze pads or other soft material.				
4	After splinting, check circulation (note color and temperature of skin, note color of nails, check pulse) to ascertain that the splint is not too tightly applied.				
5	Apply a sling to keep the arm elevated, which increases comfort and reduces swelling. *Accurately and concisely update the provider on the patient's care.*				
6	Wash hands.				
7	Document procedure in patient's chart or electronic medical record.				
Student's Total Points					
Points Possible					
Final Score (Student's Total Points/Possible Points)					

Instructor's/Evaluator's Comments and Suggestions:

_____

_____

_____

_____

_____

_____

CHECK #1	
Evaluator's Signature:	Date:

CHECK #2	
Evaluator's Signature:	Date:

CHECK #3	
Evaluator's Signature:	Date:

Work Documentation Form(s)

*Progress Note Template can be downloaded from the Premium Website

ABHES Competencies: MA.A.1.9.d Recognize and understand various treatment protocols; MA.A.1.9.e Recognize emergencies and treatments and minor office surgical procedures

CAAHEP Competency: I.P.10 Assist physician with patient care; I.A.1 Apply critical thinking skills in performing patient assessment and care; IX.P.7 Document accurately in the patient's record; XI.P.10 Perform first aid procedures

Name_____ **Date**_____ **Score**_____

⬤ **COMPETENCY ASSESSMENT**

Procedure 10-1: Develop a Personal and/or Employee Safety Plan in Case of a Disaster

Task: To develop a plan of action promoting personal safety in case of a disaster that can also be applied to both employees and patients in ambulatory care.

Conditions:
- Computer
- Clear plastic protector envelope for plan

Standards: Perform the Task within 30 minutes with a minimum score of ___ points, as determined by your instructor.

Time began: _____ **Time ended:** _____ **Total time:** _____

No.	Step	Points	Check #1	Check #2	Check #3
1	*Be proactive* by reviewing state and local recommendations for emergency preparedness. *Pay attention to detail*.				
2	*Show initiative* by gathering family members or other employees together to discuss a disaster plan.				
3	List supplies necessary for your supply kit. Be certain to include any special needs required in your supplies. Allow each person 1 personal item for the kit. Plan your needs for a minimum of 48 hours.				
4	Plan for evacuation. Where are the exits? Identify the safest route for exit. List the steps to take prior to evacuation.				
5	Determine a communication or contact plan should you be separated from others during the disaster. Where will you meet? Name a "neutral" person or friend in another location who can be a telephone contact.				
6	Schedule updates to the personal safety plan at least every quarter, *developing strategic plans to achieve your goals*.				
7	Make certain everyone has a copy of the plan. Post a copy of your plan in a prominent place where it is noticed regularly.				
Student's Total Points					
Points Possible					
Final Score (Student's Total Points/Possible Points)					

Instructor's/Evaluator's Comments and Suggestions:

_____

_____

_____

_____

_____

_____

_____

CHECK #1	
Evaluator's Signature:	Date:

CHECK #2	
Evaluator's Signature:	Date:

CHECK #3	
Evaluator's Signature:	Date:

CAAHEP Competency: XI.P.3 Develop a personal (patient and employee) safety plan

Name_____ **Date**_____ **Score**_____

● **COMPETENCY ASSESSMENT**

Procedure 10-2:   Demonstrate Proper Use of a Fire Extinguisher

Task: To demonstrate the ability to operate a fire extinguisher or help another person operate the extinguisher and to describe the precise steps to take to prevent errors and delay in operation.

Conditions: • Fire extinguisher

Standards: Perform the Task within 30 minutes with a minimum score of ___ points, as determined by your instructor.

Time began: _____ **Time ended:** _____ **Total time:** _____

No.	Step	Points	Check #1	Check #2	Check #3
1	Determine the type of fire extinguisher(s) on the premises.				
2	Examine the cylinder and carefully read any instructions supplied from the manufacturer, *paying attention to detail*.				
3	Determine if you are able to handle the weight of the extinguisher, *asking for assistance if you are unable to carry out the task*.				
4	If a fire is present, *be proactive* by calling 911 before you discharge the extinguisher.				
5	Check your nearest exit. If it is blocked, *display sound judgment* by evacuating without discharging the extinguisher.				
6	Break the seal and turn and pull the safety pin from the handle.				
7	Aim the nozzle or hose at the base of the fire and squeeze the lever to discharge the extinguishing agent.				
8	Standing several feel back from the fire, sweep side to side to put out the flames.				
9	If the fire does not respond after you have used up the fire extinguisher, *remain calm* and remove yourself to safety immediately.				
10	If the area fills with smoke, *remain calm* and leave immediately.				

No.	Step	Points	Check #1	Check #2	Check #3
11	Replace the depleted fire extinguisher immediately. Never leave an empty extinguisher where someone might believe it is ready for use.				
Student's Total Points					
Points Possible					
Final Score (Student's Total Points/Possible Points)					

Instructor's/Evaluator's Comments and Suggestions:

_____

_____

_____

_____

_____

_____

CHECK #1	
Evaluator's Signature:	Date:

CHECK #2	
Evaluator's Signature:	Date:

CHECK #3	
Evaluator's Signature:	Date:

CAAHEP Competency: *XI.P.5.b Demonstrate proper use of a fire extinguisher*

Name _____ **Date** _____ **Score** _____

● **COMPETENCY ASSESSMENT**

Procedure 11-1: Perform Routine Maintenance of Office Computers and Ancillary Equipment with Documentation

Task:　To ensure that all computers in the office are serviced according to manufacturer suggestions and that documentation is logged appropriately.

Conditions:
- Maintenance log form
- Database identifying all copyright software
- Service calendar log form
- Clipboard
- Disk defragmenter

Standards:　Perform the Task within 30 minutes with a minimum score of ___ points, as determined by your instructor.

Time began: _____　**Time ended:** _____　**Total time:** _____

No.	Step	Points	Check #1	Check #2	Check #3
1	Locate the number assigned by the office manager to identify the computer being serviced, verify serial number, manufacturer/maker, technical support phone number, warranty information, and last date of service.				
2	*Paying attention to detail,* visually inspect each piece of equipment associated with the computer setup: • *Practice risk management principles.* Check for any frayed electrical cords, loose connections, or safety issues such as tripping hazards associated with electrical cords. • Clean monitor screens, replace printer ink or toner cartridges, and refill paper trays.				
3	Remove any unnecessary data files and empty the recycle bin. Next, complete the defragmentation process.				
4	Install security patches provided by the provider of the computer software.				
5	Record updated information on the maintenance log and service calendar forms and date and initial. Report to appropriate personnel any personal copyright software that is not on the database list. Verify that the licenses are in the documentation file and properly cover the number of computers on which software is installed.				

No.	Step	Points	Check #1	Check #2	Check #3
6	Schedule equipment servicing during the current month with an appropriate vendor and let coworkers know that equipment servicing has been scheduled.				
	Student's Total Points				
	Points Possible				
	Final Score (Student's Total Points/Possible Points)				

Instructor's/Evaluator's Comments and Suggestions:

_____

_____

_____

_____

_____

_____

_____

CHECK #1	
Evaluator's Signature:	Date:

CHECK #2	
Evaluator's Signature:	Date:

CHECK #3	
Evaluator's Signature:	Date:

ABHES Competencies: MA.A.1.8.ll Apply electronic technology; MA.A.1.8.y Perform routine maintenance of administrative and clinical equipment

CAAHEP Competency: V.P.6 Use office hardware and software to maintain office systems

Work Documentation Form(s)

Maintenance Log Form

Name of Equipment	Serial Number	Mfg/ Maker	Technical Support Phone Number	Purchase Date	Service Plan	Last Serviced	Completed By
Computer #6	79031	HP	xxx–xxx–xxxx	1/20xx	On file	6/12/20xx	bql
Printer #10	80462	HP	xxx–xxx–xxxx	7/20xx	On file	6/12/20xx	bql

© Cengage Learning 2014

Service Calendar Log Form

January	February	March	April	May	June	July	August	September	October	November	December

© Cengage Learning 2014

Name _____ **Date** _____ **Score** _____

● **COMPETENCY ASSESSMENT**

Procedure 11-2:   Software Installation

Task: To add software programs to the computer system for later call-up and use.

Conditions: • Computer
                     • Software CD
                     • Software documentation

Standards: Perform the Task within 10 minutes with a minimum score of ___ points, as determined by your
                    instructor.

Time began: _____   **Time ended:** _____   **Total time:** _____

No.	Step	Points	Check #1	Check #2	Check #3
Automatic Installation					
1	Close all open programs.				
2	Insert the CD supplied with the program into your CD drive. Shortly after the light on the drive shows activity, the Installation Wizard screen will appear.				
3	Follow the instructions given by your software documentation and the Installation Wizard screens that will appear.				
4	Click FINISH and launch the program.				
Manual Installation					
1	Close all open programs.				
2	Click START. Then select RUN from the menu. The CD should already be in the drive.				
3	From My Computer, double click the icon for the CD drive. Follow the prompts in the Installation Wizard screens that appear, choosing an appropriate location for the program.				
4	Click FINISH and launch the program.				
Student's Total Points					
Points Possible					
Final Score (Student's Total Points/Possible Points)					

Instructor's/Evaluator's Comments and Suggestions:

_____
_____
_____
_____
_____
_____

CHECK #1	
Evaluator's Signature:	Date:

CHECK #2	
Evaluator's Signature:	Date:

CHECK #3	
Evaluator's Signature:	Date:

ABHES Competencies: MA.A.1.8.ll Apply electronic technology; MA.A.1.8.d Apply concepts for office procedures
CAAHEP Competency: V.P.6 Use office hardware and software to maintain office systems

Name_____   **Date**_____   **Score**_____

● COMPETENCY ASSESSMENT

Procedure 11-3:   Hardware Installation

Task: To add hardware programs to the computer system for later call-up and use.

Conditions: • Computer
                • Driver for the equipment (on CD or download)

Standards: Perform the Task within 15 minutes with a minimum score of ___ points, as determined by your instructor.

Time began: _____   **Time ended:** _____   **Total time:** _____

No.	Step	Points	Check #1	Check #2	Check #3
Using Automatic Initiation from Microsoft Windows® Installation Wizard					
1	Close all open programs.				
2	Answer questions appropriately such as: Manufacturer, Model Number, etc.				
3	Follow onscreen directions.				
Using Manual Initiation of Microsoft Windows® Installation Wizard					
1	Close all open programs.				
2	Go to START, SETTINGS, CONTROL PANEL, and double-click ADD HARDWARE.				
3	Find the hardware you wish to install and follow onscreen instructions.				
Student's Total Points					
Points Possible					
Final Score (Student's Total Points/Possible Points)					

Instructor's/Evaluator's Comments and Suggestions:

_____

_____

_____

_____

_____

_____

CHECK #1	
Evaluator's Signature:	Date:

CHECK #2	
Evaluator's Signature:	Date:

CHECK #3	
Evaluator's Signature:	Date:

ABHES Competencies: MA.A.1.8.ll Apply electronic technology; MA.A.1.8.d Apply concepts for office procedures
CAAHEP Competency: V.P.6 Use office hardware and software to maintain office systems

Name_____   **Date**_____   **Score**_____

● COMPETENCY ASSESSMENT

Procedure 12-1:   Answering and Screening Incoming Calls

Task: To answer telephone calls professionally, acquiring all necessary information from the caller, documenting it correctly, and properly acting on it.

Conditions:
- Telephone
- Computer with message screen
- Appointment book
- Calendar
- Message pad
- Pen or pencil
- Notepad

Standards: Perform the Task within 15 minutes with a minimum score of ___ points, as determined by your instructor.

Competency Assessment Information

Appropriately answer the phone and use your screening skills to determine what to do in the following situation. What should you do? (For extra practice, use the Progress Note form to document your interactions.)

Mary O'Keefe calls at 8:45 AM after her 3-year-old son Chris woke with severe ear pain. The child is pulling on his right ear and has screamed uncontrollably for 45 minutes. Chris and Mary are established patients of Dr. King.

● **Time began:** _____   **Time ended:** _____   **Total time:** _____

No.	Step	Points	Check #1	Check #2	Check #3
1	Be prepared. Have materials organized and computer with message screen up. *Implement time management principles by* answering the telephone promptly. The phone should not ring more than three times before it is answered.				
2	*Introduce the clinic and yourself* by answering the call with the preferred clinic greeting, speaking directly into the mouthpiece. The mouthpiece should be 1 to 2 inches away from the mouth. Sample greeting: "Good morning. Doctors Lewis and King. Ellen speaking. How may I help you?"				
3	Ask the name of the caller as quickly as possible, and *use sound judgment to* determine whether this is an emergency call.				
4	*Apply active listening skills.* You may need additional information to assist or direct the call appropriately.				
5	Repeat information back to the caller, *using appropriate responses/feedback.*				

No.	Step	Points	Check #1	Check #2	Check #3
6	Follow written established screening protocols for all telephone calls, **working within your scope of practice.**				
7	When using a multiline telephone as shown in Figure 12-9, it is helpful to keep a notepad by the telephone. When you answer the phone and have the caller's name, **pay attention to detail** and jot down the caller's name, which line the caller is on, and some quick notes about the content of the call. At the end of your work shift, **protect and maintain confidentiality** by shredding all notepapers with PHI.				
8	Ask if the caller has any other questions.				
9	**End the call courteously.** Say "thank you" and "good-bye" (not "bye-bye"). Allow the caller to hang up before you disconnect.				
10	Document information and record any necessary actions.				
Student's Total Points					
Points Possible					
Final Score (Student's Total Points/Possible Points)					

Instructor's/Evaluator's Comments and Suggestions:

_____

_____

_____

_____

_____

_____

CHECK #1	
Evaluator's Signature:	Date:

CHECK #2	
Evaluator's Signature:	Date:

CHECK #3	
Evaluator's Signature:	Date:

Work Documentation Form(s)

*Progress Note template can be downloaded from the Premium Website

ABHES Competencies: MA.A.1.8.ee Use proper telephone techniques; MA.A.1.8.hh Receive, organize, prioritize, and transmit information expediently

CAAHEP Competencies: IV.P.7 Demonstrate telephone techniques; IV.P.2 Report relevant information to others succinctly and accurately

Name_____ **Date**_____ **Score**_____

● **COMPETENCY ASSESSMENT**

Procedure 12-2: Taking a Telephone Message

Task: To record an accurate message and follow up as required.

Conditions:
- Telephone
- Message pad
- Black ink pen
- Notepad
- Clock or watch

Standards: Perform the Task within 5 minutes with a minimum score of ___ points, as determined by your instructor.

Competency Assessment Information

Document a phone message using the information below:

"This is Heidi from Dr. Kwiczola's office calling for Dr. Lewis. We have a new patient, Marsha Beckman, a patient in our psychiatric practice, who is experiencing symptoms of fatigue, anxiety, palpitations, and weight loss. Dr. Kwiczola suspects this patient may be suffering from hyperthyroidism. Dr. Kwiczola will be in the office tomorrow from 2:00 p.m. to 7:00 p.m. and can be reached at 555-7181."

Time began: _____ **Time ended:** _____ **Total time:** _____

No.	Step	Points	Check #1	Check #2	Check #3
1	Answer the telephone following the steps outlined in Procedure 12-1.				
2	Use a message pad or document directly into the EMR. *Pay attention to detail* when requesting the following information: • Date and time call is received • Name and correct spelling of person calling, daytime and evening telephone numbers, including area code and extension when appropriate • Ask for date of birth, clinic number, or social security number to verify correct patient • Who the call is for • The reason for the call • The action to be taken • The name or initials of the person taking the call				
3	Repeat the above information back to the caller.				
4	If the call is from an established patient or concerns an established patient, pull the medical record/chart and attach the message to it before delivering the message to the intended individual. When using EMR save the message and forward it to the intended recipient.				

No.	Step	Points	Check #1	Check #2	Check #3
5	Maintain the message book with all carbon copies intact.				
Student's Total Points					
Points Possible					
Final Score (Student's Total Points/Possible Points)					

Instructor's/Evaluator's Comments and Suggestions:

_____

_____

_____

_____

_____

_____

_____

CHECK #1	
Evaluator's Signature:	Date:

CHECK #2	
Evaluator's Signature:	Date:

CHECK #3	
Evaluator's Signature:	Date:

ABHES Competencies: MA.A.1.8.ee Use proper telephone techniques; MA.A.1.8.hh Receive, organize, prioritize, and transmit information expediently; MA.A.1.4.a Document accurately

CAAHEP Competencies: IV.P.7 Demonstrate telephone techniques; IV.P.2 Report relevant information to others succinctly and accurately; IV.P.8 Document patient care

Work Documentation Form(s): Message Pad Template

To: _____   Date: _____

From: _____   Time: _____

Telephone #: _____

Message: _____

_____

_____

Initials: _____

Attachments: _____

_____

To: _____   Date: _____

From: _____   Time: _____

Telephone #: _____

Message: _____

_____

_____

Initials: _____

Attachments: _____

_____

To: _____   Date: _____

From: _____   Time: _____

Telephone #: _____

Message: _____

_____

_____

Initials: _____

Attachments: _____

_____

Name_____ **Date**_____ **Score**_____

● COMPETENCY ASSESSMENT

Procedure 12-3:   Calling a Pharmacy to Refill an Authorized Prescription

Task: To notify a pharmacy to refill an authorized prescription.

Conditions: • Patient's chart
              • Provider authorization to refill prescription
              • Drug name, dosage and instructions for when and how to take the medication
              • Pharmacy name and telephone number
              • Telephone

Standards: Perform the Task within 15 minutes with a minimum score of ____ points.

Competency Assessment Information

Simulate calling the pharmacy using the information below. (For extra practice, use the Progress Note form and document your interactions.)

Yolanda White, (123) 344-8455, calls the clinic to request a refill for her Fosamax prescription from Dr. King.

"This is Yolanda White. I need to get my Fosamax refilled. I had several pills left from the prescription when I came for my last office visit, so I didn't get the prescription filled then. Now I've lost the prescription and I'm now out of the drug."

The pharmacy that Ms. White uses is DanMart on Polaris Drive, (123) 678-7650. Yolanda is allergic to peanuts. The provider approves the refill request: Rx for Fosamax tablets, 70 mg, take 1 tablet per week with a glass of water, one month prescription, 2 refills.

Time began: _____   **Time ended:** _____   **Total time:** _____

No.	Step	Points	Check #1	Check #2	Check #3
1	Receive patient's telephone call asking for a prescription refill. Follow appropriate telephone techniques.				
2	*Pay attention to detail.* Obtain the following information from the patient and include it on the message form or EMR message screen: • Patient's full name and correct spelling, and patient's DOB • Telephone number where the patient can be reached • Name of medication and how long patient has been taking it • Patient's symptoms and current health condition • History of this condition (last office visit) • Treatments the patient has tried • If patient is a child, ask their weight • Any known allergies • Pharmacy name, telephone number, and address if a chain				
3	Attach the completed message to the patient's chart or EMR and give it to the provider.				

No.	Step	Points	Check #1	Check #2	Check #3
4	Review comments in the chart by the provider. If the refill is authorized, call the patient's pharmacy with the refill information. Ask the pharmacy to repeat the information back to you.				
5	*Paying attention to detail,* document in the patient's chart the date and time the prescription was called to the pharmacy and the pharmacy address. Verify that the correct drug, dosage, and dosage instructions were provided to the pharmacy.				
Student's Total Points					
Points Possible					
Final Score (Student's Total Points/Possible Points)					

Instructor's/Evaluator's Comments and Suggestions:

_____

_____

_____

_____

_____

_____

CHECK #1	
Evaluator's Signature:	Date:

CHECK #2	
Evaluator's Signature:	Date:

CHECK #3	
Evaluator's Signature:	Date:

Work Documentation Form(s)

*Progress Note template can be downloaded from the Premium Website

ABHES Competencies: MA.A.1.8.dd Serve as liaison between Physician and others; MA.A.1.8.ee Use proper telephone techniques; MA.A.1.4.a Document accurately

CAAHEP Competencies: IV.P.7 Demonstrate telephone techniques; IV.P.8 Document patient care

Name_____ **Date**_____ **Score**_____

● **COMPETENCY ASSESSMENT**

Procedure 12-4:   Handling Problem Calls

Task: To handle calls in a positive and professional manner while providing necessary comfort, empathy, and information to the caller to resolve the problem.

Conditions:
- Telephone
- Message pad
- Pen or pencil

Standards: Perform the Task within 15 minutes with a minimum score of ___ points.

Competency Assessment Information

Based on the information given below, how would you handle the following calls?

1. George Ramirez calls the clinic and demands to know why his wife was seen in the clinic last week.
2. Esmeralda Jones calls the clinic and is angry because the bill she received is so high.
3. Someone calls for Dr. Lewis but refuses to identify himself.

Time began: _____   **Time ended:** _____   **Total time:** _____

No.	Step	Points	Check #1	Check #2	Check #3
1	Answer the call as outlined in Procedure 12-1.				
2	*Remain calm* and avoid becoming upset with an angry caller. Let the caller say what needs to be said without interruption (unless it is a medical emergency requiring immediate action).				
3	Lower your voice both in pitch and volume.				
4	*Listen to and acknowledge* what the caller is upset about. Paraphrase information for verification that you have understood the problem.				
5	*Be courteous, patient, and respectful.* Use the words "I understand" and show that you are interested in hearing the caller's concerns.				
6	Do not take the call personally.				
7	Offer assistance.				
8	Document the call accurately and properly.				
9	When dealing with a frightened or hysterical caller, *display a calm, caring, and professional manner* by speaking in a soothing voice; use a slower, lower tone than normal.				
10	If the call is an emergency, begin screening procedures as needed and *attend to any special needs of the patient.*				
11	Always have the caller repeat instructions.				

No.	Step	Points	Check #1	Check #2	Check #3
12	Finalize and follow through on action to be taken, whether it is confirming emergency medical personnel are on the scene or scheduling an emergency appointment.				
13	Always report problem calls to the provider or clinic manager at once.				
Student's Total Points					
Points Possible					
Final Score (Student's Total Points/Possible Points)					

Instructor's/Evaluator's Comments and Suggestions:

_____

_____

_____

_____

_____

_____

CHECK #1	
Evaluator's Signature:	Date:

CHECK #2	
Evaluator's Signature:	Date:

CHECK #3	
Evaluator's Signature:	Date:

ABHES Competencies: MA.A.1.8.ee Use proper telephone techniques; MA.A.1.8.hh Receive, organize, prioritize, and transmit information expediently; MA.A.1.4.a Document accurately

CAAHEP Competencies: IV.P.7 Demonstrate telephone techniques; IV.P.2 Report relevant information to others succinctly and accurately; IV.P.8 Document patient care

Name_____ **Date**_____ **Score**_____

● COMPETENCY ASSESSMENT

Procedure 12-5:   Preparing, Sending, and Receiving a Fax

Task: To send and receive information quickly and accurately by fax (facsimile).

Conditions:
- Fax machine
- Telephone

Standards: Perform the Task within 15 minutes with a minimum score of ___ points, as determined by your instructor.

Competency Assessment Information

Prepare a fax cover letter based on the following information, and simulate sending it.

Odetta Smith is seen in the clinic for her annual examination. After examination, Dr. Lewis would like her to have a breast ultrasound performed and refers her to Dr. Singh at Eastside Radiology. Prepare a fax cover sheet to send Ms. Smith's referral to Eastside Radiology. The fax number is (818) 555-3366 and phone number is (818) 555-3360.

Time began: _____ **Time ended:** _____ **Total time:** _____

No.	Step	Points	Check #1	Check #2	Check #3
1	*Pay attention to detail.* Prepare a cover sheet or use a preprinted cover sheet for the document to be faxed. Include the names of the sender and receiver, the number of pages being sent and whether this includes the cover sheet, and a short message if necessary.				
2	Place the document according to machine instructions.				
3	Dial the telephone or dedicated fax number of the receiver. If your fax machine has a display showing the number being faxed to, check to be sure the number you dialed is correct. Then press start.				
4	After the document passes through the fax machine, press the button requesting a receipt. Some fax machines automatically issue a report.				
5	Remove the document from the machine and, when necessary, call the recipient to be sure the fax was received.				
6	*To receive a fax:* Be sure that the fax machine is turned on and that the telephone line to the machine is not being used. Most offices have dedicated fax lines.				

No.	Step	Points	Check #1	Check #2	Check #3
7	Remove the document from the machine after it is received and immediately deliver it to the addressee.				
Student's Total Points					
Points Possible					
Final Score (Student's Total Points/Possible Points)					

Instructor's/Evaluator's Comments and Suggestions:

_____

_____

_____

_____

_____

_____

_____

CHECK #1

Evaluator's Signature:

Date:

CHECK #2

Evaluator's Signature:

Date:

CHECK #3

Evaluator's Signature:

Date:

ABHES Competencies: MA.A.1.8.hh Receive, organize, prioritize, and transmit information expediently; MA.A.1.8.a Perform basic clerical functions

CAAHEP Competency: IV.P.2 Report relevant information to others succinctly and accurately

Work Documentation Form(s)

FAX TRANSMITTAL SHEET

To: _____   Date:_____

Fax Number: _____   Time:_____

Telephone No.:_____

Number of Pages (including this one): _____

From: _____   Telephone No. _____

Note: This transmittal is intended only for the use of the individual or entity to which it is addressed and may contain information that is privileged, confidential, and exempt from disclosure under applicable law. If you are not the intended recipient, any dissemination, distribution, or photocopying of this communication is strictly prohibited. If you have received this communication in error, please notify this office immediately by telephone and return the original fax to us at the address below by U.S. Postal Service. Thank you.

Remarks:_____

_____

_____

If you cannot read this fax or if pages are missing, please contact:

INNER CITY HEALTH CARE

8600 MAIN STREET, SUITE 201 • RIVER CITY, NY 01234
OFFICE: (123) 555-0326 • FAX: (123) 555-1268

INSTRUCTIONS TO THE AUTHORIZED RECEIVER: PLEASE COMPLETE THIS STATEMENT OF RECEIPT AND RETURN TO SENDER VIA THE ABOVE FAX NUMBER.

I, _____, verify that I have received _____
(no. of pages including cover sheet)

from _____.
(sending facility's name)

Name_____ **Date**_____ **Score**_____

● COMPETENCY ASSESSMENT

Procedure 13-1: Establishing the Appointment Matrix in a Paper System

Task: To have a current and accurate record of appointment times available for scheduling patient visits, in a paper system.

Conditions: • Appointment scheduler
  • Clinic schedule
  • Provider and staff schedule
  • Office calendar

Standards: Perform the Task within 15 minutes with a minimum score of ___ points.

Competency Assessment Information

Use the following information to establish the appointment matrix in a paper system.

1. Dr. Heath will be attending a Quality Care Committee meeting at New York County Hospital on the first of every month beginning June 1, 2012 through December 31, 2012 from 9:00 a.m. to 10:00 a.m. (Note: if the first of the month is on a weekend, the meeting will be held on the next business day.)
2. Dr. Schwartz sees his patients who are residents in nursing homes every Thursday afternoon from 1:00 p.m. to 5:00 p.m.
3. Staff meetings are held biweekly on Wednesday afternoons from 1:00 p.m. to 2:00 p.m. This policy was put into place with an effective date of July 1, 2012 and will be in effect until June 30, 2013. All staff members are expected to attend.

Time began: _____   **Time ended:** _____   **Total time:** _____

No.	Step	Points	Check #1	Check #2	Check #3
1	Block off times in the appointment scheduler when patients are not to be scheduled by marking a large **X** through these time slots. This establishes the matrix.				
2	Indicate all vacations, holidays, and other clinic closures as soon as they are known. It may be helpful to indicate absences that might affect patient scheduling.				
3	*Pay attention to detail.* Note all provider meetings, hospital rounds, appointments, conferences, vacations, and other prescheduled provider commitments.				
4	If the clinic has a scheduling system for certain examinations or procedures, these can be color coded with highlighters.				
Student's Total Points					
Points Possible					
Final Score (Student's Total Points/Possible Points)					

Instructor's/Evaluator's Comments and Suggestions:

_____
_____
_____
_____
_____
_____
_____

CHECK #1 Evaluator's Signature:	Date:

CHECK #2 Evaluator's Signature:	Date:

CHECK #3 Evaluator's Signature:	Date:

ABHES Competency: MA.A.1.8.c Schedule and manage appointments

CAAHEP Competency: V.P.1 Manage appointment schedule, using established priorities

Name_____ **Date**_____ **Score**_____

● COMPETENCY ASSESSMENT

Procedure 13-2: Establishing the Appointment Matrix Using Medical Office Simulation Software (MOSS)

Task: To designate and block time for provider commitments outside the clinic on an electronic appointment matrix.

Conditions: • Computer with MOSS installed

Standards: Perform each Task within 10 minutes with a minimum score of ___ points, as determined by your instructor.

Competency Assessment Information

Use the following information to complete this procedure. The Case Study for Quality Care Committee meeting is found directly following this Competency Assessment checklist.

Today is January 15, 2013 and you are working at the front office. The Clinic Manager gives you a memorandum with the following information and asks you to block the appointment matrix as indicated below:

1. Case Study – Dr. Heath will be attending a Quality Care Committee meeting at New York County Hospital on the first of each month beginning February 1, 2013 through December 2, 2013. The meeting is from 9:00 a.m. to 10:00 a.m. in Conference Room 200. NOTE: If the first of the month is on a weekend day, the meeting will be held on the next business day.
2. Dr. Heath has requested that the calendar be blocked each Friday afternoon from 4:00 p.m. to 6:00 p.m. from February 1, 2013 through April 26, 2013. He plans to visit his patients at Retirement Inn Nursing Home every week during those three months.
3. Dr. Schwartz has requested two time blocks. The first is February 14, 2013. No patients are to be scheduled from 1:00 p.m. through closing (6:00 p.m.); he is taking the afternoon off. The second is a staff meeting for all providers on Monday, March 4, 2013 from 11 a.m. until noon. All staff doctors are to meet in the conference room.

Time began: _____ **Time ended:** _____ **Total time:** _____

No.	Step	Points	Check #1	Check #2	Check #3
1	Open MOSS and select Appointment Scheduling from the Main Menu.				
2	Using the calendar on the top right, select a date. Hint: Use the –M and +M and –Y and +Y to navigate to the correct month and year, and then click on the date.				
3	Click on the time slot in the applicable provider column and then click on *Block Calendar*.				
4	Click *Yes* to create a new calendar block. In Field 1 of the *Block Calendar* window, enter the name of the time block in the *Description* field. Complete Fields 2–9 with information as applicable to the block.				

No.	Step	Points	Check #1	Check #2	Check #3
5	Click on *Save* to post the block to the appointment matrix. A confirmation message will verify the information was posted.				
6	Check the appointment matrix to be sure the blocks are in place correctly.				
7	Close the Practice Schedule and return to the Main Menu.				
Student's Total Points					
Points Possible					
Final Score (Student's Total Points/Possible Points)					

Instructor's/Evaluator's Comments and Suggestions:

_____

_____

_____

_____

_____

_____

_____

CHECK #1

Evaluator's Signature: | Date:

CHECK #2

Evaluator's Signature: | Date:

CHECK #3

Evaluator's Signature: | Date:

ABHES Competencies: MA.A.1.7.b(2) Apply computer application skills using variety of different electronic programs including both practice management software and EMR software; MA.A.1.8.b Prepare and maintain medical records

CAAHEP Competencies: V.P.5 Execute data management using electronic healthcare records such as the EMR; V.P.6 Use office hardware and software to maintain office systems

CASE STUDY FOR QUALITY CARE COMMITTEE MEETING

No.	Step	
1	Open MOSS and select Appointment Scheduling from the Main Menu.	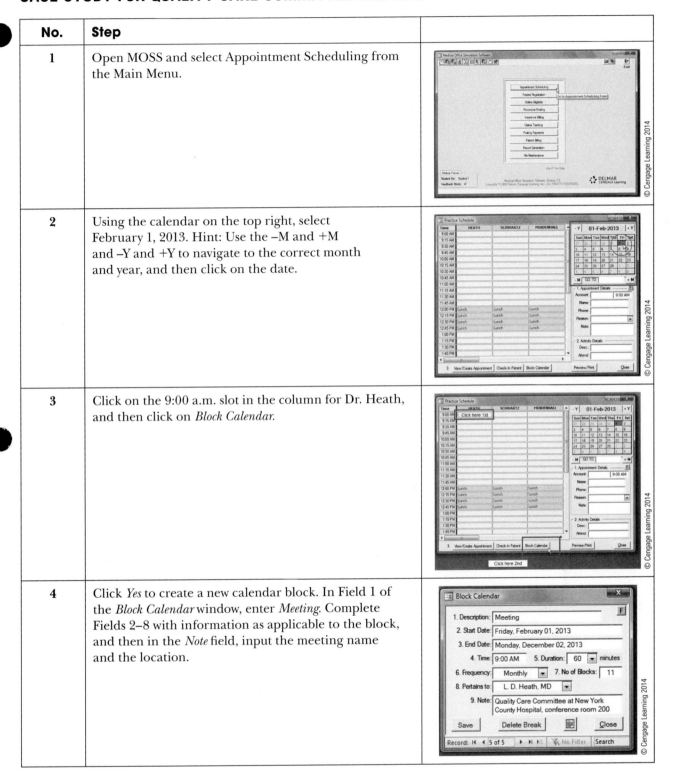
2	Using the calendar on the top right, select February 1, 2013. Hint: Use the –M and +M and –Y and +Y to navigate to the correct month and year, and then click on the date.	
3	Click on the 9:00 a.m. slot in the column for Dr. Heath, and then click on *Block Calendar*.	
4	Click *Yes* to create a new calendar block. In Field 1 of the *Block Calendar* window, enter *Meeting*. Complete Fields 2–8 with information as applicable to the block, and then in the *Note* field, input the meeting name and the location.	

© Cengage Learning 2014

No.	Step	
5	Click on *Save* to post the block to the appointment matrix. A confirmation message will verify the information was posted.	 **Block Calendar** 1. Description: Meeting 2. Start Date: Friday, February 01, 2013 3. End Date: Monday, December 02, 2013 4. Time: 9:00 AM 5. Duration: 60 minutes 6. Frequency: Monthly 7. No of Blocks: 11 8. Pertains to: L. D. Heath, MD 9. Note: Quality Care Committee at New York County Hospital Save Delete Break Close Record: ⁞ Post Break ⁞ ⁞ No Filter Search © Cengage Learning 2014
6	Check the appointment matrix to be sure the blocks are in place correctly.	
7	Close the Practice Schedule and return to the Main Menu.	

Name_____ **Date**_____ **Score**_____

⬤ COMPETENCY ASSESSMENT

Procedure 13-3: Making an Appointment Using Paper Scheduling

Task: To schedule an appointment, entering information in the appointment schedule according to clinic policy.

Conditions:
- Telephone
- Black ink pen
- Calendar
- Appointment matrix

Standards: Perform the Task within 15 minutes with a minimum score of ___ points, as determined by your instructor.

Competency Assessment Information

Use the following information to make appointments for established patients in a paper system.

1. Jordan Connell calls the clinic on June 3, 2012 because he has had a temperature of 101° F for two days. He also complains of a sore throat and ear pain. He is given a 15-minute appointment on the same day for 3:00 p.m. with Dr. Heath.
2. Ed Gormann calls the clinic on June 1, 2012 to schedule his annual physical (60-minute visit) with Dr. Heath. He agrees to be seen on September 15, 2012 at 9:00 a.m.
3. Elane Ybarra calls on June 2, 2012 because she has had persistent heartburn and indigestion along with intermittent bouts of diarrhea. She is given an appointment for June 4, 2012 at 10:15 a.m. (30-minute visit) with Dr. Schwartz.
4. Andrew Jefferson schedules an appointment on June 1, 2012 for June 5, 2012 because he has been bothered by a sore shoulder for the past 2 days. The 15-minute appointment is scheduled for 10:30 a.m. with Dr. Schwartz.
5. Eric Gordon has been experiencing problems with urination for the past week. A 15-minute appointment is scheduled for Friday, June 5, 2012 at 9:00 a.m. with Dr. Schwartz.
6. Vito Mangano calls the facility stating he has had a sore throat for the past 3 days. He is given a 15-minute appointment for June 10 at 9:00 a.m. with Dr. Heath.

Time began: _____ **Time ended:** _____ **Total time:** _____

No.	Step	Points	Check #1	Check #2	Check #3
1	In a private and quiet location, answer the ringing telephone before the third ring. *Identify the facility and yourself.*				
2	As the patient begins to speak, make notes on your personal log sheet of patient's name and reason for calling.				
3	*Apply active listening skills.* Determine if patient is new or established, provider to be seen, and reason for appointment.				
4	*Discuss with the patient any special appointment needs*, and search your appointment schedule for an available time that is convenient for the patient.				
5	Once the patient has agreed to an appropriate time, enter the patient's name in the schedule. Enter last name first, followed by the first name, telephone number, and the chief complaint. Write or print legibly with black pen in the appointment book or worksheet.				

No.	Step	Points	Check #1	Check #2	Check #3
6	Repeat the date and time for the appointment, using the patient's name. Provide any necessary instructions about coming to the facility.				
7	*End the call politely.*				
8	Make certain you transferred all necessary information from your telephone log to the appropriate appointment schedule. Draw a diagonal line through your notes on the log to indicate you have completed the task.				
Student's Total Points					
Points Possible					
Final Score (Student's Total Points/Possible Points)					

Instructor's/Evaluator's Comments and Suggestions:

_____

_____

_____

_____

_____

_____

CHECK #1	
Evaluator's Signature:	Date:

CHECK #2	
Evaluator's Signature:	Date:

CHECK #3	
Evaluator's Signature:	Date:

ABHES Competencies: MA.A.1.8.c Schedule and manage appointments; MA.A.1.8.ee Use proper telephone techniques

CAAHEP Competencies: IV.P.7 Demonstrate telephone techniques; V.P.1 Manage appointment schedule, using established priorities

Work Documentation Form(s)

APPOINTMENT RECORD

		DOCTOR			
		DATE			
		DAY			
		AM	00		
			15		
		8	30		
			45		
			00		
			15		
		9	30		
			45		
			00		
			15		
		10	30		
			45		
			00		
			15		
		11	30		
			45		
			00		
			15		
		12	30		
			45		
		PM	00		
			15		
		1	30		
			45		
			00		
			15		
		2	30		
			45		
			00		
			15		
		3	30		
			45		
			00		
			15		
		4	30		
			45		
			00		
			15		
		5	30		
			45		

Name_____ **Date**_____ **Score**_____

● COMPETENCY ASSESSMENT

Procedure 13-4: Making an Appointment Using Medical Office Simulation Software (MOSS)

Task: To schedule clinic visit appointments for new and established patients.

Conditions: • Computer with MOSS installed

Standards: Perform each Task within 15 minutes with a minimum score of ___ points, as determined by your instructor.

Competency Assessment Information

Use the following information to complete this procedure. The Case Study for Lynne Abbott is found directly following this Competency Assessment checklist.

1. Turn off *Feedback Mode* in MOSS.
2. Today is February 6, 2013, and you are working at the front office covering the scheduling desk. Schedule appointments for new and established patients for clinic visits as indicated below:

   a. Case Study – <u>New Patient</u>: Schedule Lynne Abbott for an appointment with Dr. Heath.
   Lynne A. Abbott
   DOB: 10/02/1925 SSN: 999-21-6816
   Marital Status: Other
   Address: 57213 Slate Drive, Douglasville, NY 01234
   Phone: (123) 457-7752
   Employment Status: Retired
   Appointment request: Wednesday, 2/20/2013 at 9:30 a.m. for 45 minutes
   Note: Diabetes

   <u>Established Patient</u>: Schedule Isabel Durand for an appointment with Dr. Heath.
   Appointment request: Wednesday, 2/20/2013 at 11:00 a.m. for 15 minutes
   Note: Stomach pains

   <u>Established Patient</u>: Schedule Robert Shinn for an appointment with Dr. Heath.
   Appointment request: Thursday, 2/21/2013 at 11:00 a.m. for 30 minutes
   Note: Abdominal tenderness and fever

   <u>Established Patient</u>: Schedule Anna Pinkston for an appointment with Dr. Heath.
   Appointment request: Thursday, 2/21/2013 at 11:45 a.m. for 15 minutes
   Note: Blood pressure recheck

   b. <u>New Patient</u>: Schedule Herbert VanGillis for an appointment with Dr. Schwartz.
   Herbert VanGillis
   DOB: 04/15/1972 SSN: 999-55-6218
   Marital Status: Married
   Address: 1257 Glenwood Court, Douglasville, NY 01235
   Phone: (123) 457-5162
   Employment Status: Unemployed
   Appointment request: Wednesday, 2/20/2013 at 1:00 p.m. for 60 minutes
   Note: High cholesterol

<u>Established Patient</u>: Schedule Emery Camille for an appointment with Dr. Schwartz.
Appointment request: Wednesday, 2/20/2013 at 11:00 a.m. for 30 minutes
Note: Earache

<u>Established Patient</u>: Schedule Richard Manaly for an appointment with Dr. Schwartz.
Appointment request: Thursday, 2/21/2013 at 10:00 a.m. for 15 minutes
Note: Sore Throat

c. <u>New Patient</u>: Schedule Robert Simms for an appointment with Dr. Heath.
Robert Simms
DOB: 03/05/1932 SSN: 999-16-1882
Marital Status: Married
Address: 2366 Pebble Trail, Douglasville, NY 01235
Phone: (123) 457-5162

Employment Status: Retired
Appointment request: Wednesday, 2/20/2013 at 3:00 p.m. for 60 minutes
Note: COPD and CHF

<u>Established Patient</u>: Schedule Caitlin Barryroe for an appointment with Dr. Heath.
Appointment request: Wednesday, 2/20/2013 at 9:00 a.m. for 30 minutes
Note: Allergies – stuffy nose and cough

<u>Established Patient</u>: Schedule John Conway for an appointment with Dr. Heath.
Appointment request: Thursday, 2/21/2013 at 9:00 a.m. for 30 minutes
Note: Palpitations and night sweats

Time began: _____   **Time ended:** _____   **Total time:** _____

No.	Step	Points	Check #1	Check #2	Check #3
1	Open MOSS and select Appointment Scheduling from the Main Menu.				
2	Using the calendar on the top right, select a date. Hint: Use the –M and +M and –Y and +Y to navigate to the correct month and year, and then click on the date.				
3	Click on the time slot in the applicable physician column and then click on *View/Create Appointment*. As an alternate, the time slot may be *double clicked*.				
4	Click the patient name to be scheduled, and then click *Add* from the *Appointment Scheduling* window. If a new patient, click on *Add New Patient*, and complete basic registration information and save the record before returning to scheduling.				
5	On the *Patient Appointment Form* window, enter data in the fields indicating the physician and duration in minutes and the *Reason* field with the appointment information.				
6	In the *Note* field, enter the patient's chief complaint or reason for visiting the provider.				

No.	Step	Points	Check #1	Check #2	Check #3
7	When all data is entered, click on *Save Appointment*. Check the Practice Schedule for accuracy when completed.				
8	Schedule the next patient, or close the Practice Schedule and return to the Main Menu.				
Student's Total Points					
Points Possible					
Final Score (Student's Total Points/Possible Points)					

Instructor's/Evaluator's Comments and Suggestions:

_____
_____
_____
_____
_____
_____
_____

CHECK #1 Evaluator's Signature:	Date:

CHECK #2 Evaluator's Signature:	Date:

CHECK #3 Evaluator's Signature:	Date:

ABHES Competencies: MA.A.1.7.b(2) Apply computer application skills using variety of different electronic programs including both practice management software and EMR software; MA.A.1.8.b Prepare and maintain medical records

CAAHEP Competencies: V.P.5 Execute data management using electronic healthcare records such as the EMR; V.P.6 Use office hardware and software to maintain office systems

CASE STUDY FOR LYNNE ABBOTT

No.	Step	
1	Open MOSS and select Appointment Scheduling from the Main Menu.	
2	Using the calendar on the top right, select a date. Hint: Use the –M and +M and –Y and +Y to navigate to the correct month and year, and then click on the date.	
3	Click on the 9:30 a.m. time slot in the column for Dr. Heath and then click on *View/Create Appointment.* As an alternate, the time slot may be *double clicked.*	
4	Click the patient name to be scheduled, and then click *Add* from the *Appointment Scheduling* window. Since Lynne Abbott is a new patient, click on *Add New Patient,* complete basic registration information, and save the record before returning to scheduling.	

© Cengage Learning 2014

No.	Step	
5	On the *Patient Appointment Form* window, enter data in the fields indicating the physician and duration in minutes and the *Reason* field with the appointment information.	
6	In the *Note* field, enter Lynne's chief complaint or reason for visiting the provider.	
7	When all data is entered, click on *Save Appointment*. Check the Practice Schedule for accuracy when completed.	
8	Schedule the next patient, or close the Practice Schedule and return to the Main Menu.	

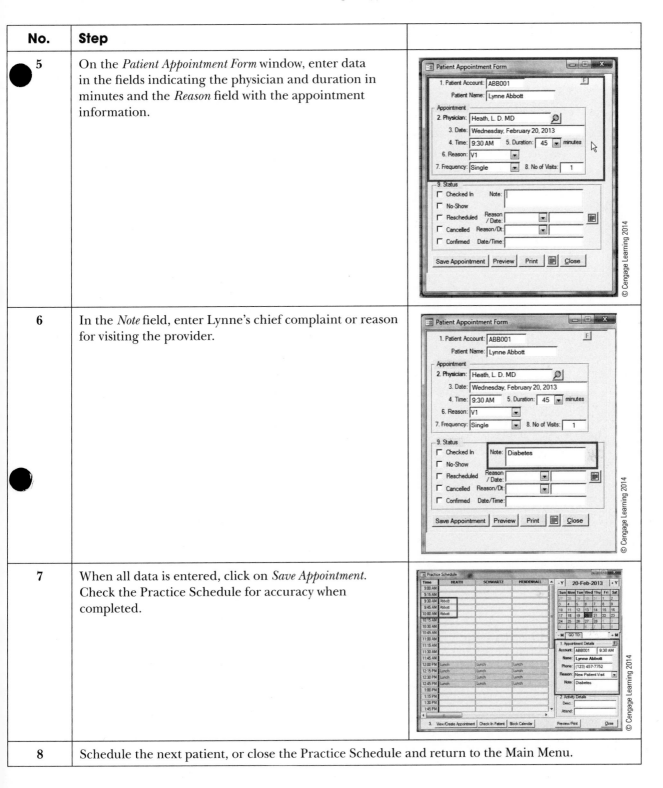

© Cengage Learning 2014

Name_____ **Date**_____ **Score**_____

COMPETENCY ASSESSMENT

Procedure 13-5:   Checking in Patients in a Paper System

Task: To ensure the patient is given prompt and proper care; to meet legal safeguards for documentation.

Conditions: • Patient chart
            • Black ink pen
            • Required forms
            • Check-in list
            • Appointment book

Standards: Perform the Task within 25 minutes with a minimum score of ___ points, as determined by your instructor.

Competency Assessment Information

Use the following information to check patients in for their appointments in a paper system. To complete appointment book page, use scheduling form provided in Procedure 13-3.

1. Jordan Connell presents in the clinic for his 3:00 p.m. appointment with Dr. Heath on June 3, 2012.
2. Elane Ybarra arrives in the clinic on June 4, 2012 for her 10:15 a.m. appointment with Dr. Schwartz.
3. Ed Gormann arrives at 9 a.m. for his physical with Dr. Heath on June 5, 2012.
4. Vito Mangano did not keep his appointment with Dr. Heath on June 10. His appointment should be marked as "no show" for record keeping purposes.

Time began: _____   **Time ended:** _____   **Total time:** _____

No.	Step	Points	Check #1	Check #2	Check #3
1	The previous evening or before opening the ambulatory care setting, prepare a list of patients to be seen and assemble the charts.				
2	Check charts to see that everything is up to date, *paying attention to detail*.				
3	*When patients arrive, acknowledge their presence.* If you cannot assist them immediately, gesture toward a chair; thank them for waiting as soon as you are available.				
4	Check in the patient and review vital information, such as address, telephone number, insurance, and reason for visit. Be certain to *protect the patient's privacy* by reviewing this information where doing so cannot be overheard by others.				
5	Use a pen to check off the patient's name from the daily worksheet if one is used for the permanent record.				
6	Politely ask the patient to be seated and indicate the appropriate wait time, if any.				

No.	Step	Points	Check #1	Check #2	Check #3
7	Following clinic policy, place the chart where it can be picked up to route the patient to the appropriate location for the visit.				
Student's Total Points					
Points Possible					
Final Score (Student's Total Points/Possible Points)					

Instructor's/Evaluator's Comments and Suggestions:

_____

_____

_____

_____

_____

_____

_____

CHECK #1	
Evaluator's Signature:	Date:

CHECK #2	
Evaluator's Signature:	Date:

CHECK #3	
Evaluator's Signature:	Date:

ABHES Competency: MA.A.1.8.c Schedule and manage appointments

CAAHEP Competencies: IV.P.2 Report relevant information to others succinctly and accurately; V.P.1 Manage appointment schedule, using established priorities

Name_____ **Date**_____ **Score**_____

● COMPETENCY ASSESSMENT

Procedure 13-6: Checking in Patients Using Medical Office Simulation Software (MOSS)

Task: To check in patients as they arrive for clinic appointments.

Conditions: • Computer with MOSS installed

Standards: Perform each Task within 5 minutes with a minimum score of ___ points, as determined by your instructor.

Competency Assessment Information

Use the following information to complete this procedure. The Case Study for Lynne Abbott is found directly following this Competency Assessment checklist.

Today is February 20, 2013, and you are working at the front office reception area. Greet patients as they arrive for appointments and check-in using MOSS as indicated below:

1. Case Study – Patient Lynne Abbott comes to the clinic and signs-in. After greeting her she is given a New Patient Information form so she can be registered. Copies/scans of her insurance cards are made. The clinic Privacy Policy is explained and the appropriate forms to be signed are given to the patient. Check in patient Abbott using MOSS.
2. Patient Barryroe arrives. As an established patient, you ask her to update her information by asking if her address, phone number, or insurance has changed since her last visit. She states the information is still the same. Check in patient Barryroe using MOSS.
3. Patients VanGillis and Simms arrive. They are new patients. Describe the information that must be obtained from these patients, and then check in both patients using MOSS.

Time began: _____ **Time ended:** _____ **Total time:** _____

No.	Step	Points	Check #1	Check #2	Check #3
1	Open MOSS and select Appointment Scheduling from the Main Menu.				
2	Using the calendar on the top right, select a date. Hint: Use the –M and +M and –Y and +Y to navigate to the correct month and year, and then click on the date.				
3	Click on the time slot for the patient's appointment and click on *View/Create Appointment*. As an alternate, the appointment time slot may be *double clicked*.				
4	On the *Patient Appointment Form* window, click in the box in front of *Checked In*. In a clinic environment, after obtaining patient information, signatures, insurance card copies and/or updating information, the patient file or electronic record is made ready for the clinical staff and provider.				

No.	Step	Points	Check #1	Check #2	Check #3
5	Click on the *Close* button to exit the *Patient Appointment Form.*				
6	Check in the next patient, or close the Practice Schedule and return to the Main Menu.				
Student's Total Points					
Points Possible					
Final Score (Student's Total Points/Possible Points)					

Instructor's/Evaluator's Comments and Suggestions:

_____

_____

_____

_____

_____

_____

_____

CHECK #1	
Evaluator's Signature:	Date:

CHECK #2	
Evaluator's Signature:	Date:

CHECK #3	
Evaluator's Signature:	Date:

ABHES Competencies: MA.A.1.7.b(2) Apply computer application skills using variety of different electronic programs including both practice management software and EMR software; MA.A.1.8.b Prepare and maintain medical records

CAAHEP Competencies: V.P.5 Execute data management using electronic healthcare records such as the EMR; V.P.6 Use office hardware and software to maintain office systems

CASE STUDY FOR LYNNE ABBOTT

No.	Step	
1	Open MOSS and select Appointment Scheduling from the Main Menu.	
2	Using the calendar on the top right, select a date. Hint: Use the –M and +M and –Y and +Y to navigate to the correct month and year, and then click on the date.	
3	Click on the time slot for Lynne Abbott's appointment and click on *View/Create Appointment.* As an alternate, the appointment time slot may be *double clicked.*	
4	On the *Patient Appointment Form* window, click in the box in front of *Checked In.* In a clinic environment, after obtaining patient information, signatures, insurance card copies and/or updating information, the patient file or electronic record is made ready for the clinical staff and provider.	
5	Click on the *Close* button to exit the *Patient Appointment Form.*	
6	Check in the next patient, or close the Practice Schedule and return to the Main Menu.	

Name_____ **Date**_____ **Score**_____

● **COMPETENCY ASSESSMENT**

Procedure 13-7: Cancelling and Rescheduling Procedures Using Paper Scheduling

Task: To protect the provider from legal complications; to free up care time for other patients; and to assure quality patient care.

Conditions:
- Patient chart
- Red ink pen
- Check-in list
- Appointment book

Standards: Perform the Task within 15 minutes with a minimum score of ___ points, as determined by your instructor.

Competency Assessment Information

Use the following information to cancel and reschedule appointments using paper scheduling.

1. Eric Gordon contacts the clinic today, June 4, 2012, because he is experiencing more acute symptoms related to his urinary problems; pain in the abdomen and burning when he urinates. His appointment for June 5 is rescheduled to today at 1:00 p.m.
2. Andrew Jefferson calls on Tuesday, June 4, 2012, to say that he cannot make the appointment tomorrow. His shoulder is no longer bothering him so he does not want to reschedule.

● **Time began:** _____ **Time ended:** _____ **Total time:** _____

No.	Step	Points	Check #1	Check #2	Check #3
1	Indicate on the appointment sheet all appointments that were changed, canceled, or did not show.				
	Changes: Note rescheduling in the appointment sheet margin and directly in the patient's chart; indicate new appointment time.				
	Cancellations: Note on both the appointment sheet and the patient's chart. Draw a single red line through canceled appointments. Date and initial cancellation in the patient chart.				
	No-shows: Note on both the appointment sheet and the patient's chart. Date and initial notations in the chart. No-shows can be indicated with a red *X* on the appointment sheet.				
	Student's Total Points				
	Points Possible				
	Final Score (Student's Total Points/Possible Points)				

Instructor's/Evaluator's Comments and Suggestions:

_____

_____

_____

_____

_____

_____

_____

CHECK #1	
Evaluator's Signature:	Date:

CHECK #2	
Evaluator's Signature:	Date:

CHECK #3	
Evaluator's Signature:	Date:

Work Documentation Form(s)

*Use using scheduling form provided in Procedure 13-3
**Progress Note template can be downloaded from the Premium Website

ABHES Competency: MA.A.1.8.c Schedule and manage appointments

CAAHEP Competencies: IV.P.8 Document patient care; V.P.1 Manage appointment schedule, using established priorities

Name_____ Date_____ Score_____

● COMPETENCY ASSESSMENT

Procedure 13-8: Cancelling a Patient Appointment Using Medical Office Simulation Software (MOSS)

Task: To cancel visits already on the practice schedule and provide a reason.

Conditions: • Computer with MOSS installed

Standards: Perform each Task within 5 minutes with a minimum score of ___ points, as determined by your instructor.

Competency Assessment Information

Use the following information to complete this procedure. The Case Study for Emery Camille is found directly following this Competency Assessment checklist.

Today is February 18, 2013, and you are working at the front office covering the scheduling desk. Cancel patient appointments as indicated below:

1. Case Study – The mother of patient Emery Camille calls to say her son's earache appears to be resolving and he feels much better. She would like to cancel the appointment on February 20, 2013.
2. Patient Ann Pinkston calls to say her children are taking her for a small vacation to their home upstate. She is not sure when she is returning. She will need to cancel her appointment on February 21, 2013, and will call at a later date to reschedule.
3. Patient Richard Manaly calls to say he wants to cancel his February 21, 2013, appointment. His sore throat is gone and he doesn't need the appointment.

Time began: _____   Time ended: _____   Total time: _____

No.	Step	Points	Check #1	Check #2	Check #3
1	Open MOSS and select Appointment Scheduling from the Main Menu.				
2	Using the calendar on the top right, select a date. Hint: Use the –M and +M and –Y and +Y to navigate to the correct month and year, and then click on the date.				
3	Click on the time slot for the patient's appointment and click on *View/Create Appointment*. As an alternate, the appointment time slot may be *double clicked*.				
4	On the *Patient Appointment Form* window, click in the box in front of *Cancelled*.				
5	Click the drop down box directly to the right and select the reason code for the patient's cancellation.				
6	In the next field to the right, enter the date of cancellation.				
7	Click on *Save Appointment*.				
8	Click on the *Close* button to exit the *Patient Appointment Form*.				

No.	Step	Points	Check #1	Check #2	Check #3
9	Cancel the next patient, or close the Practice Schedule and return to the Main Menu.				
Student's Total Points					
Points Possible					
Final Score (Student's Total Points/Possible Points)					

Instructor's/Evaluator's Comments and Suggestions:

_____

_____

_____

_____

_____

_____

_____

CHECK #1 Evaluator's Signature:	Date:

CHECK #2 Evaluator's Signature:	Date:

CHECK #3 Evaluator's Signature:	Date:

ABHES Competencies: MA.A.1.7.b(2) Apply computer application skills using variety of different electronic programs including both practice management software and EMR software; MA.A.1.8.b Prepare and maintain medical records

CAAHEP Competencies: V.P.5 Execute data management using electronic healthcare records such as the EMR; V.P.6 Use office hardware and software to maintain office systems

CASE STUDY FOR EMERY CAMILLE

No.	Step	
1	Open MOSS and select Appointment Scheduling from the Main Menu.	
2	Using the calendar on the top right, select a date. Hint: Use the –M and +M and –Y and +Y to navigate to the correct month and year, and then click on the date.	
3	Click on the time slot for the patient's appointment and click on *View/Create Appointment.* As an alternate, the appointment time slot may be *double clicked.*	
4	On the *Patient Appointment Form* window, click in the box in front of *Cancelled.*	
5	Click the drop down box directly to the right and select the reason code for the patient's cancellation.	(see screenshot for Step 4)
6	In the next field to the right, enter the date of cancellation.	(see screenshot for Step 4)

No.	Step	
7	Click on *Save Appointment*.	(see screenshot for Step 4)
8	Click on the *Close* button to exit the *Patient Appointment Form*.	
9	Cancel the next patient, or close the Practice Schedule and return to the Main Menu.	

Name_____ Date_____ Score_____

● COMPETENCY ASSESSMENT

Procedure 13-9: Rescheduling a Patient Appointment Using Medical Office Simulation Software (MOSS)

Task: To reschedule visits already on the practice schedule to another date and time.

Conditions: • Computer with MOSS installed

Standards: Perform each Task within 10 minutes with a minimum score of ___ points, as determined by your instructor.

Competency Assessment Information

Use the following information to complete this procedure. The Case Study for Isabel Durand is found directly following this Competency Assessment checklist.

Today is February 18, 2013, and you are working at the front office covering the scheduling desk. Reschedule patient appointments as indicated below:

1. Case Study – Isabel Durand calls the office to say she has to attend a meeting at work on February 20, 2013. She requests rescheduling her appointment to first thing in the morning on February 21, 2013. Change the appointment to 9:30 a.m. with Dr. Heath on February 21, 2013.
2. Robert Shinn's father calls the office to report that his son's fever is getting higher and he has missed two days of school. He would like Robert to see the doctor sooner than February 21, 2013. Reschedule his appointment for 10:00 a.m. February 18, 2013 with Dr. Heath.
3. Patient John Conway wants to reschedule his appointment from February 21, 2013, to February 19, 2013. He needs a different date, as he has another commitment to attend. Reschedule his appointment to 9:00 a.m. with Dr. Heath on February 19, 2013.

Time began: _____ **Time ended:** _____ **Total time:** _____

No.	Step	Points	Check #1	Check #2	Check #3
1	Open MOSS and select Appointment Scheduling from the Main Menu.				
2	Using the calendar on the top right, select a date. Hint: Use the –M and +M and –Y and +Y to navigate to the correct month and year, and then click on the date.				
3	Click on the time slot for the patient's appointment and click on *View/Create Appointment.* As an alternate, the appointment time slot may be *double clicked.*				
4	On the *Patient Appointment Form* window, click in the box in front of *Rescheduled.*				
5	Click the drop down box directly to the right and select the reason code for the reschedule.				
6	In the next field to the right, click on the *View Practice Reschedule* calendar icon. This will open the Practice Calendar.				

No.	Step	Points	Check #1	Check #2	Check #3
7	Select the new date, physician column, and time by double clicking in the time slot. Next, click on the *Close* button.				
8	On the *Patient Appointment Form,* click on *Save Appointment* to execute the rescheduled appointment.				
9	Click *OK* to complete the task.				
10	The updated *Patient Appointment Form* will display with the rescheduled appointment in Fields 3 and 4. Check appointment for accuracy.				
11	Click on the *Close* button to exit the *Patient Appointment Form.*				
12	Reschedule the next patient, or close the Practice Schedule and return to the Main Menu.				
Student's Total Points					
Points Possible					
Final Score (Student's Total Points/Possible Points)					

Instructor's/Evaluator's Comments and Suggestions:

_____

_____

_____

_____

_____

CHECK #1	
Evaluator's Signature:	Date:

CHECK #2	
Evaluator's Signature:	Date:

CHECK #3	
Evaluator's Signature:	Date:

ABHES Competencies: MA.A.1.7.b(2) Apply computer application skills using variety of different electronic programs including both practice management software and EMR software; MA.A.1.8.b Prepare and maintain medical records

CAAHEP Competencies: V.P.5 Execute data management using electronic healthcare records such as the EMR; V.P.6 Use office hardware and software to maintain office systems

CASE STUDY FOR ISABEL DURAND

No.	Step	
1	Open MOSS and select Appointment Scheduling from the Main Menu.	
2	Using the calendar on the top right, select a date. Hint: Use the –M and +M and –Y and +Y to navigate to the correct month and year, and then click on the date.	
3	Click on the time slot for the Patient Durand's appointment and click on *View/Create Appointment*. As an alternate, the appointment time slot may be *double clicked*.	
4	On the *Patient Appointment Form* window, click in the box in front of *Rescheduled*.	
5	Click the drop down box directly to the right and select the reason code for *Needs Different Date*.	(see screenshot for Step 4)
6	In the next field to the right, click on the *View Practice Reschedule* calendar icon. This will open the Practice Calendar.	(see screenshot for Step 4)

No.	Step	
7	Select February 21, 2013, and then double click in the time slot for 9:30 a.m. in the Dr. Heath column. Next, click on the *Close* button.	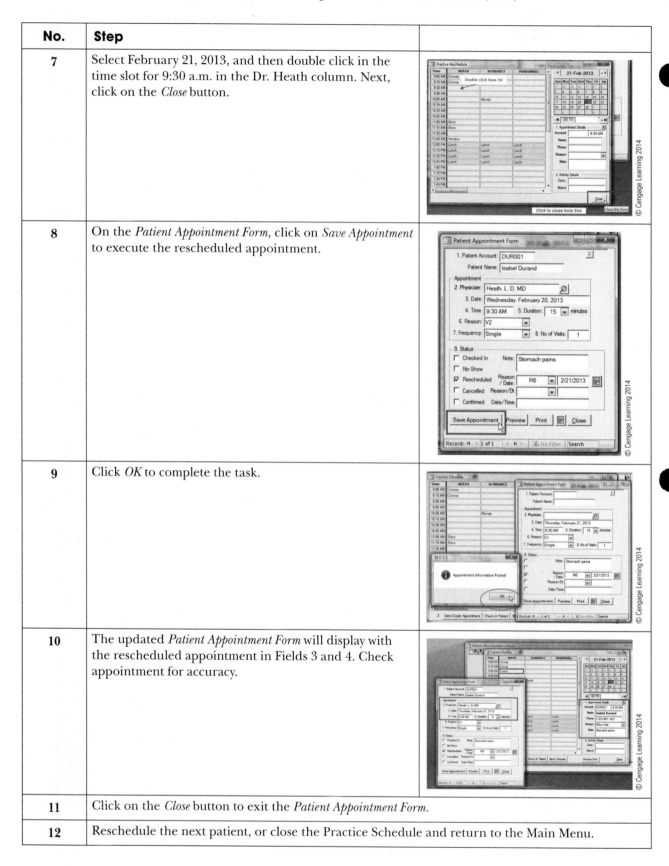
8	On the *Patient Appointment Form*, click on *Save Appointment* to execute the rescheduled appointment.	
9	Click *OK* to complete the task.	
10	The updated *Patient Appointment Form* will display with the rescheduled appointment in Fields 3 and 4. Check appointment for accuracy.	
11	Click on the *Close* button to exit the *Patient Appointment Form*.	
12	Reschedule the next patient, or close the Practice Schedule and return to the Main Menu.	

© Cengage Learning 2014

Name _____ **Date** _____ **Score** _____

● COMPETENCY ASSESSMENT

Procedure 13-10: Scheduling Inpatient and Outpatient Admissions and Procedures

Task: To assist patients in scheduling inpatient and outpatient admissions and procedures ordered by the provider.

Conditions: • Calendar
                • Black ink pen
                • Telephone
                • Referral slip
                • Patient's schedule/calendar
                • Provider's requests/orders regarding procedure/admittance

Standards: Perform the Task within 20 minutes with a minimum score of ___ points.

Competency Assessment Information

Use the following information to schedule inpatient and outpatient admissions and procedures.

1. Dr. Woo performs a nasal examination on Jose Ramirez and observes a small polyp in his left nostril. Schedule an appointment with Bayside Surgery for Mr. Ramirez to have the polyp removed on February 10 at 9 a.m.
2. Mary Petrovsky is seen in the clinic by Dr. King, who removes the cast on her left arm. He orders physical therapy as her arm is slightly atrophied. Schedule an appointment for Ms. Petrovsky on June 14 at 3 p.m.

● **Time began:** _____ **Time ended:** _____ **Total time:** _____

No.	Step	Points	Check #1	Check #2	Check #3
1	In a private and quiet location, discuss with the patient the inpatient admission or outpatient procedure ordered by the provider.				
2	If required, seek permission from the patient's insurance company for the procedure or admission.				
3	Produce a large, easily read calendar and check to see if the patient has one also.				
4	Place telephone call to the facility where the appointment is to be scheduled. Identify yourself, your provider, the clinic from where you are calling, and the reason for calling.				
5	*Display sound judgment* and identify any urgency if appropriate. Request the next available appointment for the particular appointment to be scheduled and provide the patient's diagnosis. Identify any time that is not possible for the patient.				
6	As a time is suggested, confer with the patient for an immediate response.				
7	Once the appointment has been scheduled, provide receiver with pertinent information related to the patient and request special instructions or advanced data necessary for the patient.				

No.	Step	Points	Check #1	Check #2	Check #3
8	Complete the referral slip for the patient; send or fax a copy to referred facility.				
9	If an immediate hospital admission is to be made, ***attend to special needs of patient*** by providing him or her time on the telephone to call family members to make arrangements to receive personal items and any other arrangements necessitated by the appointment.				
10	Place a reminder notice to yourself on the calendar or in a tickler file.				
11	Document the referral in the patient's chart. A copy of the referral slip and all pertinent data are to be included. Document in the chart when the appointment is completed and a report is received from the referral facility. Date and initial.				
Student's Total Points					
Points Possible					
Final Score (Student's Total Points/Possible Points)					

Instructor's/Evaluator's Comments and Suggestions:

_____

_____

_____

_____

_____

_____

_____

CHECK #1	
Evaluator's Signature:	Date:

CHECK #2	
Evaluator's Signature:	Date:

CHECK #3	
Evaluator's Signature:	Date:

Work Documentation Form(s)

*Progress Note template can be downloaded from the Premium Website

ABHES Competencies: MA.A.1.8.f Schedule inpatient and outpatient admissions; MA.A.1.8.ee Use proper telephone techniques; 8.hh Receive, organize, prioritize, and transmit information expediently

CAAHEP Competencies: IV.P.2 Report relevant information to others succinctly and accurately; IV.P.7 Demonstrate telephone techniques; V.P.2 Schedule patient admissions and/or procedures

Name _____ **Date** _____ **Score** _____

COMPETENCY ASSESSMENT

Procedure 14-1: Establishing a Paper Medical Chart for a New Patient

Task: To demonstrate an understanding of the principles for establishing a paper medical chart.

Conditions:
- File folder
- Divider pages
- Adhesive twin prong fasteners
- Twin hole punch
- Selected tabs
- Demographic patient information completed before or at the first appointment

Standards: Perform the Task within 15 minutes with a minimum score of ___ points, as determined by your instructor.

Competency Assessment Information

Use the following information to create a medical chart for a new patient in a paper system (Work Documentation).

1. Patient Registration Information for Jacalyn Dombrowski

Provider	Dr. Schwartz
Patient Contact Information	936 East Jackman Drive Douglasville, NY 12345 (123) 862-9133
Date of Birth	July 18, 1974
Social Security Number	999-82-1644
Marital Status	Married
Patient Employer Information	Regent Medical Clinic 847 Constitution Street Kensington, NY 12355 (123) 928-5475 x2198
Guarantor	Self
Insurance Information	ConsumerOne HRA 1230 Main St. Missoula, MT 08896 (800) 555-8887 ID# 463251178 Group# ADM246 Preventative visits covered at 100%
Signed HIPAA Notice of Privacy?	Yes

2. Patient Registration Information for Allen P. Boynton

Provider	Dr. Schwartz
Patient Contact Information	18 Brickyard Place, Unit #214 Douglasville, NY 12345 (123) 862-8849
Date of Birth	November 24, 1981
Social Security Number	999-33-1162
Marital Status	Single
Patient Employer Information	First Surety Investments 3175 Forest Grove Ave Ravensport, NY 12358 (123) 645-2189
Guarantor	Self
Insurance Information	Flexihealth PPO In-Network 30 W. Fifth Ave, Suite 100 New York, NY 10002 ID# 887912436 Group# 864BD $20.00 copayment
Signed HIPAA Notice of Privacy?	Yes

3. Patient Registration Information for Jessica L. McFadden

Provider	Dr. Heath
Patient Contact Information	97 Lindberg Street Douglasville, NY 12345 (123) 862-4387
Date of Birth	March 28, 1997
Social Security Number	999-76-0184
Marital Status	Single
Patient Employer Information	Full-time student at Jefferson Middle School
Guarantor	Patrick McFadden (father) SSN: 999-55-8374 Date of Birth: May 18, 1970
Guarantor's Address	Same as patient
Guarantor Employment Information	Addison-Kemp Insurance Agency 348 Main Street Douglasville, NY 12345 (123) 323-6743
Insurance Information	Signal HMO 4500 Old Town Way Lowville, NY 01453 ID# 012348756 Group# 9873
Signed HIPAA Notice of Privacy?	Yes, signed by Patrick McFadden

Time began: _____   **Time ended:** _____   **Total time:** _____

No.	Step	Points	Check #1	Check #2	Check #3
1	Assemble all supplies at a desk or table.				
2	Punch holes in the manila file folder and any necessary divider pages. Affix the adhesive twin prong fasteners.				
3	Assemble the divider pages dictated by the practice and the clinic policy in the proper location of the chart over the twin prong fasteners. Securely fasten twin prong fasteners over the divider pages.				
4	Index and code the patient's name according to the filing system to be used. Affix appropriately labeled tabs to the folder cut.				
5	Transfer demographic data in black ink pen or affix the demographic divider sheet to the inside front cover of the chart.				
6	Affix HIPAA required information, after it has been read and signed by the patient, as determined by clinic policy.				
7	Place prepared chart in proper location for pickup by the provider or clinical medical assistant.				
Student's Total Points					
Points Possible					
Final Score (Student's Total Points/Possible Points)					

Instructor's/Evaluator's Comments and Suggestions:

_____

_____

_____

_____

_____

_____

CHECK #1	
Evaluator's Signature:	Date:

CHECK #2	
Evaluator's Signature:	Date:

CHECK #3	
Evaluator's Signature:	Date:

ABHES Competencies: MA.A.1.8.a Perform basic clerical functions; MA.A.1.8.b Prepare and maintain medical records

CAAHEP Competency: V.P.3 Organize a patient's medical record

Work Documentation Form(s)

PATIENT CHART

| LAST NAME | FIRST NAME | MIDDLE NAME | BIRTH DATE | SEX | HOME PHONE |

| ADDRESS | | CITY | STATE | | ZIP CODE |

| CELL PHONE | PAGER NO. | FAX NO. | E-MAIL ADDRESS |

PATIENT'S SOC. SEC. NO.   DRIVER'S LICENSE

PATIENT'S OCCUPATION   NAME OF COMPANY

ADDRESS OF EMPLOYER   PHONE

SPOUSE OR PARENT   OCCUPATION

EMPLOYER   ADDRESS   PHONE

NAME OF INSURANCE   INSURED OR SUBSCRIBER

POLICY/CERTIFICATE NO.   GROUP NO.   REFERRED BY:

DATE	PROGRESS

Name _____ **Date** _____ **Score** _____

COMPETENCY ASSESSMENT

Procedure 14-2: Registering a New Patient Using Medical Office Simulation Software (MOSS)

Task: To register new patients using MOSS by entering information from the Patient Information Form and insurance cards.

Conditions: • Computer with MOSS installed

Standards: Perform the Task within 15 minutes with a minimum score of ___ points, as determined by your instructor.

Competency Assessment Information

Use the following information to complete this procedure. The Case Study for Lynne Abbott and all Source Documents are found directly following this Competency Assessment checklist.

1. Turn off Feedback Mode.
2. Today is February 20, 2013 and you are working at the front office reception area. After greeting and checking in patients as they arrive, new patients are registered using MOSS as indicated below:

   a. Case Study – Patient Lynne Abbott has checked in and returns her Patient Information Form and insurance cards to you. The Privacy Policy has been signed and dated by the patient. Register patient Abbott by entering this information using MOSS. HINT: Dr. Heath accepts assignment for both insurance plans, is in network, and has a signature on file for both.

   b. Patient Herbert VanGillis has checked in and returns his Patient Information Form and insurance card to you. The Privacy Policy has been signed and dated by the patient. Register patient VanGillis by entering this information using MOSS. HINT: Dr. Schwartz DOES NOT accept assignment with FlexiHealth PPO and is an out-of-network physician for that plan. No physician signatures are on file.

   c. Patient Robert Simms has checked in and returns his Patient Information Form and insurance cards to you. The Privacy Policy has been signed and dated by the patient. Register patient Simms by entering this information using MOSS. HINT: Dr. Heath accepts assignment for both insurance plans, is in network, and has a signature on file for both.

Time began: _____ **Time ended:** _____ **Total time:** _____

No.	Step	Points	Check #1	Check #2	Check #3
1	Open MOSS and select *Patient Registration* from the Main Menu.				
2	Select the patient from the *Patient Registration* window.				
3	Using the Patient Information Form, enter data for the *Patient Information Tab* from the form. When complete, click *Save.*				

No.	Step	Points	Check #1	Check #2	Check #3
4	Click on the *Primary Insurance Tab.* Enter information for the patient's primary insurance. When complete, click *Save.* Enter information about the provider accepting assignment, signature on file, and in-network status. Hint: Refer to the copy of the insurance card for other required information to enter.				
5	Click on the *Secondary Insurance Tab.* Enter information for the patient's secondary insurance. Be sure to check the box in Field 11 to bill the secondary after the primary. Enter information about the provider accepting assignment, signature on file, and in-network status. When complete, click *Save.* Hint: Refer to the copy of the insurance card for other required information to enter.				
6	Click on the *HIPAA Tab.* Check the box in front of *Yes* indicating that the HIPAA form was given and signed. Enter the date forms were signed. When complete, click *Save.*				
7	Click on the *Close* button to exit the *Patient Registration* window.				
8	Register the next patient, or close the patient selection window and return to the Main Menu.				
Student's Total Points					
Points Possible					
Final Score (Student's Total Points/Possible Points)					

Instructor's/Evaluator's Comments and Suggestions:

_____

_____

_____

_____

_____

_____

_____

CHECK #1	
Evaluator's Signature:	Date:

CHECK #2	
Evaluator's Signature:	Date:

CHECK #3	
Evaluator's Signature:	Date:

ABHES Competencies: MA.A.1.7.b(2) Apply computer application skills using variety of different electronic programs including both practice management software and EMR software; MA.A.1.8.b Prepare and maintain medical records

CAAHEP Competencies: V.P.5 Execute data management using electronic healthcare records such as the EMR; V.P.6 Use office hardware and software to maintain office systems

CASE STUDY FOR LYNNE ABBOTT

No.	Step	
1	Open MOSS and select *Patient Registration* from the Main Menu.	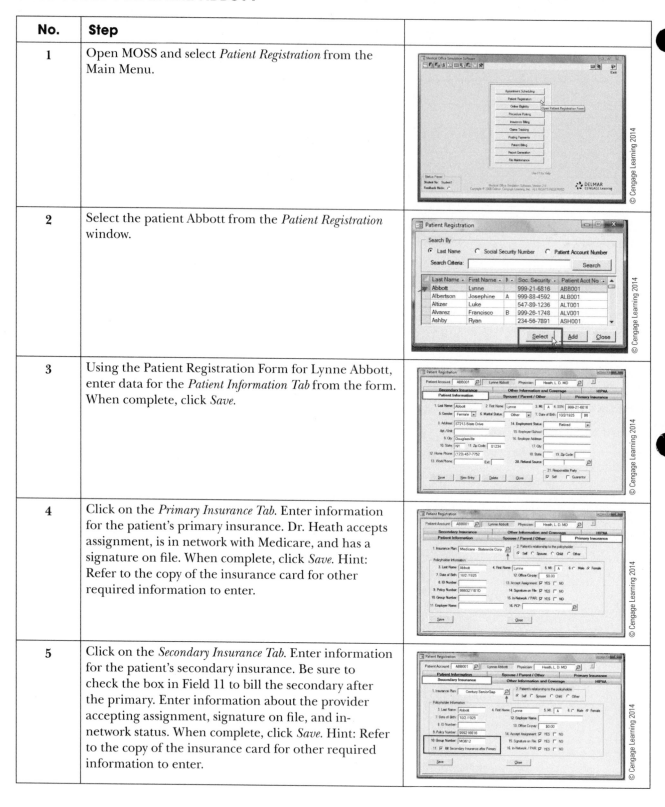
2	Select the patient Abbott from the *Patient Registration* window.	
3	Using the Patient Registration Form for Lynne Abbott, enter data for the *Patient Information Tab* from the form. When complete, click *Save*.	
4	Click on the *Primary Insurance Tab*. Enter information for the patient's primary insurance. Dr. Heath accepts assignment, is in network with Medicare, and has a signature on file. When complete, click *Save*. Hint: Refer to the copy of the insurance card for other required information to enter.	
5	Click on the *Secondary Insurance Tab*. Enter information for the patient's secondary insurance. Be sure to check the box in Field 11 to bill the secondary after the primary. Enter information about the provider accepting assignment, signature on file, and in-network status. When complete, click *Save*. Hint: Refer to the copy of the insurance card for other required information to enter.	

No.	Step	
6	Click on the *HIPAA Tab.* Check the box in front of *Yes* indicating that the HIPAA form was given and signed. Enter today's date, 02/20/2013, as received. When complete, click *Save.*	© Cengage Learning 2014
7	Click on the *Close* button to exit the *Patient Registration* window.	
8	Register the next patient, or close the patient selection window and return to the Main Menu.	

SOURCE DOCUMENTS FOR PROCEDURE 14-2: REGISTRATION FORMS

Welcome To Our Office
PLEASE PRINT

NEW PATIENT INFORMATION

Date 2/20/2013

LAST NAME Abbott	FIRST NAME Lynne	MI A	SSN 999216816		GENDER F	MARITAL STATUS Windowed	DATE OF BIRTH 10/2/25

ADDRESS 57213 State Drive		APT/UNIT	CITY Douglasville	STATE Ny	ZIP 01234	HOME PH ( ) (123) 457-7152	WORK PH ( ) EXT ( )

EMPLOYER/SCROLL Retired	EMPLOYER ADDRESS 57213 State Drive	CITY Dougtasville	STATE Ny	ZIP 01234

REFERRING PHYSICIAN (LAST NAME, FIRST NAME)	ADDRESS	CITY	STATE	ZIP	PHONE

GUARANTOR- Person responsible for payment ☒ self   ☐ spouse/other   ☐ parent   ☐ legal guardian if not "self", please complete the following:

LAST NAME	FIRST NAME	MT	SSN	GENDER	DATE OF BIRTH

ADDRESS (IF DIFFERENT FROM PATIENT)	CITY	STATE	ZIP	HOME PH ( )	ALT. PHONE

EMPLOYER NAME	EMPLOYER ADDRESS	CITY	STATE	ZIP	WORK PHONE EXT

OTHER RESPONSIBLE PARTY:

LAST NAME	FIRST NAME	MI	SSN	GENDER	DATE OF BIRTH

ADDRESS (IF DIFFERENT FROM PATIENT)	CITY	STATE	ZIP	HOME PH ( )	ALT. PHONE

EMPLOYER NAME	EMPLOYER ADDRESS	CITY	STATE	ZIP	WORK PHONE EXT

INSURANCE - PRIMARY

PLAN NAME Medicare/Statewide	PATIENT RELATIONSHIP TO INSURED: ☒ self ☐ spouse ☐ child ☐ other

POLICYHOLDER INFORMATION

LAST NAME Abbott	FIRST NAME Lynne	MI A	DATE OF BIRTH 10/2/25	ID #	POLICY # 999321181D	GROUP #

EMPLOYER NAME Retired	PCP NAME,IF APPLICABLE:

INSURANCE - SECONDARY

PLAN NAME Century Senior Gap	PATIENT RELATIONSHIP TO INSURED ☒ self ☐ spouse☐ child ☐ other

POLICYHOLDER INFORMATION

LAST NAME Abbott	FIRST NAME Lynne	MI A	DATE OF BIRTH 10/2/25	ID #	POLICY # 999216816	GROUP # ME612

EMPLOYER NAME Retired	PCP NAME, IF APPLICBLE:

ACCIDENT? ☐ YES ☐ NO IF YES, DATE OF INJURY	OCCUR AT WORK? ☐YES ☐ NO	AUTO INVOLED: ☐YES ☐NO	STATE

NAME OF ATTORNEY	PHONE NUMBER EXT.		

ALL PROFESSIONAL SERVICES RENDERED ARE CHARGED TO THE PATIENT. NECESSARY FORMS WILL BE COMPLETED TO HELP EXPEDITE INSURANCE CARRIER PAYMENTS. HOWEVER, THE PATIENT IS RESPONSIBLE FDA ALL FEES, REGARDLESS OF INSURANCE COVERAGE. IT IS ALSO CUSTOMARY TO PAY FOR SERVICES WHEN RENDERED UNLESS OTHER ARRANGEMENTS HAVE BEEN MADE IN ADVANCE WITH OUR OFFICE BOOKKEEPER.

INSURANCE AUTHORIZATION AND ASSIGNMENT

Name of Policy holder _____ Lynne Abbott _____ HIC Number _____
I request that payment of authorized Medicare/Other Insurance company benefits be made either to me or on my behalf to   Dr. Heath
for any services furnished me by that party who accepts assignment/physician. Regulations pertaining to Medicare assignment of benefits apply.
I authorize any holder of medical or other information about me to release to the Social Security Administration and CMS or its intermediaries or carriers any information needed for this or a related Medicare claim other Insurance Company claim. I permit a copy of this authorization to be used in place of the original, and request payment of medical insurance benefits either to myself or to the party who accepts assignment. I understand it is mandatory to notify the health care provider of any other party who may be responsible for paying for my treatment. (Section 1128B of the Social Security Act and 31 U.S.C. 3801–3812 provides penalties for withholding this information.) Acknowledgment of Receipt of Privacy Notice - I have been presented with a copy of this provider's Notice of Privacy Policies. detailing how my information may be used and disclosed as permitted under federal and state law. I understand the contents of the notice, and, subject to the following restriction(s) concerning my personal medical information, I agree to the disclosures named in the Notice: _____

Signature _____ Lynne Abbott _____   Date 2/20/2013 _____

Welcome To Our Office
PLEASE PRINT

NEW PATIENT INFORMATION

Date 2/20/2013

LAST NAME	FIRST NAME	MI	SSN		GENDER	MARITAL STATUS	DATE OF BIRTH
VanGillis	Herbert	-	999556218		M	Married	4/15/72

ADDRESS		APT/UNIT	CITY	STATE	ZIP	HOME PH ( )	WORK PH ( ) EXT
1257	Genwood CT		Douglasville	Ny	01235	(123) 457-5162	(123) 528-1168

EMPLOYER/SCHOOL	EMPLOYER ADDRESS	CITY	STATE	ZIP
Whole Foods	5223 Industry Way	Douglasville	Ny	01235

REFERRING PHYSICIAN (LAST NAME, FIRST NAME)	ADDRESS	CITY	STATE	ZIP	PHONE
Reed, Joseph					

GUARANTOR- Person responsible for payment ☒ self ☐ spouse/other ☐ parent ☐ legal guardian if not "self", please complete the following:

LAST NAME	FIRST NAME	MT	SSN	GENDER	DATE OF BIRTH

ADDRESS (IF DIFFERENT FROM PATIENT)	CITY	STATE	ZIP	HOME PH ( )	ALT. PHONE

EMPLOYER NAME	EMPLOYER ADDRESS	CITY	STATE	ZIP	WORK PHONE EXT

OTHER RESPONSIBLE PARTY:

LAST NAME	FIRST NAME	MI	SSN	GENDER	DATE OF BIRTH

ADDRESS (IF DIFFERENT FROM PATIENT)	CITY	STATE	ZIP	HOME PH ( )	ALT. PHONE

EMPLOYER NAME	EMPLOYER ADDRESS	CITY	STATE	ZIP	WORK PHONE EXT

INSURANCE - PRIMARY

PLAN NAME	PATIENT RELATIONSHIP TO INSURED:
Flexi Health PPO	☒ self ☐ spouse ☐ child ☐ other

POLICYHOLDER INFORMATION

LAST NAME	FIRST NAME	MI	DATE OF BIRTH	ID #	POLICY #	GROUP #
VanGills	Herbert		4/15/72		999556218	WF225

EMPLOYER NAME	PCP NAME, IF APPLICABLE:
Whole Foods	

INSURANCE - SECONDARY

PLAN NAME	PATIENT RELATIONSHIP TO INSURED ☐ self ☐ spouse ☐ child ☐ other
None	

POLICYHOLDER INFORMATION

LAST NAME	FIRST NAME	MI	DATE OF BIRTH	ID #	POLICY #	GROUP #

EMPLOYER NAME	PCP NAME, IF APPLICBLE:

ACCIDENT? ☐ YES ☐ NO IF YES, DATE OF INJURY	OCCUR AT WORK? ☐ YES ☐ NO	AUTO INVOLED: ☐ YES ☐ NO	STATE

NAME OF ATTORNEY	PHONE NUMBER EXT.		

ALL PROFESSIONAL SERVICES RENDERED ARE CHARGED TO THE PATIENT. NECESSARY FORMS WILL BE COMPLETED TO HELP EXPEDITE INSURANCE CARRIER PAYMENTS. HOWEVER, THE PATIENT IS RESPONSIBLE FDA ALL FEES, REGARDLESS OF INSURANCE COVERAGE. IT IS ALSO CUSTOMARY TO PAY FOR SERVICES WHEN RENDERED UNLESS OTHER ARRANGEMENTS HAVE BEEN MADE IN ADVANCE WITH OUR OFFICE BOOKKEEPER.

INSURANCE AUTHORIZATION AND ASSIGNMENT

Name of Policy holder____ Herbert VanGillis ____ HIC Number ____
I request that payment of authorized Medicare/Other Insurance company benefits be made either to me or on my behalf to Dr. Schwartz for any services furnished me by that party who accepts assignment/physician. Regulations pertaining to Medicare assignment of benefits apply. I authorize any holder of medical or other information about me to release to the Social Security Administration and CMS or its intermediaries or carriers any information needed for this or a related Medicare claim other Insurance Company claim. I permit a copy of this authorization to be used in place of the original, and request payment of medical insurance benefits either to myself or to the party who accepts assignment. I understand it is mandatory to notify the health care provider of any other party who may be responsible for paying for my treatment. (Section 1128B of the Social Security Act and 31 U.S.C. 3801–3812 provides penalties for withholding this information.) Acknowledgment of Receipt of Privacy Notice - I have been presented with a copy of this provider's Notice of Privacy Policies. detailing how my information may be used and disclosed as permitted under federal and state law. I understand the contents of the notice, and, subject to the following restriction(s) concerning my personal medical information, I agree to the disclosures named in the Notice;____

Signature ____ Herbert VanGillis ____   Date ____ 2/20/2013 ____

© Cengage Learning 2014

Welcome To Our Office
PLEASE PRINT

NEW PATIENT INFORMATION

Date 2/20/2013

LAST NAME Simms	FIRST NAME Robert	MI M	SSN 999161882		GENDER M	MARITAL STATUS Married	DATE OF BIRTH 3/5/32

ADDRESS 2366	APT/UNIT Pebble Trail	CITY Douglasville	STATE Ny	ZIP 01235	HOME PH ( ) (123) 457-5167	WORK PH ( ) EXT ( )

EMPLOYER/SCROOL Retired	EMPLOYER ADDRESS	CITY Douglasville	STATE Ny	ZIP 01235

REFERRING PHYSICIAN (LAST NAME, FIRST NAME) Ybarra, Elaine	ADDRESS	CITY	STATE	ZIP	PHONE

GUARANTOR- Person responsible for payment ☐ self   ☒ spouse/other   ☐ parent   ☐ legal guardian if not "self", please complete the following:

LAST NAME Simms	FIRST NAME Amelia	MT	SSN	GENDER F	DATE OF BIRTH

ADDRESS (IF DIFFERENT FROM PATIENT)	CITY	STATE	ZIP	HOME PH ( )	ALT. PHONE

EMPLOYER NAME BSA Enterprise	EMPLOYER ADDRESS	CITY	STATE	ZIP	WORK PHONE EXT (123) 528-0343

OTHER RESPONSIBLE PARTY:

LAST NAME	FIRST NAME	MI	SSN	GENDER	DATE OF BIRTH

ADDRESS (IF DIFFERENT FROM PATIENT)	CITY	STATE	ZIP	HOME PH ( )	ALT. PHONE

EMPLOYER NAME	EMPLOYER ADDRESS	CITY	STATE	ZIP	WORK PHONE EXT

INSURANCE - PRIMARY

PLAN NAME Consumerone HRA	PATIENT RELATIONSHIP TO INSURED: ☐ self ☒ spouse ☐ child ☐ other

POLICYHOLDER INFORMATION

LAST NAME Simms	FIRST NAME Amelia	MI	DATE OF BIRTH	ID #	POLICY # 99932581682R	GROUP # BSA5543

EMPLOYER NAME BSA Enterprise	PCP NAME,IF APPLICABLE:

INSURANCE - SECONDARY

PLAN NAME Medicare-Statewidecorp	PATIENT RELATIONSHIP TO INSURED ☒ self ☐ spouse ☐ child ☐ other

POLICYHOLDER INFORMATION

LAST NAME Simms	FIRST NAME Robert	MI M	DATE OF BIRTH 3/5/32	ID #	POLICY # 999161882A	GROUP #

EMPLOYER NAME Retired	PCP NAME, IF APPLICBLE:

ACCIDENT? ☐ YES ☐ NO IF YES, DATE OF INJURY	OCCUR AT WORK? ☐YES ☐ NO	AUTO INVOLED: ☐YES ☐NO	STATE

NAME OF ATTORNEY	PHONE NUMBER EXT.		

ALL PROFESSIONAL SERVICES RENDERED ARE CHARGED TO THE PATIENT. NECESSARY FORMS WILL BE COMPLETED TO HELP EXPEDITE INSURANCE CARRIER PAYMENTS. HOWEVER, THE PATIENT IS RESPONSIBLE FDA ALL FEES, REGARDLESS OF INSURANCE COVERAGE. IT IS ALSO CUSTOMARY TO PAY FOR SERVICES WHEN RENDERED UNLESS OTHER ARRANGEMENTS HAVE BEEN MADE IN ADVANCE WITH OUR OFFICE BOOKKEEPER.

INSURANCE AUTHORIZATION AND ASSIGNMENT

Name of Policy holder _____ Robert Simms _____ HIC Number_____
I request that payment of authorized Medicare/Other Insurance company benefits be made either to me or on my behalf to _____ DR. Heath _____
for any services furnished me by that party who accepts assignment/physician. Regulations pertaining to Medicare assignment of benefits apply.
I authorize any holder of medical or other information about me to release to the Social Security Administration and CMS or its intermediaries or carriers any information needed for this or a related Medicare claim other Insurance Company claim. I permit a copy of this authorization to be used in place of the original, and request payment of medical insurance benefits either to myself or to the party who accepts assignment. I understand it is mandatory to notify the health care provider of any other party who may be responsible for paying for my treatment. (Section 1128B of the Social Security Act and 31 U.S.C. 3801–3812 provides penalties for withholding this information.) Acknowledgment of Receipt of Privacy Notice - I have been presented with a copy of this provider's Notice of Privacy Policies. detailing how my information may be used and disclosed as permitted under federal and state law. I understand the contents of the notice, and, subject to the following restriction(s) concerning my personal medical information, I agree to the disclosures named in the Notice;_____

Signature _____ Robert Simms _____   Date ___ 2/20/2013 ___

SOURCE DOCUMENTS FOR PROCEDURE 14-2: INSURANCE CARDS

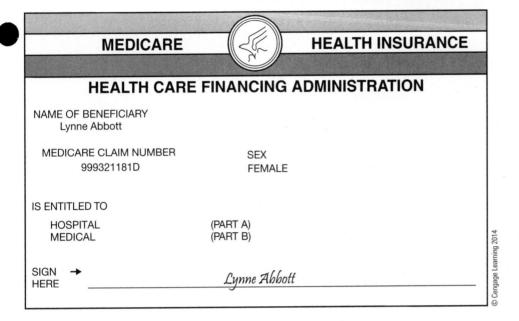

MEDICARE		HEALTH INSURANCE

HEALTH CARE FINANCING ADMINISTRATION

NAME OF BENEFICIARY
Lynne Abbott

MEDICARE CLAIM NUMBER   SEX
    999321181D   FEMALE

IS ENTITLED TO

    HOSPITAL   (PART A)
    MEDICAL   (PART B)

SIGN →
HERE   *Lynne Abbott* _____

© Cengage Learning 2014

**Century
SeniorGap**   *Medigap Plan J - region 23-5*

Insured: Lynne A. Abbott   999216816
Medigap Number: MG612

Insurer: CentSG

                               02CENT/09/TTGAP

© Cengage Learning 2014

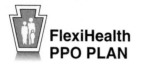

FlexiHealth
PPO PLAN

Insurer 81564

Your Health First SM

Insured: Van Gillis, Herbert
Employer: Whole Foods
Group: WF225

999556218

Network 45A-2

Physician Co-pay: $20.00
Hospital Services: $400.00 Annual deductible.
Surgery & Hospitalization: Requires preauthorization 800-123-3654

© Cengage Learning 2014

Consumer **ONE**

Benefits Card
Health Reimbursement Arrangement

Participant: Simms, Amelia
ID Number: 999325816-02R
Employer Group: BSA5543

Preventative Care: 100%
EPA – Call 800-123-8253
Level 3 - 80/20

In-Network Preferred

Plan Code GP123123

© Cengage Learning 2014

MEDICARE **HEALTH INSURANCE**

HEALTH CARE FINANCING ADMINISTRATION

NAME OF BENEFICIARY
   Robert Simms

MEDICARE CLAIM NUMBER   SEX
   999161882A   MALE

IS ENTITLED TO
   HOSPITAL   (PART A)
   MEDICAL   (PART B)

SIGN   ➜
HERE   _____ *Robert Simms* _____

© Cengage Learning 2014

Name _____ **Date** _____ **Score** _____

● **COMPETENCY ASSESSMENT**

Procedure 14-3: Correcting a Paper Medical Record

Task: To demonstrate the appropriate method to correct an error in a medical chart.

Conditions: • Document containing error
  • Document containing correction
  • Red ink pen

Standards: Perform the Task within 3 minutes with a minimum score of ___ points, as determined by your instructor.

Competency Assessment Information

Correct the following chart notes.

1. The patient's follow-up appointment should be October 16, 20XX in the chart note below.

10/14/20XX 10:00 AM	0.1 ml PPD intradermally (L) forearm. Pt given
	appointment to return 10/19/20XX to have PPT read.
	S. Jones , CMA (AAMA) ———————————

2. The patient's blood pressure should be 146/88 in right arm.

5/28/20XX 8:00 AM	T 99.6° F (R), P 104, R 20. BP 146/98 in right arm.
	C. McInnis, RMA (AMT) ———————————

Time began: _____ **Time ended:** _____ **Total time:** _____

No.	Step	Points	Check #1	Check #2	Check #3
1	Review information on correcting medical records.				
2	Draw single line through the error using a red ink pen.				
3	Write in the correct information.				
4	Write "Corr." or "Correction" above the corrected information.				
5	Initial and date the correction.				
Student's Total Points					
Points Possible					
Final Score (Student's Total Points/Possible Points)					

Instructor's/Evaluator's Comments and Suggestions:

_____

_____

_____

_____

_____

_____

_____

CHECK #1	
Evaluator's Signature:	Date:

CHECK #2	
Evaluator's Signature:	Date:

CHECK #3	
Evaluator's Signature:	Date:

Work Documentation Form(s)

*Progress Note template can be downloaded from the Premium Website

ABHES Competency: MA.A.1.8.b Prepare and maintain medical records

CAAHEP Competency: IX.P.7 Document accurately in the patient record

Name _____ **Date** _____ **Score** _____

● COMPETENCY ASSESSMENT

Procedure 14-4: Updating Patient Registration Information Using Medical Office Simulation Software (MOSS)

Task: To update patient registration information when changes are required.

Conditions: • Computer with MOSS installed

Standards: Perform the Task within 10 minutes with a minimum score of ___ points, as determined by your instructor.

Competency Assessment Information

Use the following information to complete this procedure. The Case Study for Caitlin Barryroe is found directly following this Competency Assessment checklist.

You are working at the front office reception area. Update changes to patient registration information using MOSS as indicated below:

1. Case Study – During Caitlin Barryroe's check-in on February 20, 2013, it is discovered while updating her patient information that she has changed employers and has different insurance coverage. Update the patient's registration information with the new employer and coverage:

   Employer: BSA Enterprise, 5200 Industry Way, Douglasville, NY 01235
   Insurance: ConsumerONE – HRA Policy: 999579754 Group: BSA5543 (No co-payment)

2. The clinic has had invoices returned as undeliverable by the Post Office addressed to Patient John Conway. When the patient checks in on February 19, 2013, for his visit, he is asked if his address has changed. The patient states he has moved, but all phone numbers remain the same. Update the patient's registration information with the correct address:

   7699 State Circle, Apartment 201, Douglasville, NY 01235

3. Robert Shinn's father, Karl, accompanies his son to his clinic visit. During an update at check-in on February 18, 2013, he informs that his son's phone number has changed to: (123) 457-9898. Robert Shinn will also be a full-time college student at Reginald University in New York City. He will continue to be covered on Karl Shinn's insurance until age 25. Update the patient's registration information with the correct phone number and college name.

Time began: _____   **Time ended:** _____   **Total time:** _____

No.	Step	Points	Check #1	Check #2	Check #3
1	Open MOSS and select *Patient Registration* from the Main Menu.				
2	Select the patient from the *Patient Registration* window.				
3	Select the tab(s) to display the area in which information needs to be updated, deleted, or added. Enter information as applicable.				
4	When complete, click *Save*, and then close the *Patient Registration* window.				

No.	Step	Points	Check #1	Check #2	Check #3
5	Update the next patient, or close the patient selection window and return to the Main Menu.				
Student's Total Points					
Points Possible					
Final Score (Student's Total Points/Possible Points)					

Instructor's/Evaluator's Comments and Suggestions:

CHECK #1	
Evaluator's Signature:	Date:

CHECK #2	
Evaluator's Signature:	Date:

CHECK #3	
Evaluator's Signature:	Date:

ABHES Competencies: MA.A.1.7.b(2) Apply computer application skills using variety of different electronic programs including both practice management software and EMR software; MA.A.1.8.b Prepare and maintain medical records

CAAHEP Competencies: V.P.5 Execute data management using electronic healthcare records such as the EMR; V.P.6 Use office hardware and software to maintain office systems

CASE STUDY FOR CAITLIN BARRYROE

No.	Step	
1	Open MOSS and select *Patient Registration* from the Main Menu.	
2	Select Patient Barryroe from the *Patient Registration* window.	
3	Select the tab to display the window for *Patient Information*. Update the employer information. When completed, click on *Save*.	
4	Next, select the tab to display the *Primary Insurance* and update the insurance information. When completed, click on *Save*.	
5	Close the *Patient Registration* window.	
6	Update the next patient, or close the patient selection window and return to the Main Menu.	

Name_____ **Date**_____ **Score**_____

● **COMPETENCY ASSESSMENT**

Procedure 14-5:   Steps for Manual Filing with an Alphabetic System

Task: To demonstrate an understanding of the principles of alphabetic filing.

Conditions: • Documents to be filed
                 • Dividers with guides
                 • Miscellaneous number file section
                 • Alphabetic card file and cards
                 • Accession journal, if needed

Standards: Perform the Task within 15 minutes with a minimum score of ___ points, as determined by your instructor.

Time began: _____   **Time ended:** _____   **Total time:** _____

No.	Step	Points	Check #1	Check #2	Check #3
1	Inspect and index.				
2	Sort the charts alphabetically.				
3	Create cross-reference files according to clinic policy.				
4	File the charts appropriately.				
5	Check chart placement to ensure chart is in correct location.				
Student's Total Points					
Points Possible					
Final Score (Student's Total Points/Possible Points)					

Instructor's/Evaluator's Comments and Suggestions:

_____

_____

_____

_____

_____

_____

_____

CHECK #1	
Evaluator's Signature:	Date:

CHECK #2	
Evaluator's Signature:	Date:

CHECK #3	
Evaluator's Signature:	Date:

ABHES Competencies: MA.A.1.8.a Perform basic clerical functions; MA.A.1.8.b Prepare and maintain medical records

CAAHEP Competencies: V.P.4 File medical records; V.P.8 Maintain organization by filing

Name_____ **Date**_____ **Score**_____

● **COMPETENCY ASSESSMENT**

Procedure 14-6:   Steps for Manual Filing with a Numeric System

Task: To demonstrate an understanding of the principles of the numeric filing system.

Conditions:
- Documents to be filed
- Dividers with guides
- Miscellaneous numeric file section
- Alphabetic card file and cards
- Accession journal, if needed

Standards: Perform the Task within 15 minutes with a minimum score of ___ points, as determined by your instructor.

Time began: _____ **Time ended:** _____ **Total time:** _____

No.	Step	Points	Check #1	Check #2	Check #3
1	Inspect and index.				
2	Code for filing units. Check the alphabetic card file for each piece to see if the card has already been prepared.				
3	Write the number in the upper-right corner. If no number is assigned, check the miscellaneous file. If item is ready to be assigned, make a card and note number in the right-hand corner of the card file, cross out the *M*, and make a chart file.				
4	If there is no card, make up an alphabetic card including a complete name and address, and then write either *M* or assign a number. Cross-reference if necessary and file the card properly.				
5	File in ascending order.				
Student's Total Points					
Points Possible					
Final Score (Student's Total Points/Possible Points)					

Instructor's/Evaluator's Comments and Suggestions:

_____

_____

_____

_____

_____

_____

_____

CHECK #1	
Evaluator's Signature:	Date:

CHECK #2	
Evaluator's Signature:	Date:

CHECK #3	
Evaluator's Signature:	Date:

ABHES Competencies: MA.A.1.8.a Perform basic clerical functions; MA.A.1.8.b Prepare and maintain medical records

CAAHEP Competencies: V.P.4 File medical records; V.P.8 Maintain organization by filing

Name_____ **Date**_____ **Score**_____

COMPETENCY ASSESSMENT

Procedure 14-7:   Steps for Manual Filing with a Subject Filing System

Task: To demonstrate an understanding of the principles of the subject filing system.

Conditions:
- Documents to be filed by subject
- Subject index list or index card filing listing subjects
- Alphabetic card file and cards

Standards: Perform the Task within 15 minutes with a minimum score of ___ points, as determined by your instructor.

Time began: _____   **Time ended:** _____   **Total time:** _____

No.	Step	Points	Check #1	Check #2	Check #3
1	Review the item to find the subject.				
2	Match the subject of the item with an appropriate category on the subject index list. If the item contains information that may pertain to more than one subject, decide on the proper cross-reference.				
3	If the subject title is written on the material, underline it. If the subject title is not written on the item, write it clearly in the upper right-hand corner and underline it.				
4	Use wavy underline for cross-referencing; use an *X* as with alphabetic and numeric filing.				
5	Underline the first indexing unit of the coded units.				
Student's Total Points					
Points Possible					
Final Score (Student's Total Points/Possible Points)					

Instructor's/Evaluator's Comments and Suggestions:

CHECK #1	
Evaluator's Signature:	Date:

CHECK #2	
Evaluator's Signature:	Date:

CHECK #3	
Evaluator's Signature:	Date:

ABHES Competencies: MA.A.1.8.a Perform basic clerical functions; MA.A.1.8.b Prepare and maintain medical records

CAAHEP Competencies: V.P.4 File medical records; V.P.8 Maintain organization by filing

Name _____ **Date** _____ **Score** _____

● **COMPETENCY ASSESSMENT**

Procedure 15-1: Preparing and Composing Business Correspondence Using All Components (Computerized Approach)

Task: To prepare and compose a rough draft and final copy letter using appropriate language and letter style to convey a clear and accurate message to the recipient.

Conditions:
- Computer and printer
- Printed letterhead and plan second sheet
- Dictionary, medical dictionary
- Thesaurus
- Style manual

Standards: Perform the Task within 20 minutes with a minimum score of ___ points, as determined by your instructor.

Competency Assessment Information

Go to the Premium Website to download the letterhead for Inner City Healthcare. The following patients were seen in the office and have overdue balances. Use the following information to compose letters, informing the patients that their accounts are past due and should be remitted immediately. Use March 15, 2013 as the date you are writing these letters. Remember to follow all appropriate formatting and guidelines.

1. Megan Caldwell was seen on December 14, 2012, by Dr. Schwartz, but she never paid her $20.00 co-payment. She lives at 83 Crestview Drive, Douglasville, NY 01234.
2. Justin McNamara had an office visit on December 18, 2012, and his claim was processed, indicating the balance of $64.00 to be applied to his deductible. His home address is 918 Porter Road, Compton, NY 01255.
3. Evan Lagasse had his annual physical examination on November 21, 2012. His insurance carrier processed the claim, indicating a patient deductible amount of $208.00. His address is 208 Jackman Lane, Compton, NY 01255.

Time began: _____ **Time ended:** _____ **Total time:** _____

No.	Step	Points	Check #1	Check #2	Check #3
1	Go to "Page Setup" and set document margins, paper size and source, and the layout. *Pay attention to detail*. Set the fonts to be used and paragraph parameters. Name and save the document.				
2	Organize key points to be addressed in a logical sequence. Compose a rough draft of the letter.				
3	Use language that is easily understood. State the reason for the letter in the first paragraph and encourage action in the last paragraph.				
4	Read the draft for obvious errors in grammar, spelling, and punctuation. Use the appropriate reference material to check any inaccuracies. Read again for content. Save the document again if any changes were made. Lay the letter aside and read it a third time at a later time.				
5	Choose the letter format that is customary to the ambulatory care setting.				

No.	Step	Points	Check #1	Check #2	Check #3
6	Key in the date or use the computer's auto date feature on line 15 or two to three lines below the letterhead. Key the recipient's name and address flush with the left margin beginning on line 20.				
7	On the second line below the recipient's address, key the salutation flush with the left margin. Follow the salutation with a colon unless you are using open punctuation. Key the subject of the letter on the second line below the salutation flush with the left margin, if the subject line is being used.				
8	Begin the body of the letter on the second line below the salutation or subject line.				
9	Key the complimentary closure on the second line below the body of the letter. Capitalize only the first letter of the word of the complimentary closing. Key the signature four to six lines below the complimentary closing. If reference initials are used, key the initials two lines below the keyed signature. Key the enclosure or copy notation one or two lines below the reference initials.				
10	*Pay attention to detail*. Proofread the document and make corrections as appropriate. Save the document again and print two copies.				
11	Prepare the envelope. Place the envelope flap over the letter and attach it with a paper clip.				
12	Place the letter on the provider's desk for review and signature. File a copy of the letter in an appropriate filing system.				
Student's Total Points					
Points Possible					
Final Score (Student's Total Points/Possible Points)					

Instructor's/Evaluator's Comments and Suggestions:

_____

_____

_____

_____

_____

_____

_____

CHECK #1	
Evaluator's Signature:	Date:

CHECK #2	
Evaluator's Signature:	Date:

CHECK #3	
Evaluator's Signature:	Date:

ABHES Competency: MA.A.1.8.jj Perform fundamental writing skills including correct grammar, spelling, and formatting techniques when writing prescriptions, documenting medical records

CAAHEP Competency: IV.P.10 Compose professional/business letters

Name_____ **Date**_____ **Score**_____

● **COMPETENCY ASSESSMENT**

Procedure 15-2: Addressing Envelopes According to United States Postal Service Regulations

Task: To address envelopes according to U.S. Postal Service regulations to ensure timely delivery.

Conditions:
- Computer and printer with envelope tray
- Envelopes
- Address labels
- U.S. Postal Service Publication 221, *Addressing for Success*

Standards: Perform the Task within 5 minutes with a minimum score of ___ points, as determined by your instructor.

Competency Assessment Information

Address envelopes for the patient letters created in Procedure 15-1.

1. Megan Caldwell, 83 Crestview Drive, Douglasville, NY 01234
2. Justin McNamara, 918 Porter Road, Compton, NY 01255
3. Evan Lagasse, 208 Jackman Lane, Compton, NY 01255

Time began: _____ **Time ended:** _____ **Total time:** _____

No.	Step	Points	Check #1	Check #2	Check #3
1	Insert the envelope in the printer and select the envelope format from the software program.				
2	Place the address within the proper area as directed by the U.S. Postal Service regulations.				
3	Key the address in uppercase letters. Be sure to maintain a uniform left margin on all lines. Eliminate all punctuation in the address except the hyphen in the Zip+4 code. If not using preprinted envelopes, key the return address in uppercase letters in the upper left corner of the envelope.				
4	*Pay attention to detail.* Proofread the envelope; make corrections as necessary.				
Student's Total Points					
Points Possible					
Final Score (Student's Total Points/Possible Points)					

Instructor's/Evaluator's Comments and Suggestions:

_____

_____

_____

_____

_____

_____

_____

CHECK #1	
Evaluator's Signature:	Date:

CHECK #2	
Evaluator's Signature:	Date:

CHECK #3	
Evaluator's Signature:	Date:

ABHES Competency: MA.A.1.8.a Perform basic clerical functions

Name_____ **Date**_____ **Score**_____

● **COMPETENCY ASSESSMENT**

Procedure 15-3:   Folding Letters for Standard Envelopes

Task: To fold and insert letters into envelopes so that the letters fit properly in the envelopes.

Conditions: • Letters to be mailed
                • Number 6¾ envelope, number 10 envelope, and window envelopes

Standards: Perform the Task within 2 minutes with a minimum score of ___ points, as determined by your instructor.

Competency Assessment Information

Fold the patient letters created in Procedure 15-1, for insertion into the envelopes created in Procedure 15-2.

Time began: _____   **Time ended:** _____   **Total time:** _____

No.	Step	Points	Check #1	Check #2	Check #3
1	To fit a standard-size letter into a number 6¾ envelope, fold the letter up from the bottom, leaving ¼ to ½ inch at the top, and crease it. Then fold the letter from the right edge about one third the width of the letter. Fold the left edge over to within ¼ to ½ inch of the right-edge crease. Insert the left creased edge first into the envelope.				
2	To fit a standard-size letter into a number 10 envelope, fold the letter up about one third the length of the sheet and crease it. Then fold the top of the letter down to within ¼ to ½ inch of the bottom crease, and crease the top. Insert the top creased edge first into the envelope.				
3	To fit a standard-size letter into a window envelope, turn the letter over and fold the top of the letter up about one third the length of the page so that the address is facing you. Then fold the bottom of the letter back to the first crease. Insert the letter into the envelope bottom first. *Pay attention to detail.* You should be able to read the entire address through the window.				
4	Moisten all envelopes before sealing.				
Student's Total Points					
Points Possible					
Final Score (Student's Total Points/Possible Points)					

Instructor's Evaluator's Comments and Suggestions:

_____

_____

_____

_____

_____

_____

_____

CHECK #1	
Evaluator's Signature:	Date:

CHECK #2	
Evaluator's Signature:	Date:

CHECK #3	
Evaluator's Signature:	Date:

ABHES Competency: MA.A.1.8.a Perform basic clerical functions

Name_____ **Date**_____ **Score**_____

● COMPETENCY ASSESSMENT

Procedure 15-4:   Creating a Mass Mailing Using Mail Merge

Task: To create a mass mailing using the computer's Mail Merge Helper feature contained within Microsoft Word.

Conditions: • Computer and printer
  • Composed correspondence keyed and saved as a Word document
  • A developed data source

Standards: Perform the Task within 15 minutes with a minimum score of ___ points, as determined by your instructor.

Competency Assessment Information

Go to the Premium Website to download the mail merge spreadsheet for Procedure 15-4, as well as the Inner City Health-care letterhead. Create a letter template using the information below, and then perform the mail merge.

Dr. Mendenhall will be joining the Douglasville Medicine Associates practice as of June 1, 2012. Dr. Mendenhall specializes in Allergy and Immunology. Appointments are now being accepted.

Time began: _____ **Time ended:** _____ **Total time:** _____

No.	Step	Points	Check #1	Check #2	Check #3
1	Compose and type the document.				
2	Develop a data source.				
3	Insert merge fields into the main document.				
4	Send the merged document to the printer.				
Student's Total Points					
Points Possible					
Final Score (Student's Total Points/Possible Points)					

Instructor's Evaluator's Comments and Suggestions:

_____

_____

_____

_____

_____

_____

_____

CHECK #1	
Evaluator's Signature:	Date:

CHECK #2	
Evaluator's Signature:	Date:

CHECK #3	
Evaluator's Signature:	Date:

ABHES Competencies: MA.A.1.8.a Perform basic clerical functions; MA.A.1.8.d Apply concepts for office procedures

Name_____ **Date**_____ **Score**_____

● **COMPETENCY ASSESSMENT**

Procedure 15-5:   Preparing Outgoing Mail According to United States Postal Regulations

Task: To prepare outgoing mail for expeditious delivery.

Conditions: • Manual or electronic scale
                • Postage meter or stamps
                • Envelope or package to be mailed

Standards: Perform the Task within 15 minutes with a minimum score of ___ points, as determined by your instructor.

Competency Assessment Information

Use the letters and envelopes created in Procedures 15-1, 15-2, and 15-3 to complete this exercise.

Time began: _____   **Time ended:** _____   **Total time:** _____

No.	Step	Points	Check #1	Check #2	Check #3
1	Sort the mail according to postal class.				
2	Using the manual or electronic scale, weigh the item to be mailed. *Pay attention to detail.*				
3	Affix the appropriate postage.				
4	Place the prepared mail in the area of the clinic designated for outgoing mail or deliver the mail to the post office according to clinic policy.				
Student's Total Points					
Points Possible					
Final Score (Student's Total Points/Possible Points)					

Instructor's Evaluator's Comments and Suggestions:

_____

_____

_____

_____

_____

_____

_____

CHECK #1	
Evaluator's Signature:	Date:

CHECK #2	
Evaluator's Signature:	Date:

CHECK #3	
Evaluator's Signature:	Date:

ABHES Competency: MA.A.1.8.a Perform basic clerical functions

Name_____ **Date**_____ **Score**_____

● COMPETENCY ASSESSMENT

Procedure 16-1: Transcribe Medical Referral Letters Using Medical Office Simulation Software (MOSS)

Task: Using provider's dictation, transcribe medical referral letters using MOSS.

Conditions: • Computer with MOSS installed

Standards: Perform the Task within 25 minutes with a minimum score of _____ points, as determined by your instructor.

Competency Assessment Information

Use the following information to complete this procedure. Case Study for Herbert VanGillis and all Source Documents are found directly following this Competency Assessment checklist.

Today's date is February 26, 2013. You are working in the Medical Transcription area. The clinic manager has dropped off a dictation tape in the inbox with correspondence to be transcribed today. Transcribe dictation for each patient using MOSS as indicated below:

1. Case Study – Patient VanGillis is the first patient on the tape, and the dictation is as shown on the source document. Using the Correspondence feature in MOSS, transcribe (type) the document, being sure to format the letter properly. Pay special attention to spelling, grammar, and punctuation. All transcribed documents will be placed on the provider's desk for signature. The mailing envelopes should also be prepared and be attached to any document that is to be mailed.
2. Patient Simms is next on the tape, and the dictation is as shown on the source document. Using the Correspondence feature in MOSS, transcribe the document, being sure to format the letter properly. Pay special attention to spelling, grammar, and punctuation. All transcribed documents will be placed on the provider's desk for signature. The mailing envelope should also be prepared and be attached to any document that is to be mailed.
3. Patient Abbott is next on the tape, and the dictation is as shown on the source document. Using the Correspondence feature in MOSS, transcribe the document, being sure to format the letter properly. Pay special attention to spelling, grammar, and punctuation. All transcribed documents will be placed on the provider's desk for signature. The mailing envelope should also be prepared and be attached to any document that is to be mailed.

Time began: _____ **Time ended:** _____ **Total time:** _____

No.	Step	Points	Check #1	Check #2	Check #3
1	After setting up the transcription equipment and inserting the tape, click on the *Billing* drop-down menu option in MOSS (along the top left) and click on *Patient Ledger.*				
2	Select the patient from the *Patient Account* list and click on *View.* This will display the patient's ledger. Hint: Click on the magnifying glass icon to drop down the list of patients.				
3	At the bottom left of the ledger screen, click on the *Correspondence* button.				
4	The *Output To* dialog box will open. Select a location to save your letter and name it as follows: patientlastname_letter_yourlastname. Click *OK* to save the letter.				

No.	Step	Points	Check #1	Check #2	Check #3
5	After a short pause, the letterhead for Douglasville Medicine Associates opens. Change the date of the letter to the desired date and put your own last name in the *Student No.* field.				
6	Delete the patient's name and address from the inside address area and replace with the name and address of the applicable recipient.				
7	If applicable, include a reference line with patient name before the salutation. With the cursor, click at *Type Message Here* and delete that line. Start the body of the letter at that location.				
8	Transcribe (type) the provider's dictation as shown on the source document. Be sure to format the letter, use punctuation, and use proper grammar.				
9	When complete, save the document by clicking on the *Save* button on the word processor.				
10	Print the letter so the provider may sign it and turn in a copy to your instructor. Prepare the mailing envelope(s).				
11	Close the word processor and return to the *Main Menu* in MOSS.				
Student's Total Points					
Points Possible					
Final Score (Student's Total Points/Possible Points)					

Instructor's/Evaluator's Comments and Suggestions:

_____

_____

_____

_____

_____

_____

_____

CHECK #1	
Evaluator's Signature:	Date:

CHECK #2	
Evaluator's Signature:	Date:

CHECK #3	
Evaluator's Signature:	Date:

ABHES Competencies: MA.A.1.7.b(2) Apply computer application skills using a variety of different electronic programs including both practice management software and EMR software; MA.A.1.8.b Prepare and maintain medical records

CAAHEP Competencies: V.P.5 Execute data management using electronic health care records such as the EMR; V.P.6 Use office hardware and software to maintain office systems

CASE STUDY FOR HERBERT VANGILLIS

No.	Step	
1	After setting up the transcription equipment and inserting the tape, click on the *Billing* drop-down menu option in MOSS and click on *Patient Ledger*.	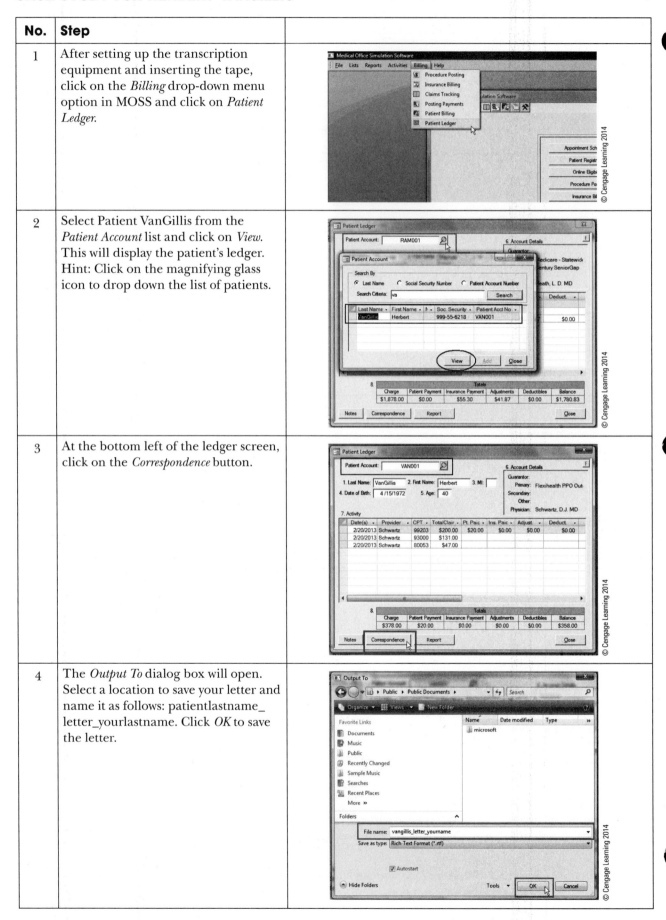
2	Select Patient VanGillis from the *Patient Account* list and click on *View*. This will display the patient's ledger. Hint: Click on the magnifying glass icon to drop down the list of patients.	
3	At the bottom left of the ledger screen, click on the *Correspondence* button.	
4	The *Output To* dialog box will open. Select a location to save your letter and name it as follows: patientlastname_letter_yourlastname. Click *OK* to save the letter.	

© Cengage Learning 2014

No.	Step	
5	After a short pause, the letterhead for Douglasville Medicine Associates opens. Change the date of the letter to the desired date and put your own last name in the *Student No.* field.	
6	Delete the patient's name from the inside address area and replace with the name and address of the applicable recipient. Hint: This letter is being sent to Dr. Kourkos.	
7	Include the reference line with patient name before the salutation, as indicated in the dictation. Next, with the cursor, click at *Type Message Here* and delete that line. Start the body of the letter at that location.	
8	Transcribe (type) the provider's dictation as shown on the source document. Be sure to format the letter, use punctuation, and use proper grammar.	(See source document for Herbert VanGillis dictation)
9	When complete, save the document by clicking on the *Save* button on the word processor.	
10	Print the letter so the provider may sign it and turn in a copy to your instructor. Prepare mailing envelopes for all recipients.	
11	Close the word processor and return to the *Main Menu* in MOSS.	

SOURCE DOCUMENTS FOR PROCEDURE 16-1: DICTATION

Patient: Herbert VanGillis

Physician: L.D. Heath, M.D.

Dictated Correspondence:

this is a letter to ... doctor matt k-o-u-r-k-o-s ... md ... at long island cardiology group ... pc ... address is four five zero zero main street in douglasville new york ... zero one two three five ... i believe it is suite three two zero ... dear doctor kourkos ... colon ... this letter is in reference to ... mister herbert vangillis ... capital v-a-n ... capital g-i-l-l-i-s ... please be sure to put a reference line with last name then first name before the salutation ... continue letter ... a new patient seen in my office on ... february ... nineteen ... two-thousand thirteen ... please check the date to be sure that was the date i saw the patient in the office ... if not put in the correct date ... mister vangillis moved to douglasville from ... hoboken ... new jersey ... and visited me to establish with a primary care physician ... new paragraph ... mister herbert is a pleasant man ... in his ... early forties and presents with a history ... of hyperlipdemia ... and mild angina pectoris ... the latter has been controlled on oral medications ... and he has lost sixty pounds within the past two years ... upon recommendation of his previous physician ... he has stopped smoking ... and participates in an exercise regimen ... four times a week ... he does have a history of ... two packs of cigarettes per day ... and started at age thirteen ... he was successful in quitting with the aid of ... a transdermal nicotine patch ... and states he has not smoked for one year ... there is a family history ... of angina ... and infarct ... for his father ... and grandfather ... the latter of which succumbed to sudden cardiac arrest at the age of ... fifty eight ... his father is also being followed by a cardiologist ... for coronary artery disease ... and had a triple bypass in his early fifties ... new paragraph ... i am referring mister vangillis to you for further evaluation ... of his cardiac health ... a chemistry metabolic panel was obtained when he was in the office ... and those results should be available by ehr in ... two days ... he also had a baseline ekg ... in the office ... with some minor abnormalities ... he did not have previous ekgs for comparison at this time ... the ekg from february twenty two thousand thirteen is attached for your review ... new paragraph ... mister herbert will be calling for ... a consultation appointment with you ... and if indicated will be ... followed for cardiac ... treatment ... with your cardiology office ... i look forward ... to receiving ... your assessment of this patients status ... sincerely yours ... l-d-heath ... md ... please send a courtesy copy of this letter to ... joseph reed ... md ... to his douglasville address ... not his office in yonkers ... one-six-zero-zero ... midway ... suite one zero two ... douglasville new york ... zero one two three four is the zip ... thank you ...

Patient: Robert Simms

Physician: L.D. Heath, M.D.

Dictated Correspondence:

this is a letter in reference to herbert ... correction ... robert ... simms ... s-i-m-m-s ... to joseph boomershine md ... pulmonary associates of douglasville ... pc ... forty five hundred main street ... suite two seven zero ... douglasville ... new york ... zero one two three five ... dear joe ... i am referring mister robert simms for evaluation of his ... c-o-p-d ... with ... cor pulmonale ... he was seen as a new patient ... in my office ... on february twenty two thousand thirteen ... mister simms has relocated to douglasville from ... hartford connecticut ... to be closer to his family and grandchildren ... new paragraph ... mister simms is an elderly gentleman with ... a history ... make that a long history ... of shortness of breath with exertion and ... requires assistance with ... everyday tasks ... he has been on long term oxygen therapy ... which he uses at all times ... at three liters per minute ... on the day of examination ... he had marked edema ... of both feet ... ankles ... and lower legs ... his height is five foot eight inches ... and weight ... weight ... is ... one hundred and ninety two pounds ... vital signs ... colon ... sorry ... vital sign sheet is misplaced ... here it is ... blood pressure one eighty two over ninety eight ... pulse one hundred two ... respirations twenty six and ... moderately labored ... there are ... audible wheezes upon auscultation ... there is a positive family history of emphysema ... and heart disease ... social history ... includes ... previous smoker up to three packs per day ... until nineteen ninety six ... he denies smoking since that time ... however ... his daughter states that he occasionally still smokes ... new paragraph ... medications include ... symbicort one sixty over four point five ... two puffs morning and night ... albuterol as needed ... two puffs every four hours ... and prednisone at flare-ups ... i do not believe mister simms has maximum benefit with his current therapy ... and have asked him to see you in consultation ... for his c-o-p-d ... he was also referred to doctor matt kourkos ... to evaluate his c-h-f ... we will follow him in this office as primary care physicians ... and look forward to co-managing mister simms health care ... with you ... thank you very much ... sincerely yours ... l-d ... heath ... md ... thank you ... no courtesy copies today

Patient: Lynne Abbott

Physician: L.D. Heath, M.D.

Dictated Correspondence:

please send this letter to … susan horwitz … md … at the northeast endocrinology center … two six two one … health drive plaza … suite five five zero … douglasville new york zero one two three five … and the letter is in reference to lynne abbott … i dont remember the date … please check our schedule and fill in the date in the body of the letter … dear doctor horwitz … missus abbott was seen in the office today … as a new patient she was born on october second nineteen twenty five and has had diabetes for over twenty five years … she … currently … lives with her daughter in … great neck … perhaps manhasset … correction … it is great neck … who has assumed … caretaker responsibilities … she uses nph and regular insulin … to maintain her blood sugars … her daughter states she was seeing an endocrinologist … at one time … but due to failing health … with joint pain … and mobility issues it is difficult for the patient … to leave home for regular doctor appointments … her last hemoglobin a-one-c … drawn several months ago was eleven point nine … blood glucose taken today was two hundred sixty … make that in the office … was two hundred sixty … new paragraph … her daughter states that the patient took … a fall … last week … but there were no apparent injuries … only minor bruising to … the knee … patient denies any pain … dizziness nausea vomiting or other neurological … abnormalities … she does have some soreness … in the hip area … but has good range of motion … and no visible injury … add strong pedal pulses after range of motion … vital signs today … colon … blood pressure one forty two over eighty-eight … heart rate eighty two … respirations sixteen … weight is one hundred thirty eight pounds height five feet four inches … she uses a walker … and has a scooter for longer distances … current medications include h-c-t-z … lisinopril … protonix … celebrex … aleve … nph … and and insulin … i have asked that missus abbott … be scheduled with you … for an evaluation of her diabetes … hopefully better control of her blood sugars can be obtained … thank you very much … sincerely yours l-d heath … md … no courtesy copies today …

Name_____ **Date**_____ **Score**_____

COMPETENCY ASSESSMENT

Procedure 17-1:   Applying Managed Care Policies and Procedures

Task: Apply managed care policies and procedures that the provider and/or medical facility has partnership agreements with.

Conditions: • Managed care contracts
                 • Managed care policies and procedures manuals
                 • Patient record
                 • Authorized forms from managed care organizations
                 • Clerical supplies

Standards: Perform the Task within 15 minutes with a minimum score of ___ points, as determined by your instructor.

Competency Assessment Information

Use the following information and the Verification of Eligibility and Benefits form (Work Documentation) to role-play a telephone call to the patient's managed care organization.

You are working in the office of Lewis & King, MD, in Northborough, Ohio.

Dr. Elizabeth M. King, NPI 1119809913
Lewis & King, MD
2501 Center Street, Northborough, OH 12345
(123) 555-7000
Dr. King participates in the FlexiHealth PPO plan.

Patient: Taye Ashton
800 Main Street, Apartment 3D
Springfield, OH 12344
(123) 557-0897
Birthday: June 30, 1986
Social Security Number: 999-56-7881
Married to Rosalee Ashton, Social Security Number: 999-48-1231

FlexiHealth **PPO PLAN**		Insurer 81564 1-800-123-3654
Insured:	Rosalee Ashton	9991234567-01
Employer:	Northborough Middle School	Network 11A-2
Group:	NMS99	
Family Plan		
Ashton, Taye E.		9991234567-02
Physician Co-pay: $20.00		
Hospital Services: $400.00 annual deductible		
Surgery & Hospitalizations: Requires preauthorization		

© Cengage Learning 2014

Time began: _____   **Time ended:** _____   **Total time:** _____

No.	Step	Points	Check #1	Check #2	Check #3
1	Determine which managed care organization the patient has contracted with.				
2	Call insurance company and obtain the correct information, including: • Verifying patient has insurance in effect and is eligible for benefits. • Confirming exclusions and noncovered services. • Determining deductibles, co-payments, or any other out-of-pocket expenses that the patient is responsible for paying. • Asking if preauthorization is required for referrals to specialists or for any procedures and/or services.				
3	Record the name, title, and telephone number and extension of the insurance person contacted.				
4	Collect any forms necessary to process the patient claims.				
5	*Pay attention to detail.* Document the information collected in the patient's medical record and on the Verification of Eligibility and Benefits form.				
6	*Show initiative* by attending seminars and workshops offered by managed care organizations or in-service training sessions.				
Student's Total Points					
Points Possible					
Final Score (Student's Total Points/Possible Points)					

Instructor's/Evaluator's Comments and Suggestions:

_____
_____
_____
_____
_____
_____
_____

CHECK #1	
Evaluator's Signature:	Date:

CHECK #2	
Evaluator's Signature:	Date:

CHECK #3	
Evaluator's Signature:	Date:

ABHES Competencies: MAA.1.8.s Obtain managed care referrals and pre-certification; MA.A.1.8.r Apply third-party guidelines

CAAHEP Competencies: VII.P.1 Apply both managed care policies and procedures; VII.P.2 Apply third party guidelines; VII.P.6 Verify eligibility for managed care services

Work Documentation Form(s)

VERIFICATION OF ELIGIBILITY & BENEFITS FORM

Patient's Name: _____

Today's Date: _____   SSN: _____   Date of Birth: _____

Primary Insurance: _____   Ph: _____

Plan ID#: _____   Group#: _____

Insured's Name: _____   SSN: _____

Is this plan a:

☐   PPO-In-Network

☐   PPO Out-of-Network

☐   Commercial/Indemnity

Insurance effective date: _____   Deductible amount: $_____

Has the deductible been met this year?   ☐ Yes   ☐ No   If no, amount remaining: $_____

Co-pay for office visits: $_____

	Is Pre-Authorization Needed? (Y/N)
Inpatient	
Surgery	
Laboratory	
Diagnostic Tests	

Where do we send the claim? _____

_____

I spoke with: _____   Phone: _____

Employee name/initials: _____

Name_____ **Date**_____ **Score**_____

● **COMPETENCY ASSESSMENT**

Procedure 17-2: Screening for Insurance

Task: Verify insurance coverage and obtain vital information required for processing and billing insurance claim forms.

Conditions:
- Patient registration forms
- Clipboard and black ink pen
- Patient's chart

Standards: Perform the Task within 15 minutes with a minimum score of ____ points, as determined by your instructor.

Competency Assessment Information

Use the following information to verify the patient's insurance.

Daniel Cho is a new patient to the practice and arrives 15 minutes before his scheduled appointment, as instructed. With another student or your instructor, role-play this exchange.

1. What form do you need to give Mr. Cho to fill out?
2. Once he returns the form, what do you need to collect from him?
3. Verify the patient's insurance coverage, using the information below. What is the phone number to call to verify eligibility?

Dr. Elizabeth M. King, NPI 1119809913
Lewis & King, MD
2501 Center Street, Northborough, OH 12345
(123) 555-7000
Dr. King participates in Medicaid.

Patient: Daniel Cho
41 Dewdrop Terrace
East Springfield, OH 12343
(123) 557-1080
Birthday: June 30, 1955
Social Security Number: 999-23-0818

OHIO DEPARTMENT OF HEALTH AND HOSPITALS
Ohio Health Choice Plan

Member ID#	111234999
Member	Daniel Cho
Card Issuance Date	January 01, 2014

Eligibility information 1-800-987-7000
Pharmacy information 1-800-987-7010
To report fraud, call 1-800-282-0889

© Cengage Learning 2014

Time began: _____   **Time ended:** _____   **Total time:** _____

No.	Step	Points	Check #1	Check #2	Check #3
1	Ask patient to bring his insurance card and arrive 15–20 minutes before appointment time to complete the patient registration form.				
2	When the patient turns in the completed registration form, review it immediately, *paying attention to detail,* to be sure that all information has been collected and that it is legible.				
3	Ask the patient for his insurance card. Make a photocopy of both sides of the card to be maintained in the patient's chart, or scan the insurance card and upload to the patient's electronic medical record.				
4	Verify proof of eligibility for Medicaid patients. The patient should have his or her proof of eligibility card with him or her, or you may need to make a telephone call directly to Medicaid or use the online electronic data exchange system to determine proof of eligibility.				
5	Each time a patient checks in, whether established or new, the following information should be verified: • Address. Confirm the patient's current address and telephone number. • Verify insurance coverage. • Ask for the patient's insurance card and verify information and effective dates. Also be sure that a photocopy of the card is maintained in the patient's chart. • Determine whether the insurance carrier covers the procedure. • Determine that the patient's PCP is performing the procedure. • Determine whether a referral is required and whether an authorization number or code is needed. • Confirm that evidence of qualifying has been secured.				
Student's Total Points					
Points Possible					
Final Score (Student's Total Points/Possible Points)					

Instructor's/Evaluator's Comments and Suggestions:

_____
_____
_____
_____
_____
_____
_____

CHECK #1	
Evaluator's Signature:	Date:

CHECK #2	
Evaluator's Signature:	Date:

CHECK #3	
Evaluator's Signature:	Date:

ABHES Competencies: MA.A.1.8.s Obtain managed care referrals and pre-certification; MA.A.1.8.r Apply third-party guidelines

CAAHEP Competencies: VII.P.1 Apply both managed care policies and procedures; VII.P.2 Apply third party guidelines; VII.P.6 Verify eligibility for managed care services

Name _____ **Date** _____ **Score** _____

● COMPETENCY ASSESSMENT

Procedure 17-3: Verify Insurance Eligibility Using Medical Office Simulation Software (MOSS)

Task: Verify insurance benefits electronically by using the Online Eligibility feature in MOSS.

Conditions: • Computer with MOSS installed

Standards: Perform each Task within 15 minutes with a minimum score of _____ points, as determined by your instructor.

Competency Assessment Information

Use the following information to complete this procedure. Case Study for Lynne Abbott is found directly following this Competency Assessment checklist.

You are working at the front office reception area on February 20, 2013. After registering new patients and inputting the patient information into MOSS, verify insurance for each patient as indicated below:

1. Case Study – Registration for Patient Lynne Abbott has been completed. Using MOSS, electronically verify benefits for Medicare and Century SeniorGap. Print the reports produced by MOSS.
2. Registration for Patient Herbert VanGillis has been completed. Using MOSS, electronically verify benefits for FlexiHealth PPO. Print the report produced by MOSS.
3. Registration for Patient Robert Simms has been completed. Using MOSS, electronically verify benefits for ConsumerONE HRA and Medicare. Print the reports produced by MOSS.

Time began: _____ **Time ended:** _____ **Total time:** _____

No.	Step	Points	Check #1	Check #2	Check #3
1	Open MOSS and select *Online Eligibility* from the Main Menu.				
2	Select the patient from the *Online Eligibility* window.				
3	Review the patient's data in the *Online Eligibility* window, and then click on the *Send to Payer* button.				
4	The *Online Eligibility Status* window will display the progress of electronically verifying the benefits. When complete, click on *View*.				
5	Review that data on the *Online Eligibility Report*, and then click on *Print (or Save, as directed by your instructor)*.				
6	Click on the *Close* button to exit the *Online Eligibility Report* window. Return to the *Main Menu*, and click on *Online Eligibility* once more.				
7	Select the patient from the *Online Eligibility* window.				
8	Verify benefits for the secondary insurance. First, click on the record bar at the bottom left to display the secondary insurance plan.				

No.	Step	Points	Check #1	Check #2	Check #3
9	Review the patient's data in the *Online Eligibility* window, and then click on the *Send to Payer* button.				
10	The *Online Eligibility Status* window will display the progress of electronically verifying the benefits. When complete, click on *View*.				
11	Review the data on the *Online Eligibility Report*, and then click on *Print (or Save, as directed by your instructor)*.				
12	Click on the *Close* button to exit the *Online Eligibility Report* window.				
13	Verify eligibility for the next patient, or return to the Main Menu.				
Student's Total Points					
Points Possible					
Final Score (Student's Total Points/Possible Points)					

Instructor's/Evaluator's Comments and Suggestions:

_____

_____

_____

_____

_____

_____

CHECK #1

Evaluator's Signature: _____ Date:

CHECK #2

Evaluator's Signature: _____ Date:

CHECK #3

Evaluator's Signature: _____ Date:

ABHES Competencies: MA.A.1.7.b(2) Apply computer application skills using variety of different electronic programs including both practice management software and EMR software; MA.A.1.8.b Prepare and maintain medical records

CAAHEP Competencies: V.P.5 Execute data management using electronic health care records such as the EMR; V.P.6 Use office hardware and software to maintain office systems

Case Study for Lynne Abbott

No.	Step	
1	Open MOSS and select *Online Eligibility* from the Main Menu.	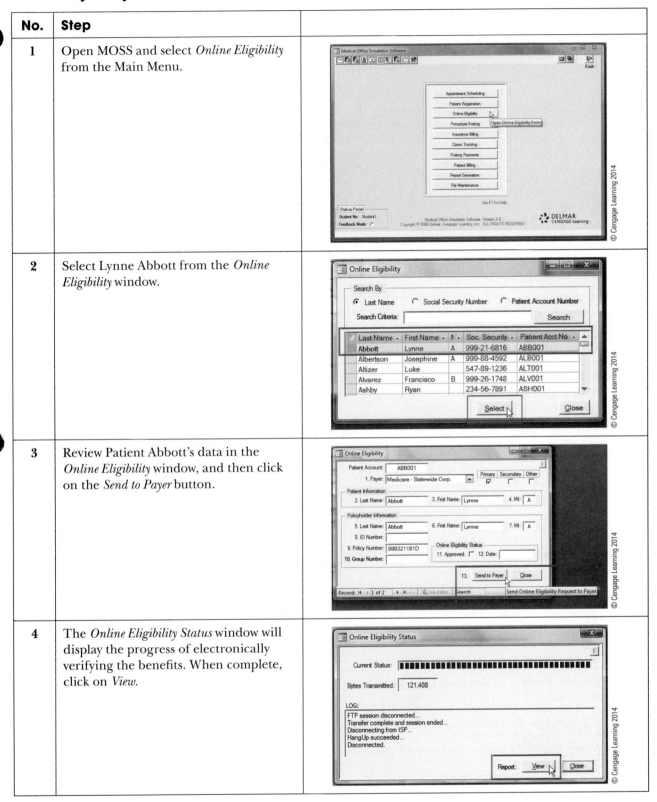
2	Select Lynne Abbott from the *Online Eligibility* window.	
3	Review Patient Abbott's data in the *Online Eligibility* window, and then click on the *Send to Payer* button.	
4	The *Online Eligibility Status* window will display the progress of electronically verifying the benefits. When complete, click on *View.*	

No.	Step	
5	Review that data on the *Online Eligibility Report,* and then click on *Print (or Save,* as directed by your instructor).	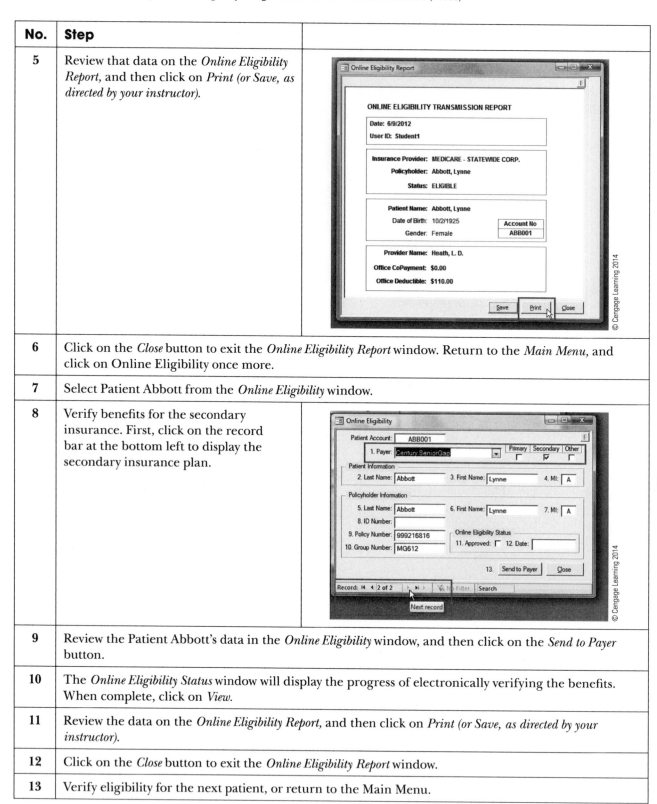
6	Click on the *Close* button to exit the *Online Eligibility Report* window. Return to the *Main Menu,* and click on Online Eligibility once more.	
7	Select Patient Abbott from the *Online Eligibility* window.	
8	Verify benefits for the secondary insurance. First, click on the record bar at the bottom left to display the secondary insurance plan.	
9	Review the Patient Abbott's data in the *Online Eligibility* window, and then click on the *Send to Payer* button.	
10	The *Online Eligibility Status* window will display the progress of electronically verifying the benefits. When complete, click on *View.*	
11	Review the data on the *Online Eligibility Report,* and then click on *Print (or Save,* as directed by your instructor).	
12	Click on the *Close* button to exit the *Online Eligibility Report* window.	
13	Verify eligibility for the next patient, or return to the Main Menu.	

© Cengage Learning 2014

Name _____   **Date** _____   **Score** _____

● COMPETENCY ASSESSMENT

Procedure 17-4:   Obtaining Referrals and Authorizations

Task: Ascertain coverage by the insurance carrier for specific medical services, hospital admissions, inpatient or outpatient surgeries, elective procedures, or when the primary care provider elects to refer the patient to another provider.

Conditions: • Patient's medical chart and copy of the patient's insurance card
               • Name of the carrier contact person and telephone number
               • Completed referral form
               • Telephone/fax machine
               • Pen/pencil

Standards: Perform the Task within 15 minutes with a minimum score of ___ points, as determined by your instructor.

Competency Assessment Information

Use the following information to complete the Treatment Authorization Request (Work Documentation).

Dr. King has ordered an MRI of the knee for Roberto Benini to confirm a diagnosis of osteomyelitis. The MRI will be done at Northborough Advanced Imaging. The patient is insured through Aetna, which requires preauthorization for this procedure.

1. Use the CPT code book and determine the correct code for MRI of the knee, without contrast material. The correct code is: _____
2. Use the ICD-9 code book and determine the correct code for acute osteomyelitis. The correct code is: _____
3. Complete the Managed Care Plan Treatment Authorization Request on the next page.

Dr. Elizabeth M. King, NPI 1119809913
Lewis & King, MD
2501 Center Street
Northborough, OH 12345
(123) 555-7000

Patient: Roberto Benini
Birth date: December 5, 1965
77 Treelawn Place
Northborough, OH 12345
(123) 555-1212

Facility: Northborough Advanced Imaging
1500 Broadway Boulevard
Northborough, OH 12345
(123) 555-8900

Time began: _____   **Time ended:** _____   **Total time:** _____

No.	Step	Points	Check #1	Check #2	Check #3
1	Collect all necessary documents and equipment. Determine the service or procedure requiring preauthorization. You will also need to know the name and telephone number of the specialist involved and the reason the request is being sought.				
2	Complete the referral form, being sure to include all pertinent information. Proofread the completed form, *paying attention to detail*.				
3	Fax the completed form to the insurance carrier. Maintain a completed copy of the referral form in the patient's chart.				
Student's Total Points					
Points Possible					
Final Score (Student's Total Points/Possible Points)					

Instructor's/Evaluator's Comments and Suggestions:

_____

_____

_____

_____

_____

_____

_____

CHECK #1	
Evaluator's Signature:	Date:

CHECK #2	
Evaluator's Signature:	Date:

CHECK #3	
Evaluator's Signature:	Date:

ABHES Competencies: MA.A.1.8.s Obtain managed care referrals and pre-certification; MA.A.1.8.r Apply third-party guidelines

CAAHEP Competencies: VII.P.4 Obtain precertification, including documentation; VII.P.5 Obtain preauthorization, including documentation

Work Documentation Form(s)

MANAGED CARE PLAN
TREATMENT AUTHORIZATION REQUEST

PATIENT INFORMATION

Patient Name _____ Date _____

M_____ F_____ DOB _____ Phone Number _____

REQUESTING PHYSICIAN INFORMATION

Primary Care Physician _____

Provider Number _____ Phone Number _____

REQUESTED SERVICE

Select service to be performed:

☐ Ambulatory Surgery/Procedure   ☐ Cardiac Rehabilitation

☐ Inpatient Services   ☐ Pain Management

☐ Medications   ☐ Durable Medical Equipment

☐ Biofeedback   ☐ Sleep Study

☐ Non-participating Provider   ☐ Physical/Occupational Therapy

Surgery/procedure/supply/med requested _____

Facility where service is to be performed _____

Facility Address _____ Phone Number _____

Facility City, State, Zip _____

Estimated length of stay_____

Procedure Code: _____ Description: _____

Procedure Code: _____ Description: _____

Diagnosis Code: _____ Description: _____

Diagnosis Code: _____ Description: _____

Signature of Requesting Physician: _____ Date: _____

TO BE COMPLETED BY UTILIZATION MANAGEMENT

Authorized _____ Not authorized _____

Deferred _____ Modified _____

Authorization Request # _____

Comments _____

Name _____ **Date** _____ **Score** _____

● COMPETENCY ASSESSMENT

Procedure 17-5: Computing the Medicare Fee Schedule

Task: Compute the Medicare allowable (MA) payment for services.

Conditions:
- CPT book
- Computer
- Calculator

Standards: Perform the Task within 15 minutes with a minimum score of ___ points, as determined by your instructor.

Competency Assessment Information

Medicare Physician Fee Schedule Formula
$[(RVUw \times GCPIw)* + (RVUe \times GCPIe) + (RVUm \times GCPI)] \times CF$

*Round product of two decimals to two places.
Conversion Factor (CF) = $37.8975.

CPT Code	Description	RVUw	RVUe	RVUm
99201	Office/Other Outpatient Visit, New Patient, Level 1	0.45	0.50	0.02
99202	Office/Other Outpatient Visit, New Patient, Level 2	0.88	0.79	0.06
99203	Office/Other Outpatient Visit, New Patient, Level 3	1.34	1.13	0.10
99204	Office/Other Outpatient Visit, New Patient, Level 4	2.00	1.51	0.12
99205	Office/Other Outpatient Visit, New Patient, Level 5	2.67	1.80	0.14

Contractor Number	Locality Number	Locality Name	GCPIw	GCPIe	GCPIm
00803	01	Manhattan, NY	1.094	1.351	1.586
00803	02	NYC Suburbs & Long Island	1.068	1.251	1.869
00803	03	Poughkeepsie/Northern NYC Suburbs, NY	1.011	1.075	1.221
14430	04	Queens, NY	1.058	1.228	1.791
56521	05	Rest of NY State	1.000	0.944	0.720

Using the information provided above, calculate the Medicare fee schedule for each of the situations below.

1. CPT 99201 in Queens, NY _____
2. CPT 99202 in Poughkeepsie, NY _____
3. CPT 99203 in Albany, NY _____
4. CPT 99204 in Buffalo, NY _____
5. CPT 99205 in Manhattan, NY _____

Time began: _____   **Time ended:** _____   **Total time:** _____

No.	Step	Points	Check #1	Check #2	Check #3
1	Using the *Current Procedural Terminology* (CPT) book, obtain the CPT code for the exact procedure or service for which a fee schedule is being computed.				
2	Using the Medicare Fee Schedule, determine the relative value units for (a) provider's time (work), (b) practice expense (PE), and (c) costs of malpractice insurance (MP) listed for the CPT code in Step 1.				
3	Using the Medicare Fee Schedule, determine the geographic practice cost index (GPCI). This factor accounts for different cost of living values for urban versus rural and geographic locations in the United States.				
4	Using the Medicare Fee Schedule, determine the Budget Neutrality Adjuster (BNA).				
5	Using the Medicare Fee Schedule, determine the relative value unit (RVU) conversion factor (CF).				
6	Compute the Medicare allowable fee for the procedure or service. Round to two decimal places.				
Student's Total Points					
Points Possible					
Final Score (Student's Total Points/Possible Points)					

Instructor's/Evaluator's Comments and Suggestions:

_____

_____

_____

_____

_____

_____

_____

CHECK #1	
Evaluator's Signature:	Date:

CHECK #2	
Evaluator's Signature:	Date:

CHECK #3	
Evaluator's Signature:	Date:

CAAHEP Competency: VII.P.1 Apply both managed care policies and procedures

Name_____ **Date**_____ **Score**_____

● COMPETENCY ASSESSMENT

Procedure 18-1: Current Procedural Terminology Coding

Task: Convert commonly accepted descriptions of medical procedures (services) and for visits of all kinds—office, hospital, nursing facility, home services—into a five-digit numeric code with two-digit numeric modifiers when required.

Conditions:
- CPT code book for the current year
- Copy of the encounter form and access to the patient's chart
- Pencil and paper

Standards: Perform the Task within 15 minutes with a minimum score of ___ points, as determined by your instructor.

Competency Assessment Information

Use the following information to determine the correct CPT codes.

1. Therapeutic or diagnostic injection (specify material injected); subcutaneous or intramuscular.
2. Aspiration of bladder by needle.

Time began: _____   **Time ended:** _____   **Total time:** _____

No.	Step	Points	Check #1	Check #2	Check #3
1	Using the CPT code book, look in the Evaluation and Management section, Office or Other Outpatient Services, New Patient. Carefully read through the options until the code matching the described scenario has been found.				
2	In the Index, find the correct code for the procedure.				
3	Now locate the code you have found in Step 2 in the Pathology and Laboratory section; ensure the description provided matches what the provider has documented in the patient's chart.				
Student's Total Points					
Points Possible					
Final Score (Student's Total Points/Possible Points)					

Instructor's/Evaluator's Comments and Suggestions:

_____

_____

_____

_____

_____

_____

_____

CHECK #1	
Evaluator's Signature:	Date:

CHECK #2	
Evaluator's Signature:	Date:

CHECK #3	
Evaluator's Signature:	Date:

ABHES Competency: MA.A.1.8.t Perform diagnostic and procedural coding

CAAHEP Competency: VIII.P.1 Perform procedural coding

Name_____   **Date**_____   **Score**_____

● **COMPETENCY ASSESSMENT**

Procedure 18-2:   International Classification of Diseases, 9th Revision, Clinical Modification Coding

Task: The ICD-9-CM code books provide a diagnostic coding system for the compilation and reporting of morbidity and mortality statistics for reimbursement purposes.

Conditions:
- Volumes I and II of the ICD-9-CM code books for the current year
- Copy of the encounter form and access to the patient's chart
- Pencil and paper

Standards: Perform the Task within 15 minutes with a minimum score of ___ points, as determined by your instructor.

Competency Assessment Information

Use the following information to determine the correct ICD-9-CM codes.

1. Anorexia nervosa.
2. Routine adult physical examination.

Time began: _____   **Time ended:** _____   **Total time:** _____

No.	Step	Points	Check #1	Check #2	Check #3
1	Using Volume II of the ICD-9-CM code books, look up the main reason or condition that brought the patient to the facility, or the specific diagnosis confirmed by test results.				
2	Using Volume I, look up the code you found in Step 1. Read all listings and determine the appropriate code having the greatest level of specificity.				
Student's Total Points					
Points Possible					
Final Score (Student's Total Points/Possible Points)					

Instructor's/Evaluator's Comments and Suggestions:

CHECK #1	
Evaluator's Signature:	Date:

CHECK #2	
Evaluator's Signature:	Date:

CHECK #3	
Evaluator's Signature:	Date:

ABHES Competency: MA.A.1.8.t Perform diagnostic and procedural coding

CAAHEP Competency: VIII.P.2 Perform diagnostic coding

Name_____ **Date**_____ **Score**_____

● **COMPETENCY ASSESSMENT**

Procedure 18-3: Applying Third-Party Guidelines

Task: Obtain written authorization to release necessary medical information to third-party payers.

Conditions: • Patient chart
                   • CMS-1500 claim form

Standards: Perform the Task within 5 minutes with a minimum score of ___ points, as determined by your instructor.

Time began: _____   **Time ended:** _____   **Total time:** _____

No.	Step	Points	Check #1	Check #2	Check #3
1	When patient signs in, check her/his chart to ascertain if an "Authorization to Release Medical Information" has been signed and is currently valid.				
2	During interaction with patient, demonstrate professional behavior, including *communicating in language the patient can understand* regarding managed care and insurance plans.				
3	If there is no record of signature on file, have the patient sign Block 12 of the CMS-1500 form.				
Student's Total Points					
Points Possible					
Final Score (Student's Total Points/Possible Points)					

Instructor's/Evaluator's Comments and Suggestions:

_____

_____

_____

_____

_____

_____

_____

CHECK #1	
Evaluator's Signature:	Date:

CHECK #2	
Evaluator's Signature:	Date:

CHECK #3	
Evaluator's Signature:	Date:

ABHES Competencies: MA.A.1.8.t Perform diagnostic and procedural coding; MA.A.1.8.r Apply third-party guidelines

CAAHEP Competency: VII.P.2 Apply third-party guidelines

Work Documentation Form(s)

1500
HEALTH INSURANCE CLAIM FORM
APPROVED BY NATIONAL UNIFORM CLAIM COMMITTEE 08/05

☐☐ PICA

PICA ☐☐

1. MEDICARE ☐ (Medicare #)   MEDICAID ☐ (Medicaid #)   TRICARE CHAMPUS ☐ (Sponsor's SSN)   CHAMPVA ☐ (Member ID#)   GROUP HEALTH PLAN ☐ (SSN or ID)   FECA BLK LUNG ☐ (SSN)   OTHER ☐ (ID)

1a. INSURED'S I.D. NUMBER   (For Program in Item 1)

2. PATIENT'S NAME (Last Name, First Name, Middle Initial)

3. PATIENT'S BIRTH DATE   MM | DD | YY   SEX   M ☐   F ☐

4. INSURED'S NAME (Last Name, First Name, Middle Initial)

5. PATIENT'S ADDRESS (No., Street)

6. PATIENT RELATIONSHIP TO INSURED   Self ☐   Spouse ☐   Child ☐   Other ☐

7. INSURED'S ADDRESS (No., Street)

CITY   STATE

8. PATIENT STATUS   Single ☐   Married ☐   Other ☐   Employed ☐   Full-Time Student ☐   Part-Time Student ☐

CITY   STATE

ZIP CODE   TELEPHONE (Include Area Code)   ( )

ZIP CODE   TELEPHONE (Include Area Code)   ( )

9. OTHER INSURED'S NAME (Last Name, First Name, Middle Initial)

10. IS PATIENT'S CONDITION RELATED TO:

11. INSURED'S POLICY GROUP OR FECA NUMBER

a. OTHER INSURED'S POLICY OR GROUP NUMBER

a. EMPLOYMENT? (Current or Previous)   YES ☐   NO ☐

a. INSURED'S DATE OF BIRTH   MM | DD | YY   SEX   M ☐   F ☐

b. OTHER INSURED'S DATE OF BIRTH   MM | DD | YY   SEX   M ☐   F ☐

b. AUTO ACCIDENT?   PLACE (State)   YES ☐   NO ☐

b. EMPLOYER'S NAME OR SCHOOL NAME

c. EMPLOYER'S NAME OR SCHOOL NAME

c. OTHER ACCIDENT?   YES ☐   NO ☐

c. INSURANCE PLAN NAME OR PROGRAM NAME

d. INSURANCE PLAN NAME OR PROGRAM NAME

10d. RESERVED FOR LOCAL USE

d. IS THERE ANOTHER HEALTH BENEFIT PLAN?   YES ☐   NO ☐   *If yes*, return to and complete item 9 a-d.

READ BACK OF FORM BEFORE COMPLETING & SIGNING THIS FORM.
12. PATIENT'S OR AUTHORIZED PERSON'S SIGNATURE I authorize the release of any medical or other information necessary to process this claim. I also request payment of government benefits either to myself or to the party who accepts assignment below.

SIGNED _____   DATE _____

13. INSURED'S OR AUTHORIZED PERSON'S SIGNATURE I authorize payment of medical benefits to the undersigned physician or supplier for services described below.

SIGNED _____

14. DATE OF CURRENT: MM | DD | YY   ◄ ILLNESS (First symptom) OR INJURY (Accident) OR PREGNANCY(LMP)

15. IF PATIENT HAS HAD SAME OR SIMILAR ILLNESS. GIVE FIRST DATE   MM | DD | YY

16. DATES PATIENT UNABLE TO WORK IN CURRENT OCCUPATION   MM | DD | YY   FROM   TO   MM | DD | YY

17. NAME OF REFERRING PROVIDER OR OTHER SOURCE

17a.
17b. NPI

18. HOSPITALIZATION DATES RELATED TO CURRENT SERVICES   MM | DD | YY   FROM   TO   MM | DD | YY

19. RESERVED FOR LOCAL USE

20. OUTSIDE LAB?   YES ☐   NO ☐ $ CHARGES

21. DIAGNOSIS OR NATURE OF ILLNESS OR INJURY (Relate Items 1, 2, 3 or 4 to Item 24E by Line)

1. |___ . ____   3. |___ . ____
2. |___ . ____   4. |___ . ____

22. MEDICAID RESUBMISSION CODE   ORIGINAL REF. NO.

23. PRIOR AUTHORIZATION NUMBER

24. A. DATE(S) OF SERVICE						B. PLACE OF SERVICE	C. EMG	D. PROCEDURES, SERVICES, OR SUPPLIES (Explain Unusual Circumstances)		E. DIAGNOSIS POINTER	F. $ CHARGES	G. DAYS OR UNITS	H. EPSDT Family Plan	I. ID. QUAL.	J. RENDERING PROVIDER ID. #
From MM	DD	YY	To MM	DD	YY			CPT/HCPCS	MODIFIER						
1														NPI	
2														NPI	
3														NPI	
4														NPI	
5														NPI	
6														NPI	

25. FEDERAL TAX I.D. NUMBER   SSN ☐ EIN ☐

26. PATIENT'S ACCOUNT NO.

27. ACCEPT ASSIGNMENT? (For govt. claims, see back)   YES ☐   NO ☐

28. TOTAL CHARGE $

29. AMOUNT PAID $

30. BALANCE DUE $

31. SIGNATURE OF PHYSICIAN OR SUPPLIER INCLUDING DEGREES OR CREDENTIALS (I certify that the statements on the reverse apply to this bill and are made a part thereof.)

SIGNED _____   DATE _____

32. SERVICE FACILITY LOCATION INFORMATION

a. NPI   b.

33. BILLING PROVIDER INFO & PH # ( )

a. NPI   b.

NUCC Instruction Manual available at: www.nucc.org

APPROVED OMB-0938-0999 FORM CMS-1500 (08-05)

Side labels: CARRIER / PATIENT AND INSURED INFORMATION / PHYSICIAN OR SUPPLIER INFORMATION

Name_____ **Date**_____ **Score**_____

● COMPETENCY ASSESSMENT

Procedure 18-4:   Completing a Medicare CMS-1500 (08-05) Claim Form

Task: Complete the CMS-1500 insurance claim form for reimbursement.

Conditions: • Patient information
                  • Patient account or ledger card
                  • Copy of patient's insurance card
                  • Computer and printer
                  • CMS-1500 Claim Form

Standards: Perform the Task within 30 minutes with a minimum score of ___ points, as determined by your
                  instructor.

Competency Assessment Information

1. Jordan Connell had an appointment on June 3, 2012, with Dr. Heath. Dr. Heath is billing for an established patient level 3 visit (99213, $111.00) and a rapid strep test (87880, $46.00). The diagnoses indicated by Dr. Heath are as follows: Strep Throat (034.0) and Otitis Media (382.9). Patient reference number is 100.
2. Ed Gormann came in for his physical with Dr. Heath on September 15, 2012. This visit will be billed using the preventive medicine procedure code 99396 ($266.00) and diagnosis code V70.0. Patient reference number is 101.
3. Elane Ybarra's appointment was on June 4, 2012, with Dr. Schwartz. Dr. Schwartz has submitted a superbill indicating that he is billing for an established patient level 4 visit (99214, $180.00). He has also indicated the following diagnosis: Gastroenteritis (558.9). Patient reference number is 102.

Time began: _____   **Time ended:** _____   **Total time:** _____

No.	Step	Points	Check #1	Check #2	Check #3
1	Correctly complete the Carrier section, in the upper portion of the form.				
2	Correctly complete the Patient and Insured section of the form, Blocks 1–13.				
3	Correctly complete the Provider or Supplier section of the form, Blocks 14–33.				
4	Proofread the form to ensure information is correct.				
Student's Total Points					
Points Possible					
Final Score (Student's Total Points/Possible Points)					

Instructor's/Evaluator's Comments and Suggestions:

_____

_____

_____

_____

_____

_____

CHECK #1	
Evaluator's Signature:	Date:

CHECK #2	
Evaluator's Signature:	Date:

CHECK #3	
Evaluator's Signature:	Date:

ABHES Competencies: MA.A.1.8.t Perform diagnostic and procedural coding; MA.A.1.8.u Prepare and submit insurance claims

CAAHEP Competency: VIII.P.2 Perform diagnostic coding

Work Documentation Form(s)

CARRIER

1500
HEALTH INSURANCE CLAIM FORM
APPROVED BY NATIONAL UNIFORM CLAIM COMMITTEE 08/05

PICA   PICA

1. MEDICARE MEDICAID TRICARE CHAMPUS CHAMPVA GROUP HEALTH PLAN FECA BLK LUNG OTHER	1a. INSURED'S I.D. NUMBER (For Program in Item 1)

(Medicare #)   (Medicaid #)   (Sponsor's SSN)   (Member ID#)   (SSN or ID)   (SSN)   (ID)

2. PATIENT'S NAME (Last Name, First Name, Middle Initial)

3. PATIENT'S BIRTH DATE MM | DD | YY   SEX   M   F

4. INSURED'S NAME (Last Name, First Name, Middle Initial)

5. PATIENT'S ADDRESS (No., Street)

6. PATIENT RELATIONSHIP TO INSURED   Self   Spouse   Child   Other

7. INSURED'S ADDRESS (No., Street)

CITY   STATE

8. PATIENT STATUS   Single   Married   Other

CITY   STATE

ZIP CODE   TELEPHONE (Include Area Code) ( )

Employed   Full-Time Student   Part-Time Student

ZIP CODE   TELEPHONE (Include Area Code ( )

9. OTHER INSURED'S NAME (Last Name, First Name, Middle Initial)

10. IS PATIENT'S CONDITION RELATED TO:

11. INSURED'S POLICY GROUP OR FECA NUMBER

a. OTHER INSURED'S POLICY OR GROUP NUMBER

a. EMPLOYMENT? (Current or Previous)   YES   NO

a. INSURED'S DATE OF BIRTH MM | DD | YY   SEX   M   F

b. OTHER INSURED'S DATE OF BIRTH MM | DD | YY   SEX   M   F

b. AUTO ACCIDENT?   PLACE (State)   YES   NO

b. EMPLOYER'S NAME OR SCHOOL NAME

c. EMPLOYER'S NAME OR SCHOOL NAME

c. OTHER ACCIDENT?   YES   NO

c. INSURANCE PLAN NAME OR PROGRAM NAME

d. INSURANCE PLAN NAME OR PROGRAM NAME

10d. RESERVED FOR LOCAL USE

d. IS THERE ANOTHER HEALTH BENEFIT PLAN?   YES   NO   **If yes,** return to and complete item 9 a-d.

READ BACK OF FORM BEFORE COMPLETING & SIGNING THIS FORM.
12. PATIENT'S OR AUTHORIZED PERSON'S SIGNATURE I authorize the release of any medical or other information necessary to process this claim. I also request payment of government benefits either to myself or to the party who accepts assignment below.

SIGNED _____ DATE _____

13. INSURED'S OR AUTHORIZED PERSON'S SIGNATURE I authorize payment of medical benefits to the undersigned physician or supplier for services described below.

SIGNED _____

PATIENT AND INSURED INFORMATION

14. DATE OF CURRENT: MM | DD | YY   ILLNESS (First symptom) OR INJURY (Accident) OR PREGNANCY(LMP)

15. IF PATIENT HAS HAD SAME OR SIMILAR ILLNESS. GIVE FIRST DATE MM | DD | YY

16. DATES PATIENT UNABLE TO WORK IN CURRENT OCCUPATION MM | DD | YY   FROM   TO   MM | DD | YY

17. NAME OF REFERRING PROVIDER OR OTHER SOURCE   17a.   17b. NPI

18. HOSPITALIZATION DATES RELATED TO CURRENT SERVICES MM | DD | YY   FROM   TO   MM | DD | YY

19. RESERVED FOR LOCAL USE

20. OUTSIDE LAB?   YES   NO $ CHARGES

21. DIAGNOSIS OR NATURE OF ILLNESS OR INJURY (Relate Items 1, 2, 3 or 4 to Item 24E by Line)
1. |___ . ___|
2. |___ . ___|
3. |___ . ___|
4. |___ . ___|

22. MEDICAID RESUBMISSION CODE   ORIGINAL REF. NO.

23. PRIOR AUTHORIZATION NUMBER

24. A. DATE(S) OF SERVICE From MM DD YY To MM DD YY	B. PLACE OF SERVICE	C. EMG	D. PROCEDURES, SERVICES, OR SUPPLIES (Explain Unusual Circumstances) CPT/HCPCS MODIFIER	E. DIAGNOSIS POINTER	F. $ CHARGES	G. DAYS OR UNITS	H. EPSDT Family Plan	I. ID. QUAL.	J. RENDERING PROVIDER ID. #
1								NPI	
2								NPI	
3								NPI	
4								NPI	
5								NPI	
6								NPI	

PHYSICIAN OR SUPPLIER INFORMATION

25. FEDERAL TAX I.D. NUMBER   SSN   EIN

26. PATIENT'S ACCOUNT NO.

27. ACCEPT ASSIGNMENT? (For govt. claims, see back)   YES   NO

28. TOTAL CHARGE $

29. AMOUNT PAID $

30. BALANCE DUE $

31. SIGNATURE OF PHYSICIAN OR SUPPLIER INCLUDING DEGREES OR CREDENTIALS (I certify that the statements on the reverse apply to this bill and are made a part thereof.)

SIGNED _____ DATE _____

32. SERVICE FACILITY LOCATION INFORMATION
a. NPI   b.

33. BILLING PROVIDER INFO & PH # ( )
a. NPI   b.

NUCC Instruction Manual available at: www.nucc.org

APPROVED OMB-0938-0999 FORM CMS-1500 (08-05)

Name_____ Date_____ Score_____

● COMPETENCY ASSESSMENT

Procedure 19-1: Recording/Posting Patient Charges, Payments, and Adjustments in a Manual System

Task: Record information including services rendered, fees charged, any adjustments made, and balances pertaining to a patient's visit to the provider's and the patient's account.

Conditions: • Calculator
• Patient's account or ledger

Standards: Perform the Task within 15 minutes with a minimum score of _____ points, as determined by your instructor.

Competency Assessment Information

Using the information below, post the charges to the appropriate patient accounts. Use the Patient Ledger form (Work Documentation) to complete this procedure.

1. Jordan Connell had an appointment on June 3, 2012, with Dr. Heath. Dr. Heath is billing for an established patient level 3 visit (99213, $111.00) and a rapid strep test (87880, $46.00). The diagnoses indicated by Dr. Heath are as follows: strep throat (034.0) and otitis media (382.9). Patient reference number is 100.
2. FlexiHealth PPO In-Network reimbursed the practice on October 20, 2012, for Ed Gormann's physical performed on September 15, 2012. The plan allowable was $200.56 minus a $20.00 patient co-payment that was not collected at the time of service. The net amount the plan paid for the visit totals $180.56.
3. Ed Gormann came in for his physical with Dr. Heath on September 15, 2012. This visit will be billed using the preventive medicine procedure code 99396 ($266.00) and diagnosis code V70.0. Patient reference number is 101.
4. Payment is received from ConsumerOne HRA on July 31, 2012, for Jordan Connell's visit on June 3, 2012, in the amount of $71.76 for the office visit (99213) and $11.04 for the strep test (87880). Write off any remaining balance as an insurance adjustment.
5. Elane Ybarra's appointment was on June 4, 2012, with Dr. Schwartz. Dr. Schwartz has submitted a superbill indicating that he is billing for an established patient level 4 visit (99214, $180.00). He has also indicated the following diagnosis: gastroenteritis (558.9). Patient reference number is 102.
6. For Elane Ybarra's visit on June 4, 2012, her insurer, FlexiHealth PPO In-Network, reimbursed the practice on August 10, 2012, in the amount of $89.06. The EOB indicates that the patient has a $22.26 coinsurance that was not collected at the time of the visit. Dr. Schwartz is not a participating provider in this plan.

Time began: _____   Time ended: _____   Total time: _____

No.	Step	Points	Check #1	Check #2	Check #3
1	Check the patient's account before the patient's appointment to make certain it is current.				
2	When the patient arrives, check for name, address, telephone numbers, and any charges regarding medical insurance. Make any changes in the account or on the ledger.				

No.	Step	Points	Check #1	Check #2	Check #3
3	On the encounter form or superbill, complete any necessary items such as the date of service and the responsible party's name. Then attach it to the patient's medical chart that is now ready for the clinical medical assistant to take with the patient to the examination room. When the provider completes the treatment or examination, he or she will check the procedures and diagnosis on the encounter form.				
4	When the patient returns to the front desk, refer to the provider's fee schedule, enter the charge next to each procedure, and calculate the total. If the procedure description is not indicated, one is to be provided. A description is necessary for each service. Check to see if the codes match the services provided. If they do not match, refer it back to the provider or licensed caregiver for correction.				
5	In the *manual pegboard system*, post each service or procedure as a charge or debit. Post any payments received today in the payment column as a credit.				
6	If any adjustment applies to the account, enter the amount in the adjustment column. If there is no adjustment column and the adjustment will *reduce* the bill, enter the amount in the payment column enclosed by parentheses. If the adjustment will *increase* the bill, place the amount in the charge column (no parentheses) with an explanation in the description column. In the *manual system*, the adjustment amount will be either added or subtracted from the totaled figures.				
7	Determine current balance by adding credits and subtracting debits to the running balance and determine the amount in the current balance.				
8	If the recording is a payment from the patient, place a restrictive endorsement on the check.				
9	Enter the amount in the payment column. In the description column, identify as cash, check, or insurance payment. If payment is a check, enter the number of the check.				
10	Place the cash or processed check in the appointed secure place awaiting deposit.				
Student's Total Points					
Points Possible					
Final Score (Student's Total Points/Possible Points)					

Instructor's/Evaluator's Comments and Suggestions:

_____

_____

_____

_____

_____

_____

_____

CHECK #1	
Evaluator's Signature:	Date:

CHECK #2	
Evaluator's Signature:	Date:

CHECK #3	
Evaluator's Signature:	Date:

ABHES Competencies: MA.A.1.8.h Post entries on a day sheet; MA.A.1.8.i Perform billing and collection procedures; MA.A.1.8.m Post adjustments; MA.A.1.8.w Use manual and computerized bookkeeping systems

CAAHEP Competencies: VI.P.2.a Post entries on a day sheet; VI.P.2.b Perform billing procedures; VI.P.2.d Post adjustments

Work Documentation Form(s): Patient Ledger

STATEMENT
DOUGLASVILLE MEDICINE ASSOCIATES.
5076 Brand Blvd., Suite 401
Douglasville, NY 01234
TEL: (123) 456-7890
FAX: (123) 456-7891

Patient Name:
Address:

Phone No.(H)_____(W)_____Birthdate_____
Insurance Co._____ Policy No._____

DATE	REFERENCE	DESCRIPTION	CHARGES	CREDITS		BALANCE	
				Pymnt s.	Adj.		
		BALANCE FORWARD					

Name_____ **Date**_____ **Score**_____

● COMPETENCY ASSESSMENT

Procedure 19-2: Balancing Day Sheets in a Manual System

Task: Verify that all entries to the day sheet are correct and that the totals balance.

Conditions:
- Day sheet
- Calculator

Standards: Perform the Task within 15 minutes with _____ points, as determined by your instructor.

Time began: _____ **Time ended:** _____ **Total time:** _____

No.	Step	Points	Check #1	Check #2	Check #3
1	Total columns A, B_1, B_2, C, and D, and enter the total for each column in the boxes marked "Totals This Page." Then add the column totals to the figures entered in the "Previous Page" column boxes to arrive at the "Month to Date" totals, which provide the total charges, credits, and so forth entered from the first working day of the month to the present.				
2	Correctly complete Proof of Posting box. • Enter today's column D total, which shows the sum of all the previous balances entered when the transactions were posted. • Add this to the column A total of all charges for that day, to arrive at a subtotal. Enter the amount where indicated in the box. • Add columns B_1 and B_2 together and enter them in the box labeled "Less Cols B_1 and B_2"; the total of credits is subtracted from the subtotal. If all entries and addition are correct in the posting area, the result should equal the amount in column C and the transactions for that day are balanced.				
3	Correctly complete Accounts Receivable Control box. • Carry the column A and column B totals straight across from the Proof of Posting box to the corresponding blanks in the A/R Control box. • Add the amount already entered in the Previous Day's Total space to the Column A amount to arrive at a subtotal. • Subtract the amount carried over from the "Less Columns B_1 and B_2" box to find the new A/R amount.				

No.	Step	Points	Check #1	Check #2	Check #3
4	Correctly complete Accounts Receivable Proof box. If all posting and addition are correct, the Total A/R amounts in the A/R Control and A/R Proof boxes will match and the day is balanced. • Enter the amount from column A (month-to-date) where shown. • Add the column A amount to the "A/R 1st of Month" figure and enter the sum in the subtotal space. • Enter the B_1 and B_2 month-to-date amounts and subtract from the subtotal. This amount goes in the Total A/R space.				
5	Correctly calculate the Total Deposit and enter in the appropriate field.				
6	Correctly complete the Business Analysis Summary, if used, and total each column in the summary section.				
7	Complete the transfer of balances. • Take out a new day sheet for the next day. • Transfer the "Month-To-Date" column totals to the "Previous Page" columns boxes on the new sheet. • Enter the Total A/R amount from the last day sheet in the "Previous Day's Total" space of the A/R Control box on the new day sheet. • Enter the A/R 1st of Month Amount in the A/R Proof box on the new sheet.				
Student's Total Points					
Points Possible					
Final Score (Student's Total Points/Possible Points)					

Instructor's/Evaluator's Comments and Suggestions:

_____

_____

_____

_____

_____

_____

_____

CHECK #1 Evaluator's Signature:	Date:

CHECK #2 Evaluator's Signature:	Date:

CHECK #3 Evaluator's Signature:	Date:

ABHES Competencies: MA.A.1.8.h. Post entries on a day sheet; MA.A.1.8.w. Use manual or computerized book-keeping systems

CAAHEP Competency: VI.P.2.a Post entries on a day sheet

Work Documentation Form(s): Day Sheet

DAYSHEET (RECORD OF CHARGES AND RECEIPTS)

PAGE NO _____ OF _____ DATE _____

RECORD OF DEPOSITS

DATE	REFERENCE	DESCRIPTION	CHARGES	GREDITS		BALANCE	PREVIOUS BALANCE	√	NAME	RECEIPT NUMBER
				PYMNTS.	ADJ.					

CREDITS: Col. A | Col. B-1 | Col. B-2 | Col. C | Col. D

RECORD OF DEPOSITS — DATE: | CASH | CHECKS

Receipt rows numbered 1–28

PREPARED BY

TOTAL CASH
TOTAL CHECKS
TOTAL DEPOSIT

TOTALS THIS PAGE
PREVIOUS PAGE
MONTH-TO-DATE

PROOF OF POSTING

COL. D TOTAL	$
PLUS COL. A TOTAL	$
SUB TOTAL	$
LESS COLS. B-1 & B-2	$
MUST EQUAL COL. C	$

ACCOUNTS RECEIVABLE CONTROL

PREVIOUS DAY'S TOTAL	$
PLUS COL. A	$
SUB TOTAL	$
LESS COLS. B-1 & B-2	$
TOTAL ACCTS. REC.	$

ACCOUNTS RECEIVABLE PROOF

ACCTS. REC. 1ST OF MONTH	$
PLUS COL. A - MONTH TO DATE	$
SUB TOTAL	$
LESS B-1 & B-2 MO. TO DATE	$
TOTAL ACCTS. REC.	$

CASH PAID OUT

	$
	$

CASH CONTROL

Beginning Cash On Hand	$
Receipts Today (Col. B-1)	$
Total	$
Less Paid Outs	$
Less Bank Deposit	$
Closing Cash On Hand	$

BUSINESS ANALYSIS SUMMARIES (OPTIONAL)

RB40BC-6-96

Name_____ **Date**_____ **Score**_____

● COMPETENCY ASSESSMENT

Procedure 19-3: Posting Procedure Charges and Payments Using Medical Office Simulation Software (MOSS)

Task: Post service charges to a patient account and apply a payment during the check out.

Conditions: • Computer with MOSS installed

Standards: Perform each Task within 15 minutes with a minimum score of _____ points, as determined by your instructor.

Competency Assessment Information

Use the following information to complete this procedure. Case Study and all Source Documents are found directly following this Competency Assessment checklist.

You are working at the front office reception area. Apply charges and payments to patient accounts using MOSS as indicated below:

1. Case Study – Patient VanGillis arrives at the reception area after his appointment. Post the charges as shown on his Encounter Form (see Source Document) using MOSS for services rendered on February 20, 2013. He pays with check number 2244 in the amount of $20.00 for his co-payment. Post the payment using MOSS.
2. Patient Durand arrives at the reception area after her appointment. Post the charges as shown on her Encounter Form (see Source Document) using MOSS for services rendered on February 21, 2013. She has Medicare and will not be making a payment today.
3. Patient Barryroe arrives at the reception area after her appointment. Post the charges as shown on her Encounter Form (see Source Document) using MOSS for services rendered on February 20, 2013. She pays with check number 845 in the amount of $76.00. Post the payment using MOSS.

Time began: _____ **Time ended:** _____ **Total time:** _____

No.	Step	Points	Check #1	Check #2	Check #3
1	Open MOSS and select *Procedure Posting* from the *Main Menu.*				
2	Select the patient from the *Procedure Posting* patient list, and then click *Add.*				
3	Enter the Encounter Form Reference Number in Field 1. Hint: See Encounter Form.				
4	Enter the Date of Service in Field 5. Hint: See Encounter Form.				
5	Enter the first CPT service code in Field 8. Hint: See Encounter Form.				
6	Enter the ICD (diagnostic codes) in Field 12, using up to four codes as applicable.				
7	Click *Post* to apply the charges to the patient account.				
8	Enter additional services in the same manner until all service charges have been posted.				
9	Click the *Post Payment* button to apply a payment during the time of procedure posting.				

No.	Step	Points	Check #1	Check #2	Check #3
10	Click on the line item for the required procedure, and then click on the *Select/Edit* button.				
11	Enter the date of posting in Field 3 and the payment information in Fields 4 through 12 as applicable to the payment.				
12	Click on *Post* to apply the payment.				
13	Click on the *View Ledger* button.				
14	Review all postings on the patient's ledger.				
15	Click *Close* to close all open windows and return to the *Procedure Posting* patient selection window.				
16	Post charges for the next patient, or close the Posting Procedures patient selection window and return to the *Main Menu*.				
Student's Total Points					
Points Possible					
Final Score (Student's Total Points/Possible Points)					

Instructor's/Evaluator's Comments and Suggestions:

_____

_____

_____

_____

_____

_____

_____

CHECK #1	
Evaluator's Signature:	Date:

CHECK #2	
Evaluator's Signature:	Date:

CHECK #3	
Evaluator's Signature:	Date:

ABHES Competencies: MA.A.1.7.b(2) Apply computer application skills using variety of different electronic programs including both practice management software and EMR software; MA.A.1.8.b Prepare and maintain medical records

CAAHEP Competencies: V.P.5 Execute data management using electronic health care records such as the EMR; V.P.6 Use office hardware and software to maintain office systems

CASE STUDY FOR HERBERT VANGILLIS

No.	Step	
1	Open MOSS and select *Procedure Posting* from the Main Menu.	
2	Select the Patient VanGillis from the *Patient Posting* patient list, and then click *Add* (to add procedures).	
3	Enter the Encounter Form Reference Number in Field 1. Hint: See Encounter Form.	
4	Enter the Date of Service in Field 5, 02/20/2013. Hint: See Encounter Form.	(see figure in Step 3)
5	Enter the first CPT service code, 99203, in Field 8. Hint: See Encounter Form.	(see figure in Step 3)
6	Enter the ICD (diagnostic codes) in Field 12, 413.9 and 272.0.	(see figure in Step 3)
7	Click *Post* to apply the charges to the patient account.	

No.	Step	
8	Enter and post service charges for CPT 80053 in the same manner.	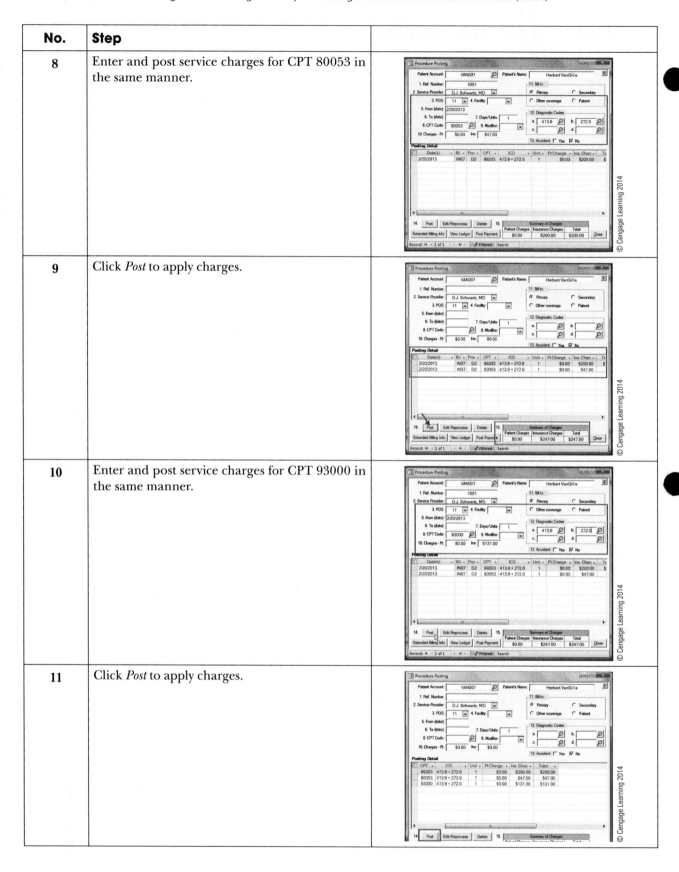
9	Click *Post* to apply charges.	
10	Enter and post service charges for CPT 93000 in the same manner.	
11	Click *Post* to apply charges.	

© Cengage Learning 2014

No.	Step
12	Click the *Post Payment* button to apply a payment during the time of procedure posting.
13	Click on the line item for procedure 99203, and then click on the *Select/Edit* button.
14	Enter the date of posting, 02/20/2013, in Field 3. Enter the type of payment in Field 7, under *Patient Payment*, select PATCHECK. Next, enter the check number and amount in Fields 8 and 9.
15	Click on *Post* to apply the payment.
16	Click on the *View Ledger* button.

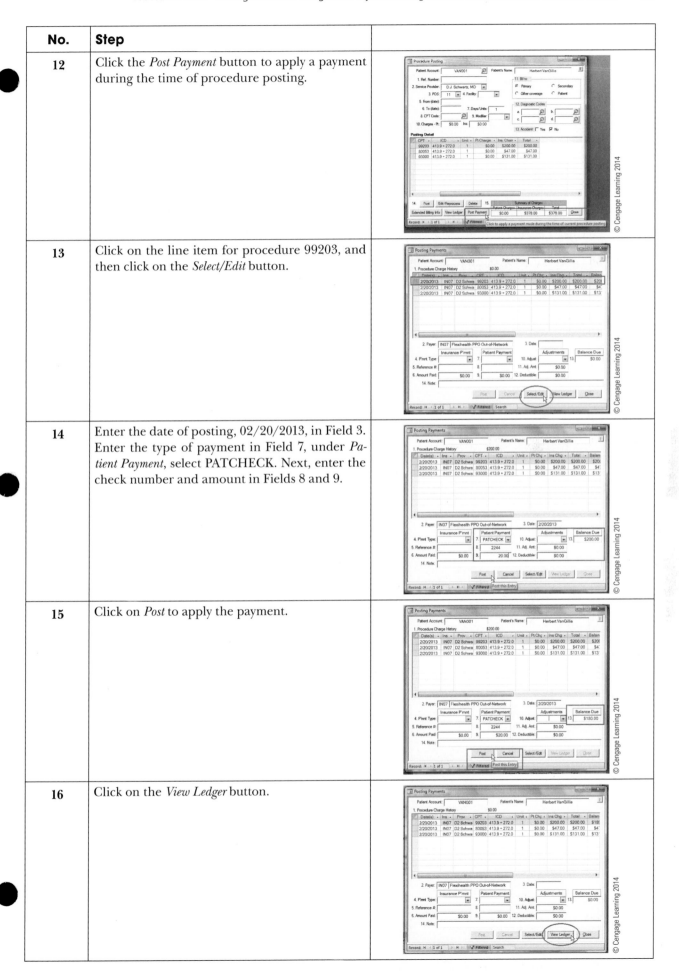

© Cengage Learning 2014

No.	Step	
17	Review all postings on the Patient VanGillis Ledger.	
18	Click *Close* to close all open windows and return to the *Procedure Posting* patient selection window.	
19	Post charges for the next patient, or close the Posting Procedures patient selection window and return to the Main Menu.	

SOURCE DOCUMENTS FOR PROCEDURE 19-3

PATIENT'S LAST NAME	FIRST	INITIAL	BIRTHDATE		SEX		TODAY'S DATE
Van Gillis	Herbert		4/5/72		[X] MALE ☐ FEMALE		2/20/2013

PATIENT INFORMATION

ADDRESS		CITY	STATE	ZIP	RELATIONSHIP TO SUBSCRIBER		INJURY DATE

SUBSCRIBER OR POLICYHOLDER	INSURANCE PAYER
	Flexi Health PPO

ADDRESS	CITY	STATE	ZIP	INS. I.D.	COVERAGE CODE	GROUP

ASSIGNMENT AND RELEASE: I HEREBY AUTHORIZE MY INSURANCE BENEFITS TO BE PAID DIRECTLY TO THE UNDERSIGNED PHYSICIAN. I AM FINANCIALLY RESPONSIBLE FOR NON-COVERED SERVICES. I ALSO AUTHORIZE THE PHYSICIAN TO RELEASE ANY INFORMATION REQUIRED.

OTHER HEALTH COVERAGE YES ☐ NO [X] IDENTIFY

DISABILITY RELATED TO:
☐ ACCIDENT ☐ INDUSTRIAL [X] ILLNESS ☐ OTHER

SIGNED (PATIENT, OR PARENT, IF MINOR) Herbert Van Gillis Date 2/20/2013

DATE SYMPTOMS APPEARED, INCEPTION OF PREGNANCY, OR ACCIDENT OCCURRED:

✓	DESCRIPTION	CPT/MD	FEE	✓	DESCRIPTION	CPT/MD	FEE	✓	DESCRIPTION	CPT/MD	FEE
	OFFICE VISITS	NEW PT			LABORATORY (Cont'd.)				PROCEDURES		
✓	Level III	99203			Wet Mount	87210		✓	EKG (93000)	93005	
	Level IV	99204			Pap Smear	88141			Resp. Function Test	94010	
	Level V	99205			Handling	99000			Ear Lavage	69210	
	OFFICE VISITS	EST. PT			Hemoccult Stool	82270			Injection Inter. Jt.	20605	
	Level I	99211			Glucose	82948			Injection Major Jt.	20610	
	Level II	99212			INJECTIONS				Anoscopy	46600	
	Level III	99213			Vitamin B12/B Complex	J3420			Sigmoidoscopy	45355	
	Level IV	99214			ACTH	J0800			I & D	10060	
	Level V	99215			Depo-Estradiol	J1000			Electrocautery	17000	
	CONSULTATIONS	OFFICE			Depo Testosterone	J1070			Thromb Hemor.	46320	
	Level III	99243			Imferon	J1750			Inj. Tendon	20550	
	Level IV	99244		✓	Vertabolic Panel	86053					
	HOME	EST. PT			Influenza Vaccine - Flu	90658			MISCELLANEOUS		
	Level II	99348			Pneumococcal Vaccine	90732			Drugs, Supplies, Materials	99070	
	ER				TB Tine Test	86585			Special Reports	99080	
	Level III	99283			Aminophyllin	J0280			Services After Hrs.	99050	
	Level IV	99284			Terbutaline Sulf.	J3105			Services 10pm - 8am	99052	
	LABORATORY				Demerol HCL	J2175			Services Sun. & Holidays	99054	
	Urinalysis - Complete	81000			Compazine	J0780			Counseling	99403	
	Hemoglobin	85018			Injection Therapeutic	90782					
	Culture, Strep/Monilia	87081			Estrone Susp.	J1410					

DIAGNOSIS:

☐ Allergic Rhinitis	477.9	☐ CHF	428.0	☐ Gout	274.9	☐ Parkinsonism	332.0	
☐ Anemia	280.9	☐ Cholecystitis	575.10	☐ HCVD	429.2	☐ Peripheral Vascular Dis	443.9	
☐ Angina Pectoris	413.9	☐ Chronic Fatigue Synd.	300.5	☐ Headache, Vascular	784.0	☐ Pharyngitis	462	
☐ Anxiety	300.00	☐ COPD	496	☐ Headache, Migraine	346.90	☐ Pneumonia, Bacterial	482.9	
☐ Aortic Stenosis	424.1	☐ Costochondritis	733.99	☐ Hemorrhoids	455.6	☐ Pneumonia, Viral	480.9	
☐ ASCVD	429.2	☐ CVA	431	☐ Hiatal Hernia	553.3	☐ Rectal Bleeding	569.3	
☐ ASHD	414.9	☐ Cystitis	595.9	☐ Hiatal Hernia & Reflux	530.10	☐ Renal Failure, Chronic	585	
☐ Asthma	493.90	☐ Deg. Disc. Disease, CX	722.4	☐ HVD	402.10	☐ Rheumatoid Arthritis	714.0	
☐ Atrial Fibrillation	427.31	☐ Deg. Disc. Dis., Lumbar	722.52	☐ Hyperlipidemia	272.4	☐ Sinusitis	461.9	
☐ Bigeminy	427.89	☐ Depression, Endogenous	296.20	☐ Hypothyroidism	244.9	☐ Supraventr. Tachycardia	427.0	
☐ BPH	600._	☐ Dermatitis	692.9	☐ Impacted Cerumen	380.4	☐ T.I.A.	435.9	
☐ Bronchitis, Acute	466.11	☐ Diabetes Mellitus, Adult	250.00	☐ Influenza, Viral	487.1	☐ Tachycardia	426.89	
☐ Bronchitis, Chronic	491.9	☐ Diarrhea	558.9	☐ Irritable Bowel Syndrome	564.1	☐ Tendinitis	726.90	
☐ Bursitis	726._	☐ Diverticulitis	562.11	☐ Laryngitis	464.00	☐ Tonsillitis	463	
☐ Cardiomyopathy	425.4	☐ Esophagitis	530.10	☐ Menopausal Syndrome	627.2	☐ URI	465.9	
☐ Carotid Artery Disease	433.10	☐ Fibrocystic Breast Disease	610.1	☐ Mitral Insufficiency	396.2	☐ UTI	599.0	
☐ Cerebral Vascular Disease	437.9	☐ Fissure in Ano	565.0	☐ Neuritis	729.2	☐ Vaginitis	616.10	
		☐ Gastroenteritis	558.9	☐ Otitis Media	382.9	☐ Vertigo	780.4	

DIAGNOSIS: (IF NOT CHECKED ABOVE)	REF. DR. & #
Hypercholesterolemia 272.0	1001

DOCTOR'S SIGNATURE / DATE	NO SERVICES PURCHASED	SERVICE PERFORMED	ACCEPT ASSIGNMENT	TODAY'S FEE	
Dr. Heath 2/20/2013					

INSTRUCTIONS TO PATIENT FOR FILING INSURANCE CLAIMS

MAIL THIS FORM DIRECTLY TO YOUR INSURANCE COMPANY.
ATTACH YOUR OWN INSURANCE COMPANY'S FORM.

PLEASE REMEMBER THAT PAYMENT IS YOUR OBLIGATION, REGARDLESS OF INSURANCE OR OTHER THIRD PARTY INVOLVEMENT.

OFFICE ☑	YES ☐	AMT. REC'D TODAY $20.00
E.R. ☐	NO ☑	
HOME ☐		TOTAL DUE

Courtesy of Bibbero Systems, Inc., Petaluma, CA 800-242-2376, http://www.bibbero.com

PATIENT INFORMATION

PATIENT'S LAST NAME	FIRST	INITIAL	BIRTHDATE		SEX	TODAY'S DATE
Durand	Isabel				☐ MALE ☒ FEMALE	2/21/2013

ADDRESS	CITY	STATE	ZIP	RELATIONSHIP TO SUBSCRIBER	INJURY DATE

SUBSCRIBER OR POLICYHOLDER	INSURANCE PAYER
	Medicare-Statewide

ADDRESS	CITY	STATE	ZIP	INS. I.D.	COVERAGE CODE	GROUP

ASSIGNMENT AND RELEASE: I HEREBY AUTHORIZE MY INSURANCE BENEFITS TO BE PAID DIRECTLY TO THE UNDERSIGNED PHYSICIAN. I AM FINANCIALLY RESPONSIBLE FOR NON-COVERED SERVICES. I ALSO AUTHORIZE THE PHYSICIAN TO RELEASE ANY INFORMATION REQUIRED.

OTHER HEALTH COVERAGE   YES ☒   NO ☐   IDENTIFY

DISABILITY RELATED TO:
☐ ACCIDENT   ☐ INDUSTRIAL   ☒ ILLNESS   ☐ OTHER

SIGNED (PATIENT, OR PARENT, IF MINOR)   Isabel Durand   Date 2/21/2013

DATE SYMPTOMS APPEARED, INCEPTION OF PREGNANCY, OR ACCIDENT OCCURRED:

✓	DESCRIPTION	CPT/MD	FEE	✓	DESCRIPTION	CPT/MD	FEE	✓	DESCRIPTION	CPT/MD		FEE
	OFFICE VISITS	NEW PT			LABORATORY (Cont'd.)				PROCEDURES			
	Level III	99203			Wet Mount	87210			EKG	93000	93005	
	Level IV	99204			Pap Smear	88141			Resp. Function Test	94010		
	Level V	99205			Handling	99000			Ear Lavage	69210		
	OFFICE VISITS	EST. PT			Hemoccult Stool	82270			Injection Inter. Jt.	20605		
	Level I	99211			Glucose	82948			Injection Major Jt.	20610		
✓	Level II	99212			INJECTIONS				Anoscopy	46600		
	Level III	99213			Vitamin B12/B Complex	J3420			Sigmoidoscopy	45355		
	Level IV	99214			ACTH	J0800			I & D	10060		
	Level V	99215			Depo-Estradiol	J1000			Electrocautery	17000		
	CONSULTATIONS	OFFICE			Depo Testosterone	J1070			Thromb Hemor.	46320		
	Level III	99243			Imferon	J1750			Inj. Tendon	20550		
	Level IV	99244										
	HOME	EST. PT			Influenza Vaccine - Flu	90658			MISCELLANEOUS			
	Level II	99348			Pneumococcal Vaccine	90732			Drugs, Supplies, Materials	99070		
	ER				TB Tine Test	86585			Special Reports	99080		
	Level III	99283			Aminophyllin	J0280			Services After Hrs.	99050		
	Level IV	99284			Terbutaline Sulf.	J3105			Services 10pm - 8am	99052		
	LABORATORY				Demerol HCL	J2175			Services Sun. & Holidays	99054		
	Urinalysis - Complete	81000			Compazine	J0780			Counseling	99403		
	Hemoglobin	85018			Injection Therapeutic	90782						
	Culture, Strep/Monilia	87081			Estrone Susp.	J1410						

DIAGNOSIS:

☐ Allergic Rhinitis	477.9	☐ CHF	428.0	☐ Gout	274.9	☐ Parkinsonism	332.0	
☐ Anemia	280.9	☐ Cholecystitis	575.10	☐ HCVD	429.2	☐ Peripheral Vascular Dis	443.9	
☐ Angina Pectoris	413.9	☐ Chronic Fatigue Synd.	300.5	☐ Headache, Vascular	784.0	☐ Pharyngitis	462	
☐ Anxiety	300.00	☐ COPD	496	☐ Headache, Migraine	346.90	☐ Pneumonia, Bacterial	482.9	
☐ Aortic Stenosis	424.1	☐ Costochondritis	733.99	☐ Hemorrhoids	455.6	☐ Pneumonia, Viral	480.9	
☐ ASCVD	429.2	☐ CVA	431	☐ Hiatal Hernia	553.3	☐ Rectal Bleeding	569.3	
☐ ASHD	414.9	☐ Cystitis	595.9	☐ Hiatal Hernia & Reflux	530.10	☐ Renal Failure, Chronic	585	
☐ Asthma	493.90	☐ Deg. Disc. Disease, CX	722.4	☐ HVD	402.10	☐ Rheumatoid Arthritis	714.0	
☐ Atrial Fibrillation	427.31	☐ Deg. Disc. Dis., Lumbar	722.52	☐ Hyperlipidemia	272.4	☐ Sinusitis	461.9	
☐ Bigeminy	427.89	☐ Depression, Endogenous	296.20	☐ Hypothyroidism	244.9	☐ Supraventr. Tachycardia	427.0	
☐ BPH	600._	☐ Dermatitis	692.9	☐ Impacted Cerumen	380.4	☐ T.I.A.	435.9	
☐ Bronchitis, Acute	466.11	☐ Diabetes Mellitus, Adult	250.00	☐ Influenza, Viral	487.1	☐ Tachycardia	426.89	
☐ Bronchitis, Chronic	491.9	☐ Diarrhea	558.9	☐ Irritable Bowel Syndrome	564.1	☐ Tendinitis	726.90	
☐ Bursitis	726._	☐ Diverticulitis	562.11	☐ Laryngitis	464.00	☐ Tonsillitis	463	
☐ Cardiomyopathy	425.4	☐ Esophagitis	530.10	☐ Menopausal Syndrome	627.2	☐ URI	465.9	
☐ Carotid Artery Disease	433.10	☐ Fibrocystic Breast Disease	610.1	☐ Mitral Insufficiency	396.2	☐ UTI	599.0	
☐ Cerebral Vascular Disease	437.9	☒ Fissure in Ano / Gastroenteritis	565.0 / 558.9	☐ Neuritis	729.2	☐ Vaginitis	616.10	
				☐ Otitis Media	382.9	☐ Vertigo	780.4	

DIAGNOSIS: (IF NOT CHECKED ABOVE)

REF. DR. & #   1002

DOCTOR'S SIGNATURE / DATE	NO SERVICES PURCHASED	SERVICE PERFORMED	ACCEPT ASSIGNMENT	TODAY'S FEE	
Dr. Heath					

INSTRUCTIONS TO PATIENT FOR FILING INSURANCE CLAIMS

MAIL THIS FORM DIRECTLY TO YOUR INSURANCE COMPANY.
ATTACH YOUR OWN INSURANCE COMPANY'S FORM.

PLEASE REMEMBER THAT PAYMENT IS YOUR OBLIGATION, REGARDLESS OF INSURANCE OR OTHER THIRD PARTY INVOLVEMENT.

OFFICE ☒   YES ☒   AMT. REC'D TODAY   0

E.R. ☐   NO ☐

HOME ☐   TOTAL DUE

PATIENT'S LAST NAME: Barryroe	FIRST: Caitlin	INITIAL	BIRTHDATE	SEX: ☐ MALE ☒ FEMALE	TODAY'S DATE: 02/20/2013

ADDRESS | CITY | STATE | ZIP | RELATIONSHIP TO SUBSCRIBER | INJURY DATE

SUBSCRIBER OR POLICYHOLDER | INSURANCE PAYER: Consumer One

ADDRESS | CITY | STATE | ZIP | INS. I.D. | COVERAGE CODE | GROUP

ASSIGNMENT AND RELEASE: I HEREBY AUTHORIZE MY INSURANCE BENEFITS TO BE PAID DIRECTLY TO THE UNDERSIGNED PHYSICIAN. I AM FINANCIALLY RESPONSIBLE FOR NON-COVERED SERVICES. I ALSO AUTHORIZE THE PHYSICIAN TO RELEASE ANY INFORMATION REQUIRED.

OTHER HEALTH COVERAGE YES ☐ NO ☒   IDENTIFY

DISABILITY RELATED TO: ☐ ACCIDENT ☐ INDUSTRIAL ☒ ILLNESS ☐ OTHER

SIGNED (PATIENT, OR PARENT, IF MINOR): Caitlin Barryroe Date 02/20/2013

DATE SYMPTOMS APPEARED, INCEPTION OF PREGNANCY, OR ACCIDENT OCCURRED:

✓	DESCRIPTION	CPT/MD	FEE	✓	DESCRIPTION	CPT/MD	FEE	✓	DESCRIPTION	CPT/MD	FEE
	OFFICE VISITS	NEW PT			LABORATORY (Cont'd.)				PROCEDURES		
	Level III	99203			Wet Mount	87210			EKG 93000	93005	
	Level IV	99204			Pap Smear	88141			Resp. Function Test	94010	
	Level V	99205			Handling	99000			Ear Lavage	69210	
	OFFICE VISITS	EST. PT			Hemoccult Stool	82270			Injection Inter. Jt.	20605	
✓	Level I	99211			Glucose	82948			Injection Major Jt.	20610	
	Level II	99212			INJECTIONS				Anoscopy	46600	
	Level III	99213			Vitamin B12/B Complex	J3420			Sigmoidoscopy	45355	
	Level IV	99214			ACTH	J0800			I & D	10060	
	Level V	99215			Depo-Estradiol	J1000			Electrocautery	17000	
	CONSULTATIONS	OFFICE			Depo Testosterone	J1070			Thromb Hemor.	46320	
	Level III	99243			Imferon	J1750			Inj. Tendon	20550	
	Level IV	99244									
	HOME	EST. PT			Influenza Vaccine - Flu	90658			MISCELLANEOUS		
	Level II	99348			Pneumococcal Vaccine	90732			Drugs, Supplies, Materials	99070	
	ER				TB Tine Test	86585			Special Reports	99080	
	Level III	99283			Aminophyllin	J0280			Services After Hrs.	99050	
	Level IV	99284			Terbutaline Sulf.	J3105			Services 10pm - 8am	99052	
	LABORATORY				Demerol HCL	J2175			Services Sun. & Holidays	99054	
	Urinalysis - Complete	81000			Compazine	J0780			Counseling	99403	
	Hemoglobin	85018			Injection Therapeutic	90782		✓	CBC with DIFF	85031	
	Culture, Strep/Monilia	87081			Estrone Susp.	J1410					

DIAGNOSIS:
☒ Allergic Rhinitis ... 477.9
☐ Anemia ... 280.9
☐ Angina Pectoris ... 413.9
☐ Anxiety ... 300.00
☐ Aortic Stenosis ... 424.1
☐ ASCVD ... 429.2
☐ ASHD ... 414.9
☐ Asthma ... 493.90
☐ Atrial Fibrillation ... 427.31
☐ Bigeminy ... 427.89
☐ BPH ... 600.__
☐ Bronchitis, Acute ... 466.11
☐ Bronchitis, Chronic ... 491.9
☐ Bursitis ... 726.__
☐ Cardiomyopathy ... 425.4
☐ Carotid Artery Disease ... 433.10
☐ Cerebral Vascular Disease ... 437.9

☐ CHF ... 428.0
☐ Cholecystitis ... 575.10
☐ Chronic Fatigue Synd. ... 300.5
☐ COPD ... 496
☐ Costochondritis ... 733.99
☐ CVA ... 431
☐ Cystitis ... 595.9
☐ Deg. Disc. Disease, CX ... 722.4
☐ Deg. Disc. Dis., Lumbar ... 722.52
☐ Depression, Endogenous ... 296.20
☐ Dermatitis ... 692.9
☐ Diabetes Mellitus, Adult ... 250.00
☐ Diarrhea ... 558.9
☐ Diverticulitis ... 562.11
☐ Esophagitis ... 530.10
☐ Fibrocystic Breast Disease ... 610.1
☐ Fissure in Ano ... 565.0
☐ Gastroenteritis ... 558.9

☐ Gout ... 274.9
☐ HCVD ... 429.2
☐ Headache, Vascular ... 784.0
☐ Headache, Migraine ... 346.90
☐ Hemorrhoids ... 455.6
☐ Hiatal Hernia ... 553.3
☐ Hiatal Hernia & Reflux ... 530.10
☐ HVD ... 402.10
☐ Hyperlipidemia ... 272.4
☐ Hypothyroidism ... 244.9
☐ Impacted Cerumen ... 380.4
☐ Influenza, Viral ... 487.1
☐ Irritable Bowel Syndrome ... 564.1
☐ Laryngitis ... 464.00
☐ Menopausal Syndrome ... 627.2
☐ Mitral Insufficiency ... 396.2
☐ Neuritis ... 729.2
☐ Otitis Media ... 382.9

☐ Parkinsonism ... 332.0
☐ Peripheral Vascular Dis ... 443.9
☐ Pharyngitis ... 462
☐ Pneumonia, Bacterial ... 482.9
☐ Pneumonia, Viral ... 480.9
☐ Rectal Bleeding ... 569.3
☐ Renal Failure, Chronic ... 585
☐ Rheumatoid Arthritis ... 714.0
☒ Sinusitis ... 461.9
☐ Supraventr. Tachycardia ... 427.0
☐ T.I.A. ... 435.9
☐ Tachycardia ... 426.89
☐ Tendinitis ... 726.90
☐ Tonsillitis ... 463
☐ URI ... 465.9
☐ UTI ... 599.0
☐ Vaginitis ... 616.10
☐ Vertigo ... 780.4

DIAGNOSIS: (IF NOT CHECKED ABOVE)

REF. DR. & # 1005

DOCTOR'S SIGNATURE / DATE: Dr. Heath

NO SERVICES PURCHASED

INSTRUCTIONS TO PATIENT FOR FILING INSURANCE CLAIMS
MAIL THIS FORM DIRECTLY TO YOUR INSURANCE COMPANY.
ATTACH YOUR OWN INSURANCE COMPANY'S FORM.
PLEASE REMEMBER THAT PAYMENT IS YOUR OBLIGATION, REGARDLESS OF INSURANCE OR OTHER THIRD PARTY INVOLVEMENT.

SERVICE PERFORMED: OFFICE ☒ E.R. ☐ HOME ☐
ACCEPT ASSIGNMENT: YES ☒ NO ☐
TODAY'S FEE
AMT. REC'D TODAY $76.00
TOTAL DUE

Courtesy of Bibbero Systems, Inc., Petaluma, CA 800-242-2376, http://www.bibbero.com

Name_____ **Date**_____ **Score**_____

● COMPETENCY ASSESSMENT

Procedure 19-4:   Insurance Billing Using Medical Office Simulation Software (MOSS)

Task: Submit claims electronically to insurance carriers using MOSS.

Conditions: • Computer with MOSS installed

Standards: Perform each Task within 10 minutes with a minimum score of _____ points, as determined by your instructor.

Competency Assessment Information

Use the following information to complete this procedure. Case Study is found directly following this Competency Assessment checklist.

You are working in the Patient Accounts office on February 25, 2013. Submit electronic claims for last week's services using MOSS as indicated below:

1. Case Study – Submit claims electronically for ConsumerOne HRA insurance for the week from 02/18/2013 through 02/22/2013. Print the Prebilling Worksheet Report and the Claims Submission Report.
2. Submit claims electronically for Medicare—Statewide for the week from 02/18/2013 through 02/22/2013. Print the Prebilling Worksheet Report and the Claims Submission Report.
3. Submit all remaining claims for the week from 02/18/2013 through 02/22/2013. Hint: Select *All* in the *Payer* field. Print the Prebilling Worksheet Report and the Claims Submission Report.

●

Time began: _____   **Time ended:** _____   **Total time:** _____

No.	Step	Points	Check #1	Check #2	Check #3
1	Open MOSS and select *Insurance Billing* from the Main Menu.				
2	In the *Claim Preparation* window, drop down the list for Field 1 and select *Patient Name.*				
3	In Field 2, *Settings,* select the specific provider name or *ALL,* enter the *From/Through* Service dates, and select an individual patient or *ALL* for *Patient Name* and *Patient Account.*				
4	In Field 3, *Transmit Type,* click in front of the box for the type of claim to be submitted, *Electronic* or *Paper (1500).*				
5	In Field 4, *Billing Options,* select whether claim is primary insurance, secondary, or other.				
6	In Field 5, click on the insurance carrier to be billed, or *All.*				
7	Click on the *Prebilling Worksheet* button.				
8	Review claims to be billed on the *Prebilling Worksheet* report.				

●

No.	Step	Points	Check #1	Check #2	Check #3
9	Print the *Prebilling Worksheet* report.				
10	Close the *Prebilling Worksheet* report and return to the *Claims Preparation* window. Hint: Be careful not to close the entire MOSS software program.				
11	Click on the *Generate Claims* button.				
12	Before sending the claims electronically or printing paper claims, preview the CMS 1500 claims forms for each patient. Hint: Use the record bar at the bottom left to see each patient's claim.				
13	Click on *Transmit EMC* (or *Print Forms* for paper claims) to execute the claims submissions.				
14	After the electronic transmission is completed, click on *View* to review the *Transmission Report*, or collect printed claim forms from printer, as applicable.				
15	Print the *Claims Submission Report*, or prepare mailing envelopes for the paper claims, as applicable.				
16	Close the *Claims Submission Report* and click *Close* to exit the *Transmission* window, or return to the *Main Menu* if paper claims were printed by closing all windows. Hint: Be careful not to close the entire MOSS software program.				
Student's Total Points					
Points Possible					
Final Score (Student's Total Points/Possible Points)					

Instructor's/Evaluator's Comments and Suggestions:

_____

_____

_____

_____

_____

_____

_____

CHECK #1	
Evaluator's Signature:	Date:

CHECK #2	
Evaluator's Signature:	Date:

CHECK #3	
Evaluator's Signature:	Date:

ABHES Competencies: MA.A.1.7.b(2) Apply computer application skills using variety of different electronic programs including both practice management software and EMR software; MA.A.1.8.b Prepare and maintain medical records

CAAHEP Competencies: V.P.5 Execute data management using electronic health care records such as the EMR; V.P.6 Use office hardware and software to maintain office systems

CASE STUDY FOR CONSUMERONE HRA INSURANCE

No.	Step	
1	Open MOSS and select *Insurance Billing* from the Main Menu.	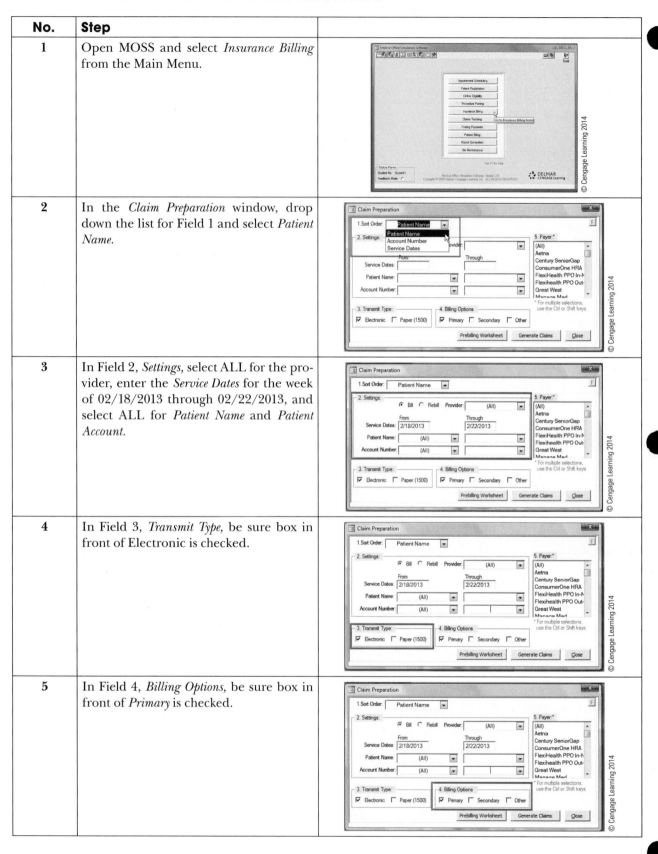
2	In the *Claim Preparation* window, drop down the list for Field 1 and select *Patient Name*.	
3	In Field 2, *Settings,* select ALL for the provider, enter the *Service Dates* for the week of 02/18/2013 through 02/22/2013, and select ALL for *Patient Name* and *Patient Account.*	
4	In Field 3, *Transmit Type,* be sure box in front of Electronic is checked.	
5	In Field 4, *Billing Options,* be sure box in front of *Primary* is checked.	

No.	Step	
6	In Field 5, *Payer*, select *ConsumerOne HRA*.	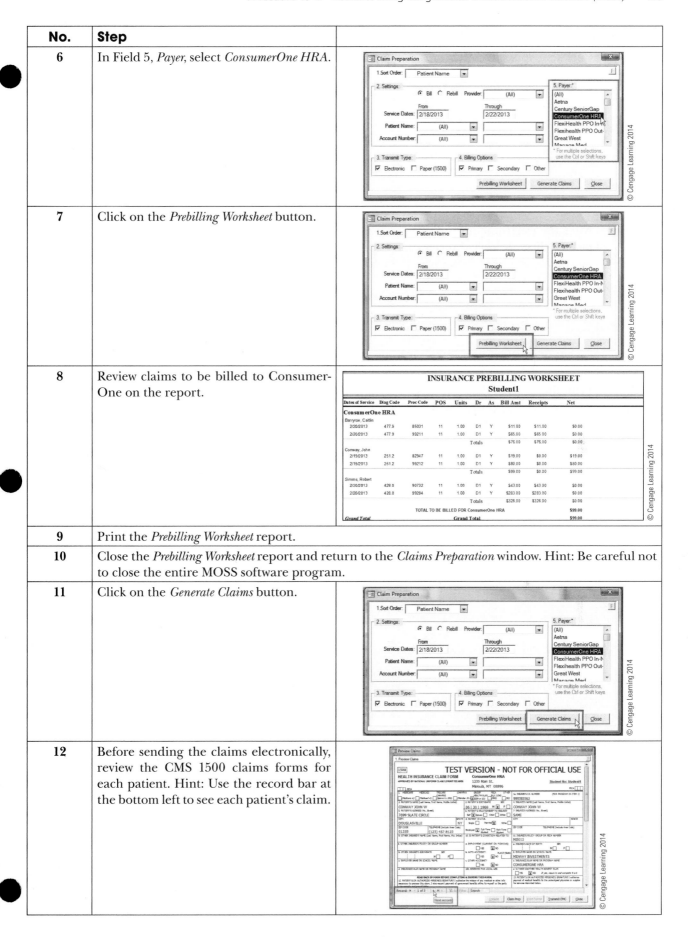
7	Click on the *Prebilling Worksheet* button.	
8	Review claims to be billed to Consumer-One on the report.	
9	Print the *Prebilling Worksheet* report.	
10	Close the *Prebilling Worksheet* report and return to the *Claims Preparation* window. Hint: Be careful not to close the entire MOSS software program.	
11	Click on the *Generate Claims* button.	
12	Before sending the claims electronically, review the CMS 1500 claims forms for each patient. Hint: Use the record bar at the bottom left to see each patient's claim.	

No.	Step	
13	Click on *Transmit EMC* (or *Print Forms* for paper claims) to execute the claims submissions.	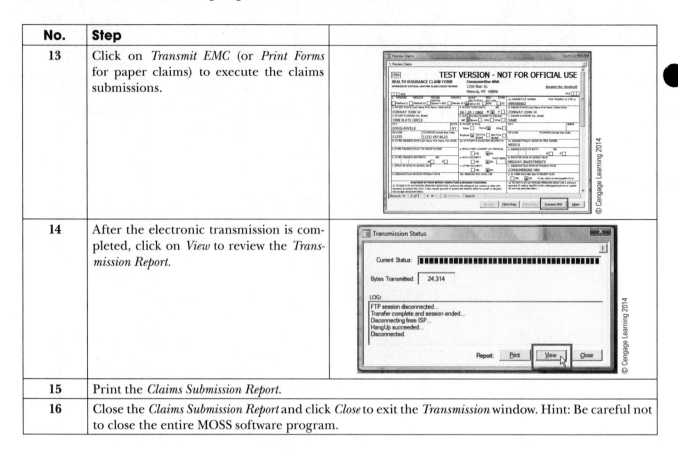
14	After the electronic transmission is completed, click on *View* to review the *Transmission Report*.	
15	Print the *Claims Submission Report*.	
16	Close the *Claims Submission Report* and click *Close* to exit the *Transmission* window. Hint: Be careful not to close the entire MOSS software program.	

Name_____ **Date**_____ **Score**_____

● COMPETENCY ASSESSMENT

Procedure 19-5:   Posting Insurance Payments and Adjustments Using Medical Office Simulation Software (MOSS)

Task: Post insurance payments and adjustments to patient accounts using MOSS.

Conditions: • Computer with MOSS installed

Standards: Perform each Task within 10 minutes with a minimum score of _____ points, as determined by your instructor.

Competency Assessment Information

Use the following information to complete this procedure. Case Study and all Source Documents are found directly following this Competency Assessment checklist.

You are working in the Patient Accounts office on March 21, 2013. Post payments and adjustments to patient accounts using MOSS as indicated below:

1. Case Study – Refer to the Explanation of Benefits (EOB) for Caitlin Barryroe (see Source Document). Post payments and adjustments as applicable to the patient account.
2. Refer to the EOB for Herbert VanGillis (see Source Document). Post payments and adjustments as applicable to the patient account.
3. Refer to the RA for Isabel Durand (see Source Document). Post payments and adjustments as applicable to the patient account. Use the ICN as the reference number.

Time began: _____   **Time ended:** _____   **Total time:** _____

No.	Step	Points	Check #1	Check #2	Check #3
1	Read the EOB/RA from the insurance carrier and prepare information before applying a payment to the patient's account. Use the guidelines below to read the EOB/RA: • How much did the insurance allow? • How much was disallowed? • How much did the insurance pay?				
2	Click on the *Posting Payments* button on the *Main Menu*. Select the patient and then click *Apply Payment*.				
3	Click on the line item for the date and procedure for which a payment shall be posted in the *Procedure Charge History* area (Field 1), and then click on the *Select/Edit* button. Make certain Field 13 shows the correct *Balance Due*.				

No.	Step	Points	Check #1	Check #2	Check #3
4	Input the date of posting and the insurance payment information as follows: • Payment by insurance, Field 4; click the drop-down box. • Reference #, Field 5; enter claim number, check number, or other reference number. • Amount of payment, Field 6. • Press Enter when finished to update the *Balance Due* in Field 13.				
5	Input the disallowed amount as an insurance adjustment as follows: • Select *Adjustment Insurance*, Field 10, and then enter the *Adjustment Amount* in Field 11. • Press Enter when finished to update the *Balance Due* in Field 13.				
6	Click *Post* when payment is ready to be posted to the account.				
7	If there is more than one service on the EOB/RA, prepare the information for the next service before applying a payment to the patient's account. Use the guidelines below: • How much did the insurance allow? • How much was disallowed? • How much did the insurance pay?				
8	Enter the payment information as before for the next service. Hint: Click on the line item for the applicable date and procedure.				
9	Click *Post* when payment is ready to be posted to the account.				
10	Click *View Ledger* to review payment posting.				
11	When complete, either view and print a report or click on *Close* and return to the patient selection window.				
12	Post payment for the next patient or return to the *Main Menu*.				
Student's Total Points					
Points Possible					
Final Score (Student's Total Points/Possible Points)					

Instructor's/Evaluator's Comments and Suggestions:

_____

_____

_____

_____

_____

_____

_____

CHECK #1	
Evaluator's Signature:	Date:

CHECK #2	
Evaluator's Signature:	Date:

CHECK #3	
Evaluator's Signature:	Date:

ABHES Competencies: MA.A.1.7.b(2) Apply computer application skills using variety of different electronic programs including both practice management software and EMR software; MA.A.1.8.b Prepare and maintain medical records

CAAHEP Competencies: V.P.5 Execute data management using electronic health care records such as the EMR; V.P.6 Use office hardware and software to maintain office systems

CASE STUDY FOR CAITLIN BARRYROE

No.	Step	
1	Read the EOB from ConsumerONE HRA (see Source Document) for Caitlin Barryroe. Prepare information before applying a payment to the patient's account. Use the guidelines below to read the EOB: • How much did the insurance allow? $55.00 • How much was disallowed? $10.00 • How much did the insurance pay? $44.00	
2	Click on the *Posting Payments* button on the *Main Menu.*	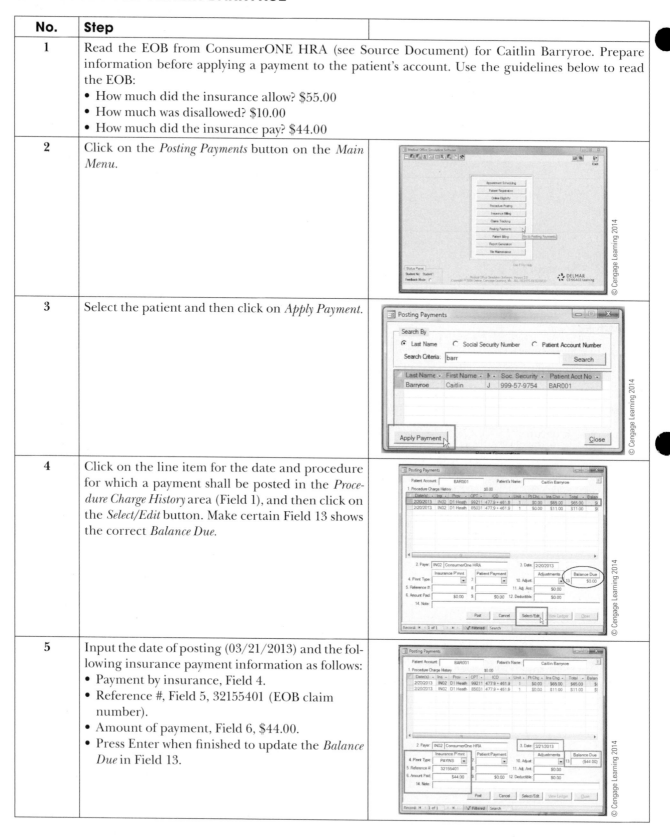
3	Select the patient and then click on *Apply Payment.*	
4	Click on the line item for the date and procedure for which a payment shall be posted in the *Procedure Charge History* area (Field 1), and then click on the *Select/Edit* button. Make certain Field 13 shows the correct *Balance Due.*	
5	Input the date of posting (03/21/2013) and the following insurance payment information as follows: • Payment by insurance, Field 4. • Reference #, Field 5, 32155401 (EOB claim number). • Amount of payment, Field 6, $44.00. • Press Enter when finished to update the *Balance Due* in Field 13.	

No.	Step	
6	Input the disallowed amount as an insurance adjustment as follows: • Select *Adjustment Insurance* from the drop-down box, Field 10, and then enter the *Adjustment Amount* in Field 11, $10.00. • Press Enter when finished to update the *Balance Due* in Field 13.	
7	Click *Post* when payment is ready to be posted to the account.	
8	If there is more than one service on the EOB, prepare the information for the next service before applying a payment to the patient's account. Use the guidelines below: • How much did the insurance allow? $9.50 • How much was disallowed? $1.50 • How much did the insurance pay? $7.60	
9	Enter the payment information as before for the next service. Hint: Click on the line item for the applicable date and procedure for which a payment shall be posted.	
10	Click *Post* when payment is ready to be posted to the account.	(see Figure in Step 7)
11	Click *View Ledger* to review payment posting.	

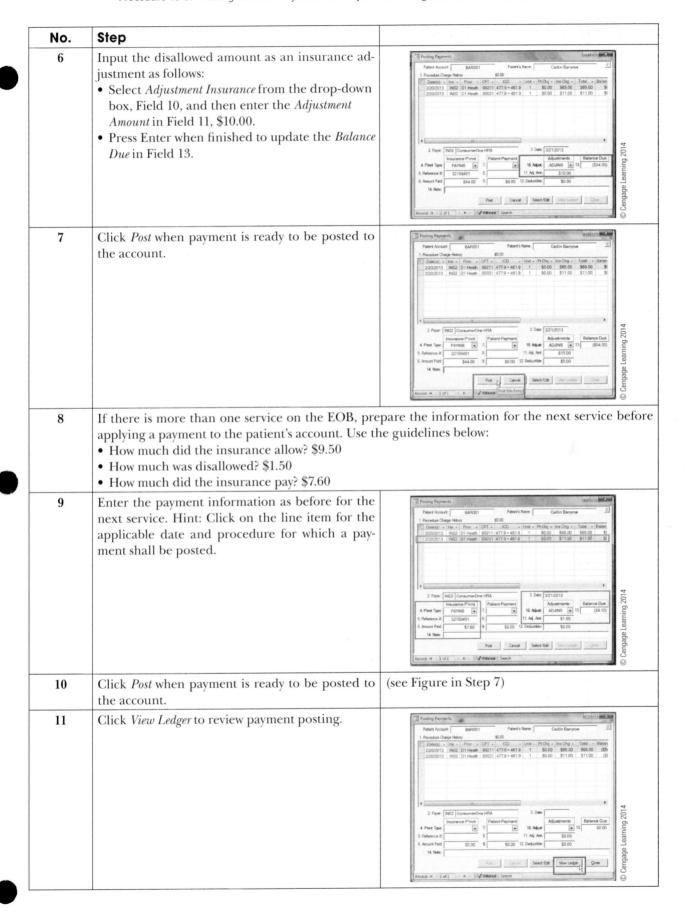

© Cengage Learning 2014

No.	Step	
12	When complete, either view and print a report or click on *Close* and return to the patient selection window.	
13	Post payment for the next patient or return to the *Main Menu*.	

SOURCE DOCUMENTS FOR PROCEDURE 19-5

Service Detail – Consumer ONE HRA
EXPLANATION OF BENEFITS

Date(s) of Service	Amount Charged	Amount Allowed	Amount Disallowed	Level One	Level Two	Level Three	Preventative Care	Patient Responsibility	Benefit Paid by HRA	*Remark Codes
Patient: CAITLIN BARRYROE			**Claim #: 32155401**			**Provider: HEATH**		**Douglasville Medicine Associates**		
02/20/2013	$65.00	$55.00	$10.00	$0.00	$0.00	$55.00	$0.00	$11.00	$44.00	003
02/20/2013	$11.00	$9.50	$1.50	0.00	0.00	$9.50	$0.00	$1.90	$7.60	003
TOTALS	$76.00	$64.50	$11.50	$0.00	$0.00	$64.50	$0.00	$12.90	$51.60	*

*Remark Codes:

001 Level One EPA – Disallowed amount is an in-network provider write-off.

002 Level Two – Patient out-of-pocket responsibility up to $300.00; EPA exhausted

003 Level Three – In-Network 80/20 HRA reimbursement agreement.

Source Document 19-3_1_BARRYROE

TOTALS:

$65.00 – Service 99211

$55.00 – Amount Allowed

$10.00 – Amount Disallowed

$11.00 – Patient Responsibility

$44.00 – Consumer ONE Paid Amount

$11.00 – Service 85031

$ 9.50 – Amount Allowed

$1.50 – Amount Disallowed

$ 1.90 – Patient Responsibility

$ 7.60 – ConsumerONE Paid Amount

Explanation of Medical Benefits   **FlexiHealth PPO Plan**

Service Date	Type of Service	Charge(s) Submitted	Not Covered or Discount	Amount Covered	Patient Co-payment Co-insurance Deductible	Covered Balance	Plan Liability	See Note
Insured Name **HERBERT VANGILLIS**		Insured/Patient ID **999556218**			Patient Name **HERBERT VANGILLIS**			
Provider Name: DJ SCHWARTZ, MD – **Out-of-Network Provider** Reference Number: 9871233								
02/20/2013	99203 Ext Prob Foc	$200.00	$ 30.20	$169.80	$0.00	$169.80	$169.80	A
02/20/2013	80053 Metabolic Panel	$47.00	$ 0.00	$ 47.00	$0.00	$ 47.00	$ 47.00	A
02/20/2013	93000 Electrocardiogram	$131.00	$ 18.60	$112.40	$0.00	$112.40	$112.40	A
						Total Paid:	**$329.20**	

Notes on Benefit Determination:

A – Patient has met out of pocket maximum for 2013; services covered 100%

Source Document 19-3_2_VANGILLIS

TOTALS

$200.00 – Service 99203
$169.80 – Amount Covered
$30.20 – Amount Not Covered
$ 0.00 – Patient Responsibility
$169.80 – Plan Liability, Paid by FlexiHealth PPO

$ 47.00 – Service 80053
$ 47.00 – Amount Covered
$ 0.00 – Amount Not Covered
$ 0.00 – Patient Responsibility
$ 47.00 – Plan Liability, Paid by FlexiHealth PPO

$131.00 – Service 93000
$112.40 – Amount Covered
$ 18.60 – Amount Not Covered
$ 0.00 – Patient Responsibility
$112.40 – Plan Liability, Paid by FlexiHealth PPO

```
Medicare Remittance Advice (MOSS Sample)

------------------------------------------------------------------------
 03-12-2013 MEDICARE CLAIMS SUBMITTED FOR L.D. Heath, MD  999501
------------------------------------------------------------------------
------------------------------------------------------------------------
DURAND,ISABEL              BILLED ALLOWED  DEDUCT   COINS PROV-PD  MC-ADJUSTMENT

  HIC 999621132D          ASG Y  ICN  973333578
  ACNT CAR001

0221  022113  11  99212    80.00 60.00      0      12.00  48.00    20.00
            CLAIM TOTALS:  80.00 60.00      0      12.00  48.00    20.00

TOTAL PAID TO PROVIDER:  $48.00


_____


Source Document 19-3_6_DURAND



TOTALS

$ 80.00 - Service 99212
$ 60.00 - Amount Allowed
$ 20.00 - Amount Disallowed
$ 12.00 - Patient Responsibility (or bill to secondary)
$ 48.00 - Medicare Paid Amount (to Provider)
```

Name_____ **Date**_____ **Score**_____

COMPETENCY ASSESSMENT

Procedure 19-6: Processing Credit Balances and Refunds Using Medical Office Simulation Software (MOSS)

Task: Post overpayment refunds to patient accounts with a credit balance.

Conditions: • Computer with MOSS installed

Standards: Perform each Task within 10 minutes with a minimum score of _____ points, as determined by your instructor.

Competency Assessment Information

Use the following information to complete this procedure. Case Study is found directly following this Competency Assessment checklist.

You are working in the Patient Accounts office on March 21, 2013. Post refunds to patients with credit balances as indicated below using MOSS:

1. Case Study – Patient Barryroe paid $76.00 at the time of service on 02/20/2013. Her insurance, ConsumerONE HRA, paid $51.60 for services on that date, and $11.50 was adjusted as the disallowed amount. As a result, the patient has a credit of $63.10 on her account. Post an overpayment refund to the account; the office will return the money to the patient by check.
2. Patient VanGillis paid a $20.00 co-payment at the time of service on 02/20/2013. His insurance, FlexiHealth PPO, paid $329.20 for services on that date, and $48.80 was adjusted as the discount amount. He has met his out-of-pocket expenses for the year and his charges are being paid at 100% of the covered balance, with no co-payment due. As a result, the patient has a credit of $20.00 on his account. Post an overpayment refund to the account; the office will return the money to the patient by check.
3. Patient Albertson has a credit balance of $20.00 on her account since 7/10/2009. She is now asking for the money back. Post an overpayment refund to the account; the office will return the money to the patient by check.

Time began: _____ **Time ended:** _____ **Total time:** _____

No.	Step	Points	Check #1	Check #2	Check #3
1	Click on the *Posting Payments* button on the *Main Menu*. Select the patient and then click *Apply Payment*.				
2	Select the patient and then click *Apply Payment*.				
3	Click on the line item for the date and procedure for which a refund shall be posted in the *Procedure Charge History* area (Field 1), and then click on the *Select/Edit* button. Make certain Field 13 shows the correct *Balance Due.* Hint: If more than one service needs to be refunded, apply it to each separately.				
4	In Field 10, drop down the list of adjustment types and select *Refund Overpayment*.				
5	In Field 11, enter the amount to be refunded. Press enter to apply the refund to the balance. Make certain Field 13 shows the correct *Balance Due - $0.00* (or balance if only a portion was refunded).				

No.	Step	Points	Check #1	Check #2	Check #3
6	Click *Post* to enter the refund to the account.				
7	If applicable, apply a refund to the next service. Click on the line item for the procedure (Field 1), and then click on the *Select/Edit* button. Make certain Field 13 shows the correct *Balance Due*.				
8	In Field 10, drop down the list of adjustment types and select *Refund Overpayment*.				
9	In Field 11, enter the amount to be refunded. Press enter to apply the refund to the balance. Make certain Field 13 shows the correct *Balance Due - $0.00* (or balance if only a portion was refunded).				
10	Click *Post* to enter the refund to the account.				
11	When complete, click *Close* and select the next patient, or return to the *Main Menu*.				
Student's Total Points					
Points Possible					
Final Score (Student's Total Points/Possible Points)					

Instructor's/Evaluator's Comments and Suggestions:

CHECK #1	
Evaluator's Signature:	Date:

CHECK #2	
Evaluator's Signature:	Date:

CHECK #3	
Evaluator's Signature:	Date:

ABHES Competencies: MA.A.1.7.b(2) Apply computer application skills using variety of different electronic programs including both practice management software and EMR software; MA.A.1.8.b Prepare and maintain medical records

CAAHEP Competencies: V.P.5 Execute data management using electronic health care records such as the EMR; V.P.6 Use office hardware and software to maintain office systems

CASE STUDY FOR CAITLIN BARRYROE

No.	Step	
1	Click on the *Posting Payments* button on the *Main Menu.*	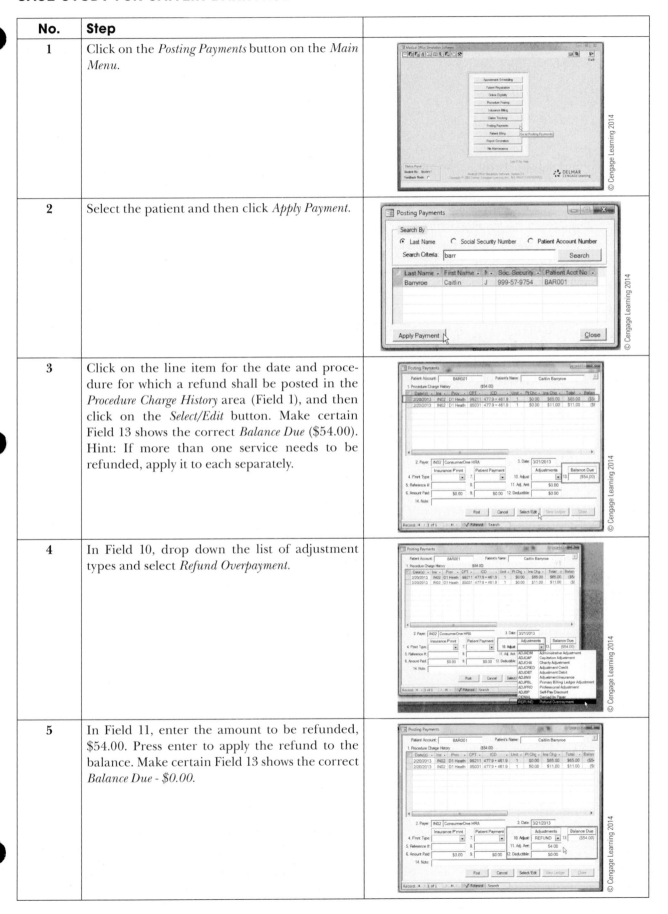
2	Select the patient and then click *Apply Payment.*	
3	Click on the line item for the date and procedure for which a refund shall be posted in the *Procedure Charge History* area (Field 1), and then click on the *Select/Edit* button. Make certain Field 13 shows the correct *Balance Due* ($54.00). Hint: If more than one service needs to be refunded, apply it to each separately.	
4	In Field 10, drop down the list of adjustment types and select *Refund Overpayment.*	
5	In Field 11, enter the amount to be refunded, $54.00. Press enter to apply the refund to the balance. Make certain Field 13 shows the correct *Balance Due - $0.00.*	

No.	Step	
6	Click *Post* to enter the refund to the account.	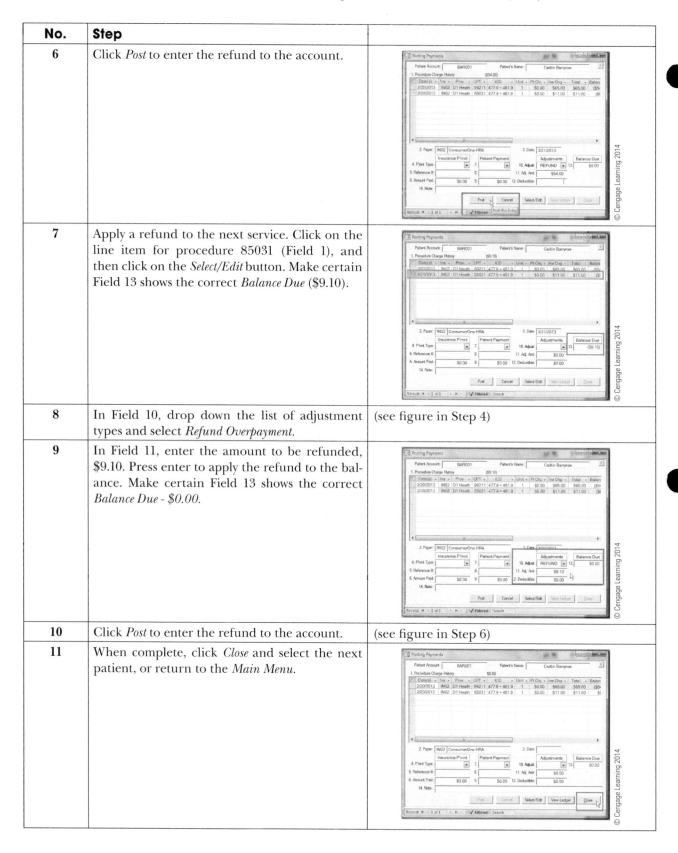
7	Apply a refund to the next service. Click on the line item for procedure 85031 (Field 1), and then click on the *Select/Edit* button. Make certain Field 13 shows the correct *Balance Due* ($9.10).	
8	In Field 10, drop down the list of adjustment types and select *Refund Overpayment*.	(see figure in Step 4)
9	In Field 11, enter the amount to be refunded, $9.10. Press enter to apply the refund to the balance. Make certain Field 13 shows the correct *Balance Due - $0.00.*	
10	Click *Post* to enter the refund to the account.	(see figure in Step 6)
11	When complete, click *Close* and select the next patient, or return to the *Main Menu.*	

Name _____ **Date** _____ **Score** _____

● COMPETENCY ASSESSMENT

Procedure 19-7:   Preparing a Deposit

Task: Create a deposit slip for the day's receipts.

Conditions:
- New deposit slip
- Check endorsement stamp
- Calculator
- Cash and checks received for the day, day sheet

Standards: Perform the Task within 15 minutes with a minimum score of _____ points, as determined by your instructor.

Competency Assessment Information

Using the information below, prepare a deposit for the medical office. Use the Deposit Slip form (Work Documentation) to complete this procedure.

On October 15, 20XX, the day's receipts were:

Cash: (2) $20 bills, (1) $5 bill (no coins)
Checks: $25.00; $76.31; $20.00; $10.00; $36.34; $124.78; $25.00; $40.00

Time began: _____   **Time ended:** _____   **Total time:** _____

No.	Step	Points	Check #1	Check #2	Check #3
1	Separate all checks from currency (paper money).				
2	Count all currency to be deposited and enter the amount in the space provided. Gather bills facing the same direction in order (i.e., 50s, 20s, 10s, and so on).				
3	Count all coins to be deposited and enter the amount in the space provided. Coins may need to be wrapped.				
4	On the back of the deposit slip, list each check separately. Include the patient name in the left-hand column and enter the amount of the check in the right-hand column.				
5	Total the checks listed and copy the total on the front where it is indicated to place the total from the other side.				
6	The sum of currency, coins, and checks should always equal the total in the Payments column on that day's day sheet.				
7	Attach the top copy of the deposit slip to the deposit, leaving the carbon on the pad.				
8	Enter the date and amount of the deposit in the space provided on the checkbook stubs.				

No.	Step	Points	Check #1	Check #2	Check #3
9	Add the amount of the deposit to the checkbook balance.				
10	Deposit at the bank, either in person or at the night deposit.				
Student's Total Points					
Points Possible					
Final Score (Student's Total Points/Possible Points)					

Instructor's/Evaluator's Comments and Suggestions:

CHECK #1	
Evaluator's Signature:	Date:

CHECK #2	
Evaluator's Signature:	Date:

CHECK #3	
Evaluator's Signature:	Date:

ABHES Competency: MA.A.1.8.g. Prepare and reconcile a bank statement and deposit record

CAAHEP Competency: VI.P.1 Prepare a bank deposit

Work Documentation Form(s): Deposit Slip

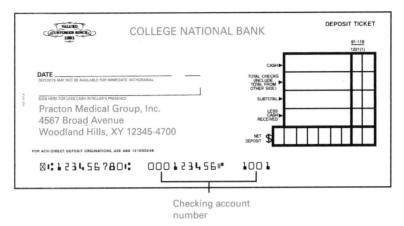

Checking account number

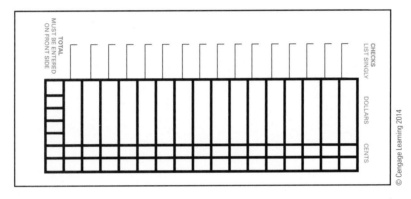

Name_____ **Date**_____ **Score**_____

● **COMPETENCY ASSESSMENT**

Procedure 19-8:   Recording a Nonsufficient Funds Check in a Manual System

Task: Perform bookkeeping functions that keep account in proper balance.

Conditions: • The practice's account balance
                 • Manual day sheet
                 • Manual ledger
                 • NSF check

Standards: Perform the Task within 15 minutes with a minimum score of _____ points, as determined by your instructor.

Time began: _____   **Time ended:** _____   **Total time:** _____

No.	Step	Points	Check #1	Check #2	Check #3
1	Follow the clinic policy for notifying the patient of the returned check.				
2	When the NSF check has been returned the second time, deduct the check amount from the account balance of the practice.				
3	Add the amount of the NSF check back into the patient's ledger. Place the amount in parentheses in the paid column and increase the total by the same amount. In a manual system, the entry and math are performed by the medical assistant.				
4	Place a brief explanation in the description of the column such as "NSF 12/09/2012."				
Student's Total Points					
Points Possible					
Final Score (Student's Total Points/Possible Points)					

Instructor's/Evaluator's Comments and Suggestions:

_____

_____

_____

_____

_____

_____

_____

CHECK #1	
Evaluator's Signature:	Date:

CHECK #2	
Evaluator's Signature:	Date:

CHECK #3	
Evaluator's Signature:	Date:

ABHES Competency: MA.A.1.8.p. Post nonsufficient funds (NSF)

CAAHEP Competency: VI.P.2.g Post nonsufficient fund (NSF) checks

Name_____   **Date**_____   **Score**_____

● COMPETENCY ASSESSMENT

Procedure 19-9:   Writing a Check

Task: Write a check to pay for expenses incurred and provide proof of payment.

Conditions: • Checkbook
                 • Check register
                 • Pen with black ink
                 • Calculator

Standards: Perform the Task within 15 minutes with a minimum score of _____ points, as determined by your instructor.

Competency Assessment Information

Using the information below, write checks for the medical office. Use the check forms (Work Documentation) to complete this procedure.

1. $54.99 for case of printer paper to Landau Products.
2. $450.00 for last month's janitorial services to Mjb Services.
3. $1,335.38 for clinical supplies to Redding Medical Supply House.
4. $687.19 to Atlantic Electric for last month's heat and electricity.
5. $350 to American Association of Medical Assistants for AAMA membership for the four medical assistants in the clinic.

● **Time Began:** _____   **Time Ended:** _____   **Total Time:** _____

No.	Step	Points	Check #1	Check #2	Check #3
1	Gather all invoices to be paid.				
2	For the check register, use black ink: a. Enter check number 101 in the register if not preprinted. b. Enter the current date and year (usually in numbers, i.e., 02/14/2012). c. Enter the individual or company the check is to be paid to: Landau Products. d. Enter the amount to be paid on the check: $54.99. e. Subtract check amount from the present balance. Total $7,243.36 appears as the available balance.				
3	To write the check, use black ink: a. Enter check number 101 if not preprinted. b. Enter the current date and year (usually written out, i.e., February 14, 2012). c. Enter the individual or company the check is to be paid to: Landau Products. d. Enter the amount to be paid on the check: $54.99. Do not leave spaces between numbers or between the dollar sign and the first number.				

No.	Step	Points	Check #1	Check #2	Check #3
	e. Write out the amount to be paid by check (Fifty-four dollars and 99/100). Fill in any space left between the last number or word and draw a wiggly line over to the amount entered in numbers. f. Describe what the check is written for in the bottom left corner (Printer paper, case). g. If you have check-writing authority in the clinic, sign the check with your name the same as indicated on the bank's records. If you do not have check-writing authority, hold this check and the others to give to the individual with that authority.				
4	Continue writing checks for items 2 through 5 in the Check Writing Exercises, being certain to number checks consecutively and to subtract each check amount from the balance.				
Student's Total Points					
Points Possible					
Final Score (Student's Total Points/Possible Points)					

Instructor's/Evaluator's Comments and Suggestions:

_____

_____

_____

_____

_____

_____

_____

CHECK #1	
Evaluator's Signature:	Date:

CHECK #2	
Evaluator's Signature:	Date:

CHECK #3	
Evaluator's Signature:	Date:

ABHES Competency: MA.A.1.8.J Perform accounts payable procedures

Work Documentation Form(s): Checks

PRACTON MEDICAL GROUP, INC.
4567 Broad Avenue
Woodland Hills, XY 12345-4700

FOR INSTRUCTIONAL USE ONLY

DATE	ITEM	AMOUNT

479   3-2/310

PAY _____ DOLLARS

PAY TO THE ORDER OF	DATE	GROSS	DISC.	CHECK AMOUNT
				$.

NOT VALID

THE FIRST NATIONAL BANK – Woodland Hills, XY 12345-4700
RB40BC-4-96

⑆123450⑆ 000123456⑈   0479

PRACTON MEDICAL GROUP, INC.
4567 Broad Avenue
Woodland Hills, XY 12345-4700

FOR INSTRUCTIONAL USE ONLY

DATE	ITEM	AMOUNT

480   3-2/310

PAY _____ DOLLARS

PAY TO THE ORDER OF	DATE	GROSS	DISC.	CHECK AMOUNT
				$.

NOT VALID

THE FIRST NATIONAL BANK – Woodland Hills, XY 12345-4700
RB40BC-4-96

⑆123450⑆ 000123456⑈   0480

PRACTON MEDICAL GROUP, INC.
4567 Broad Avenue
Woodland Hills, XY 12345-4700

FOR INSTRUCTIONAL USE ONLY

DATE	ITEM	AMOUNT

481   3-2/310

PAY _____ DOLLARS

PAY TO THE ORDER OF	DATE	GROSS	DISC.	CHECK AMOUNT
				$.

NOT VALID

THE FIRST NATIONAL BANK – Woodland Hills, XY 12345-4700
RB40BC-4-96

⑆123450⑆ 000123456⑈   0481

Name_____ **Date**_____ **Score**_____

● COMPETENCY ASSESSMENT

Procedure 19-10: Reconciling a Bank Statement

Task: Verify that the balance listed in the checkbook agrees with the balance shown by the bank.

Conditions:
- Checkbook
- Bank statement
- Calculator

Standards: Perform the Task within 15 minutes with a minimum score of _____ points, as determined by your instructor.

Competency Assessment Information

Using the Bank Statement Reconciliation Worksheet (Work Documentation), reconcile your checkbook with your monthly bank statement.

Time began: _____ **Time ended:** _____ **Total time:** _____

No.	Step	Points	Check #1	Check #2	Check #3
1	Make sure the balance in the checkbook is current.				
2	If a service charge is listed on the statement, subtract that amount from the last balance listed in the checkbook.				
3	In the checkbook, check off each check listed on the statement and verify the amount against the check stub.				
4	In the checkbook, check off each deposit listed on the statement.				
5	The back of the statement contains a worksheet to be used for balancing. Copy the ending balance from the front of the statement to the area indicated on the back.				
6	Go through the check stubs and list on the back of the statement in the area provided any checks that have not cleared and any deposits that were not shown as received on the statement.				
7	Total the checks not cleared on the statement worksheet.				
8	Total the deposits not credited on the worksheet.				
9	Add together the statement balance and the total of deposits not credited.				
10	Subtract the total of checks not cleared. This amount should agree with the balance in the checkbook. If so, the checkbook is balanced and the statement should be filed in the appropriate place.				
	Student's Total Points				
	Points Possible				
	Final Score (Student's Total Points/Possible Points)				

Instructor's/Evaluator's Comments and Suggestions:

_____

_____

_____

_____

_____

_____

_____

CHECK #1	
Evaluator's Signature:	Date:

CHECK #2	
Evaluator's Signature:	Date:

CHECK #3	
Evaluator's Signature:	Date:

ABHES Competency: MA.A.1.8.g Prepare and reconcile a bank statement and deposit record

Work Documentation Form(s)

BANK STATEMENT RECONCILIATION

FOUR EASY STEPS TO HELP YOU BALANCE YOUR CHECKBOOK

1. UPDATE YOUR CHECKBOOK
   - Compare and check off each transaction recorded in your check register with those listed on this statement. These include checks, direct deposits, direct debits, deposits, ATM transactions, etc.
   - Add interest and subtract service charges.

2. DETERMINE OUTSTANDING ITEMS
   - Use the charts below to list transactions shown in your check register but not included on this statement.
   - Include any from previous months.

OUTSTANDING CHECKS OR OTHER WITHDRAWALS				DEPOSITS NOT CREDITED	
CHECK NO.	AMOUNT	CHECK NO.	AMOUNT	DATE	AMOUNT
	$		$		$
		TOTAL	$	TOTAL	$

3. BALANCE YOUR ACCOUNT
   - Enter Ending Statement Balance shown on this statement. $ _____
   - Add deposits listed in your register and not shown on this statement.   + _____
   - Subtract outstanding checks/withdrawals.   - _____
   - **ADJUSTED TOTAL** (should agree with your checkbook balance) $ _____

4. IF THE BALANCE IN YOUR CHECKBOOK DOES NOT AGREE WITH THE ADJUSTED TOTAL, THEN
   - Check all addition and subtraction.
   - Make sure all outstanding checks, withdrawals, and deposits have been listed in the appropriate chart above.
   - Compare the amount of each check, withdrawal, and deposit in your checkbook with the amounts on this statement.
   - Review the figures on last month's statement.

IN CASE OF ERRORS OR QUESTIONS ABOUT YOUR ELECTRONIC TRANSFERS, telephone us at the telephone number shown on this statement, or write us at: P.O. Box 30987, City of Industry, CA 91896-7987 as soon as you can if you think your statement or receipt is wrong or if you need more information about a transfer on the statement or receipt. We must hear from you no later than 60 days after we sent you the FIRST statement on which the error or problem appeared. Tell us your name and account number, and describe the error or the transfer you are unsure about. Please explain as clearly as you can why you believe there is an error or why you need more information. You must also tell us the exact dollar amount of the suspected error. If you tell us orally, we require that you send us your complaint or question in writing within 10 business days. If you do not put your complaint or questions in writing or we do not receive it within 10 business days, we may not recredit your account. If we decide that there was no error, we will send you a written explanation within 3 business days after we finish our investigation. You may ask for copies of the documents that we used in our investigation. For purposes of error resolution, our business days are Monday through Friday, 8:30 a.m. to 5:00 p.m., Pacific Time. We are closed Saturdays, Sundays, and federal holidays.

All Non-POS, MasterMoney™ or Foreign Transactions
We will tell you the results of our investigation within 10 business days after we receive your written complaint and will correct any error promptly. If we need more time, however, we may take up to 45 days to investigate your complaint or questions. If we decide we need additional time, we will recredit your account within 10 business days for the amount you think is in error, so that you will have the use of the money during the time it takes us to complete our investigation.

POS, MasterMoney™ and Foreign Transactions
If the transfer results from a point-of-sale transaction, MasterMoney™ transaction, or a transfer initiated outside the United States, we will still correct any error promptly. However, we may take up to 20 business days after we receive your written complaint to tell you the results of our investigation. If we need more time, we may use an additional 90 days. Should we take this additional time, we will recredit your account within 20 business days for the amount you think is in error. This will allow you to have the use of this money while we complete our investigation.

CF 5299F (5/96)

Name_____ **Date**_____ **Score**_____

COMPETENCY ASSESSMENT

Procedure 19-11:   Establishing and Maintaining a Petty Cash Fund

Task: Establish and maintain a petty cash fund for incidental expenses making certain that receipts match the difference between the beginning and ending balance of the fund.

Conditions: • Petty cash box with cash balance
                 • Vouchers
                 • Calculator

Standards: Perform the Task within 15 minutes with a minimum score of _____ points, as determined by your instructor.

Competency Assessment Information

Using the information below, write checks for the medical office. Use the Petty Cash Voucher form and the Check Template form (Work Documentation) to complete this procedure.

1. Write a check for $100 cash at the bank.
2. Vouchers are made for the following incidentals:
   A. $20 to staff employee to purchase coffee supplies. Actual amount for supplies is $13.87; employee returns $6.13 cash.
   B. $2.24 for postage due to postal employee.
   C. $3.18 to postal employee for guaranteed forwarding address.
   D. $35.00 to Shannon's Pizza delivery for staff meeting lunch.

Time began: _____   **Time ended:** _____   **Total time:** _____

No.	Step	Points	Check #1	Check #2	Check #3
1	Correctly prepare a check for $100, written to "Cash."				
2	Receive the cash and place in cash box.				
3	Using the Petty Cash Exercises, correctly prepare vouchers for the amounts needed. Remove the appropriate cash from the cash box.				
4	After the purchases, place receipts for the purchases in the cash box.				
5	Correctly balance the Petty Cash fund by counting the money remaining and totaling the receipts.				
6	Correctly prepare a check for the amount that was used, bringing the total of the Petty Cash fund back to $100.				
Student's Total Points					
Points Possible					
Final Score (Student's Total Points/Possible Points)					

Instructor's/Evaluator's Comments and Suggestions:

_____

_____

_____

_____

_____

_____

_____

CHECK #1 Evaluator's Signature:	Date:

CHECK #2 Evaluator's Signature:	Date:

CHECK #3 Evaluator's Signature:	Date:

ABHES Competency: MA.A.1.8.1 Establish and maintain a petty cash fund

Work Documentation Form(s)

PETTY CASH RECEIPT ENVELOPE

From _____ **20XX To** _____ **20XX**   **Paid by Check No.** _____

Entered		Audited	Approved		Paid	

Date	No.	Paid to:	Item	Account	Amount	

Office Fund Amount	$ _____	**Receipts Paid**	$ _____
Total Receipts and Cash	$ _____	**Cash on Hand**	$ _____
(Over or Short)	$ _____	**TOTAL**	$ _____

DISTRIBUTION OF PETTY CASH

										Totals

PRACTON MEDICAL GROUP, INC.
4567 Broad Avenue
Woodland Hills, XY 12345-4700

FOR INSTRUCTIONAL USE ONLY

DATE	ITEM	AMOUNT

479

3-2
310

PAY _____ DOLLARS

PAY TO THE ORDER OF	DATE	GROSS	DISC.	CHECK AMOUNT
				$.

NOT VALID

THE FIRST NATIONAL BANK – Woodland Hills, XY 12345-4700
RB40BC-4-96

⑈123450⑈ 000123456⑈   0479

PRACTON MEDICAL GROUP, INC.
4567 Broad Avenue
Woodland Hills, XY 12345-4700

FOR INSTRUCTIONAL USE ONLY

DATE	ITEM	AMOUNT

480

3-2
310

PAY _____ DOLLARS

PAY TO THE ORDER OF	DATE	GROSS	DISC.	CHECK AMOUNT
				$.

NOT VALID

THE FIRST NATIONAL BANK – Woodland Hills, XY 12345-4700
RB40BC-4-96

⑈123450⑈ 000123456⑈   0480

PRACTON MEDICAL GROUP, INC.
4567 Broad Avenue
Woodland Hills, XY 12345-4700

FOR INSTRUCTIONAL USE ONLY

DATE	ITEM	AMOUNT

481

3-2
310

PAY _____ DOLLARS

PAY TO THE ORDER OF	DATE	GROSS	DISC.	CHECK AMOUNT
				$.

NOT VALID

THE FIRST NATIONAL BANK – Woodland Hills, XY 12345-4700
RB40BC-4-96

⑈123450⑈ 000123456⑈   0481

Name_____ **Date**_____ **Score**_____

● **COMPETENCY ASSESSMENT**

Procedure 20-1: Explaining Fees in the First Telephone Interview

Task: To establish rapport with patients; to discuss providers' fees; to identify patient's responsibility before the first visit.

Conditions:
- Fee schedule
- Appointment schedule
- Telephone
- Note pad

Standards: Perform the Task within 15 minutes with a minimum score of ___ points, as determined by your instructor.

Competency Assessment Information

Go to the Premium Website to download a sample fee schedule for Procedure 20-1. Use the information below to role-play a telephone call.

Diana Goeltz, a potential new patient, calls the Douglasville Medicine Associates to inquire about an appointment with Dr. Schwartz. She has Flexihealth PPO In-Network.

- Dr. Schwartz is a participating provider with Medicare, Flexihealth PPO In-Network, ConsumerOne HRA, and Signal HMO.
- Dr. Schwartz is a nonparticipating provider with Flexihealth PPO Out of Network and Medicaid.
- Clinic policy requires any copayment and coinsurance to be paid at the time of the visit.

Time began: _____   **Time ended:** _____   **Total time:** _____

No.	Step	Points	Check #1	Check #2	Check #3
1	Place the providers' fee schedule and the appointment schedule close to the telephone.				
2	Answer the phone before the third ring. *Identify the name of the clinic and yourself.*				
3	*Acknowledge the patient* and offer assistance.				
4	After the patient is identified as a new patient and the nature of the visit is determined appropriate, discuss possible dates for the appointment.				
5	Tell the patient that you will be discussing clinic policies briefly now and will mail the Patient Information Brochure before the appointment.				
6	Ask about medical insurance. If insured, get the identification number, the name of the subscriber, employer, and a telephone number of the insurance carrier if possible.				
7	Explain that the clinic policy requires any co-payment and coinsurance to be paid at the time of the visit.				

No.	Step	Points	Check #1	Check #2	Check #3
8	Check to see if the patient has transportation and knows how to get to the clinic, and provide directions if necessary.				
9	Request that the patient arrive about 15 minutes before the appointment to complete some forms.				
10	After closing the telephone interview, promptly mail the Patient Information Brochure.				
Student's Total Points					
Points Possible					
Final Score (Student's Total Points/Possible Points)					

Instructor's/Evaluator's Comments and Suggestions:

_____

_____

_____

_____

_____

_____

CHECK #1	
Evaluator's Signature:	Date:

CHECK #2	
Evaluator's Signature:	Date:

CHECK #3	
Evaluator's Signature:	Date:

ABHES Competencies: MA.A.1.8.ee Use proper telephone techniques; MA.A.1.8.v Use physician fee schedule

CAAHEP Competencies: IV.P.2 Report relevant information to others succinctly and accurately; IV.P.4 Explain general office policies; IV.P.7 Demonstrate telephone techniques

Name_____ **Date**_____ **Score**_____

● COMPETENCY ASSESSMENT

Procedure 20-2:   Prepare Itemized Patient Accounts for Billing in a Manual System

Task: To notify patients of the fees for services rendered and collect on those accounts.

Conditions:
- Computer or typewriter
- Calculator
- Patient account or ledger cards
- Billing statement forms

Standards: Perform the Task within 20 minutes with a minimum score of ___ points, as determined by your instructor.

Competency Assessment Information

In Procedures 19-3 and 19-5, you created patient ledger cards and posted payments to the ledger cards for three patients. Now prepare itemized statements for billing, using the Patient Statement Template Form (Work Documentation).

1. Prepare a statement for Herbert VanGillis.
2. Prepare a statement for Isabel Durand.
3. Prepare a statement for Caitlin Barryroe.

Time began: _____ **Time ended:** _____ **Total time:** _____

No.	Step	Points	Check #1	Check #2	Check #3
1	Gather all accounts and ledgers with outstanding balances.				
2	Separate any accounts that are labeled as overdue.				
3	*Pay attention to detail*, and for each account, perform the following: a. Verify the name and address of the patient and the person responsible for payment. b. Place current date on the statement. c. Scan the account information for any possible errors. d. Itemize the procedures in terms patients understand and indicate charges. e. Identify and subtract any payments (co-payment, coinsurance, down payment) that have been made. f. Use the calculator to verify the unpaid balance that is carried forward and is due.				
4	*Discuss with the clinic manager* any action to be taken on past-due accounts. Follow through with those instructions.				
5	Place statements in envelopes and mail.				
Student's Total Points					
Points Possible					
Final Score (Student's Total Points/Possible Points)					

Instructor's/Evaluator's Comments and Suggestions:

_____

_____

_____

_____

_____

CHECK #1	
Evaluator's Signature:	Date:

CHECK #2	
Evaluator's Signature:	Date:

CHECK #3	
Evaluator's Signature:	Date:

ABHES Competencies: MA.A.1.8.i Perform billing and collection procedures; MA.A.1.8.j Perform accounts payable procedures; MA.A.1.8.k Perform accounts receivable procedures

CAAHEP Competency: VI.P.2.c Perform collections procedures

WORK DOCUMENTATION FORM(S): PATIENT STATEMENT

STATEMENT
DOUGLASVILLE MEDICINE ASSOCIATES
5076 Brand Blvd., Suite 401
Douglasville, NY 01234
TEL: (123) 456-7890
FAX: (123) 456-7891

Patient Name:
Address:

Phone No.(H)_____**(W)**_____**Birthdate**_____
Insurance Co. _____**Policy No.**_____

| DATE | REFERENCE | DESCRIPTION | CHARGES | CREDITS | | BALANCE |
				PYMNTS.	ADJ.	
		BALANCE FORWARD ⟶				

RB40BC-2-96   PLEASE PAY LAST AMOUNT IN BALANCE COLUMN ↗

THIS IS A COPY OF YOUR ACCOUNT AS IT APPEARS ON OUR RECORDS

Name_____ **Date**_____ **Score**_____

COMPETENCY ASSESSMENT

Procedure 20-3: Identifying Accounts Receivable Using Medical Office Simulation Software (MOSS)

Task: To identify accounts receivable for patient billing or secondary insurance billing.

Conditions: • Computer with MOSS installed

Standards: Perform each Task within 10 minutes with a minimum score of ___ points, as determined by your instructor.

Competency Assessment Information

Use the following information to complete this procedure. The Case Study is found directly following this Competency Assessment checklist.

You are working in the Patient Accounts office. Generate a report and identify patients as indicated below using MOSS:

1. Case Study – Generate and print a *Billing and Payment Report* for February 2013 using start and end dates: 02/02/2013 through 02/28/2013. Review all patients and the balances due from each.
2. Use the report printed in step 1 above, or generate and print another report for February 2013. Review the patients and identify those who have balances and also have secondary insurances pending billing and payment of those balances. Hint: Use the patient ledger.
3. Use the report printed in step 1 above, or generate and print another report for February 2013. Review the patients and identify those who have balances that will need to be paid by the patient. Hint: Use the patient ledger.

Time began: _____ **Time ended:** _____ **Total time:** _____

No.	Step	Points	Check #1	Check #2	Check #3
1	Click on the *Report Generation* button on the *Main Menu.*				
2	Select the *Billing and Payment Report,* option 5.				
3	Enter start date of the report needed, then click *OK.*				
4	Enter end date of the report needed, then click *OK.*				
5	Size the report to a comfortable viewing size.				
6	Print the *Billing and Payment Report.*				
7	Review the report and identify all patients and the balance due for each.				
8	When necessary to view the patient ledger while analyzing the report, click on *Billing* from the drop-down menu along the top left of MOSS, and select *Patient Ledger.*				

No.	Step	Points	Check #1	Check #2	Check #3
9	Select the patient name in the ledger to view details of the financial transactions against the *Billing and Payment Report.*				
10	Close the report and return to the *Main Menu.* Hint: Be careful to close the report only, and not the entire MOSS software.				
Student's Total Points					
Points Possible					
Final Score (Student's Total Points/Possible Points)					

Instructor's/Evaluator's Comments and Suggestions:

_____

_____

_____

_____

_____

_____

CHECK #1	
Evaluator's Signature:	Date:

CHECK #2	
Evaluator's Signature:	Date:

CHECK #3	
Evaluator's Signature:	Date:

ABHES Competencies: MA.A.1.7.b(2) Apply computer application skills using variety of different electronic programs including both practice management software and EMR software; MA.A.1.8.b Prepare and maintain medical records

CAAHEP Competencies: V.P.5 Execute data management using electronic healthcare records such as the EMR; V.P.6 Use office hardware and software to maintain office systems

CASE STUDY FOR GENERATING AND PRINTING A BILLING AND PAYMENT REPORT

No.	Step	
1	Click on the *Report Generation* button on the *Main Menu*.	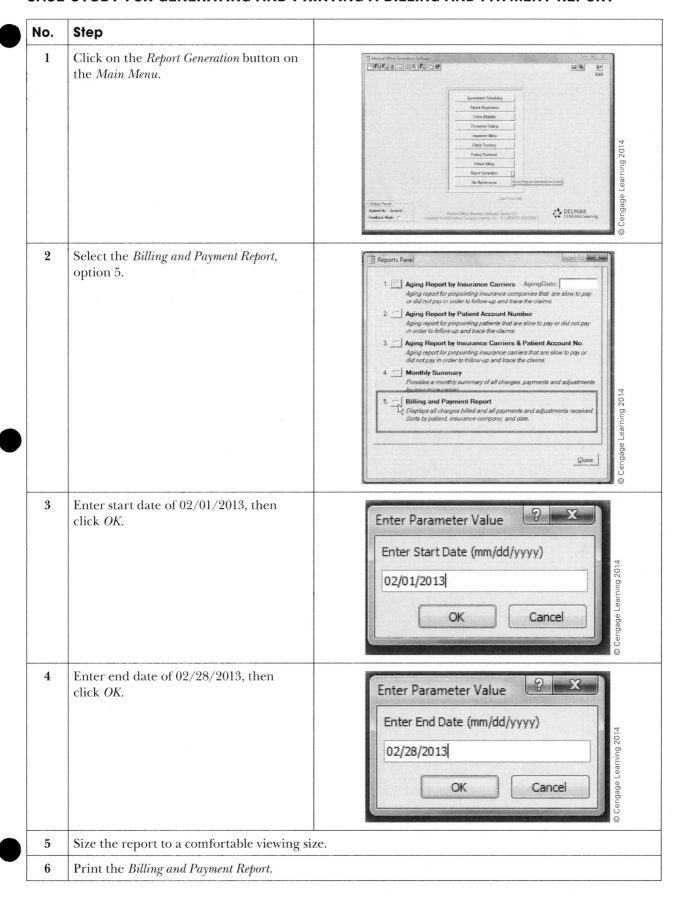
2	Select the *Billing and Payment Report*, option 5.	
3	Enter start date of 02/01/2013, then click *OK*.	
4	Enter end date of 02/28/2013, then click *OK*.	
5	Size the report to a comfortable viewing size.	
6	Print the *Billing and Payment Report*.	

No.	Step	
7	Review the report and identify all patients and the balance due for each.	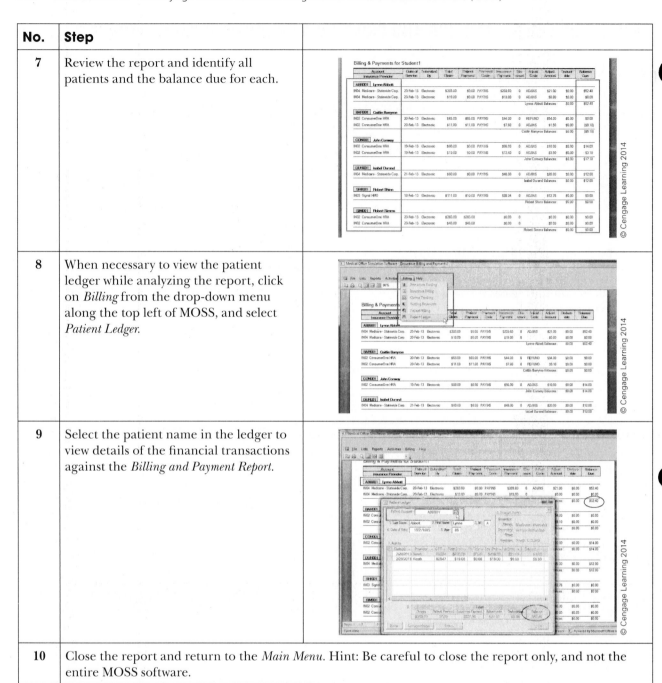
8	When necessary to view the patient ledger while analyzing the report, click on *Billing* from the drop-down menu along the top left of MOSS, and select *Patient Ledger*.	
9	Select the patient name in the ledger to view details of the financial transactions against the *Billing and Payment Report*.	
10	Close the report and return to the *Main Menu*. Hint: Be careful to close the report only, and not the entire MOSS software.	

© Cengage Learning 2014

Name_____ **Date**_____ **Score**_____

●COMPETENCY ASSESSMENT

Procedure 20-4: Preparing Itemized Patient Statements Using Medical Office Simulation Software (MOSS)

Task: To prepare statements for patients with balances due on account.

Conditions: • Computer with MOSS installed

Standards: Perform each Task within 10 minutes with a minimum score of ___ points, as determined by your instructor.

Competency Assessment Information

Use the following information to complete this procedure. The Case Study for patient Robert Shinn is found directly following this Competency Assessment checklist.

You are working in the Patient Accounts office on March 22, 2013. Post charges for NSF to patient accounts as indicated below, using MOSS:

1. Case Study – Prepare a 30-60-90 Standard Statement for Patient Robert Shinn, who had an NSF check charged back to his account, including bank fees. The check number was 4699 and the original amount of the check was $10.00; the bank fee was $35.00. Provide a dunning message explaining the statement balance and print the statement for mailing. Prepare a mailing envelope to the patient.
2. Prepare a 30-60-90 Standard Statement for Patient Isabel Durand. She has secondary insurance that will be billed for the remaining balance. Provide a dunning message explaining that insurance payment is still pending from the secondary payer. Prepare a mailing envelope to the patient.
3. Prepare a Remainder Statement for Patient John Conway. His primary insurance has paid its portion and the remaining balance is the patient's responsibility. Provide a dunning message for the patient explaining the balance due. Prepare a mailing envelope.

Time began: _____ **Time ended:** _____ **Total time:** _____

No.	Step	Points	Check #1	Check #2	Check #3
1	Click on the *Patient Billing* button on the *Main Menu*.				
2	Select the following items on the *Patient Billing* window: • Field 1: 30-60-90 Standard Statement (or Remainder Statement, as applicable) • Field 2: Provider: All • Field 3: Service Dates: Enter from/through dates • Field 3: Report Date: Date of billing • Field 3: Patient Name: Select Patient • Field 3: Account Number: Select Account Number				
3	In Field 6, enter the dunning message, if required to explain the balance.				
4	In Field 7, select the patient name(s) from the list of accounts that will get the dunning message.				
5	Click *Process* to produce the statement(s).				

No.	Step	Points	Check #1	Check #2	Check #3
6	Print the statement(s) and prepare mailing envelopes.				
7	Close the statement window and return to the *Patient Billing* window. Input data for another statement, or close the window and return to the *Main Menu*.				
Student's Total Points					
Points Possible					
Final Score (Student's Total Points/Possible Points)					

Instructor's/Evaluator's Comments and Suggestions:

_____

_____

_____

_____

_____

_____

_____

CHECK #1	
Evaluator's Signature:	Date:

CHECK #2	
Evaluator's Signature:	Date:

CHECK #3	
Evaluator's Signature:	Date:

ABHES Competencies: MA.A.1.7.b(2) Apply computer application skills using variety of different electronic programs including both practice management software and EMR software; MA.A.1.8.b Prepare and maintain medical records

CAAHEP Competencies: V.P.5 Execute data management using electronic healthcare records such as the EMR; V.P.6 Use office hardware and software to maintain office systems

CASE STUDY FOR ROBERT SHINN

No.	Step	
1	Click on the *Patient Billing* button on the *Main Menu*.	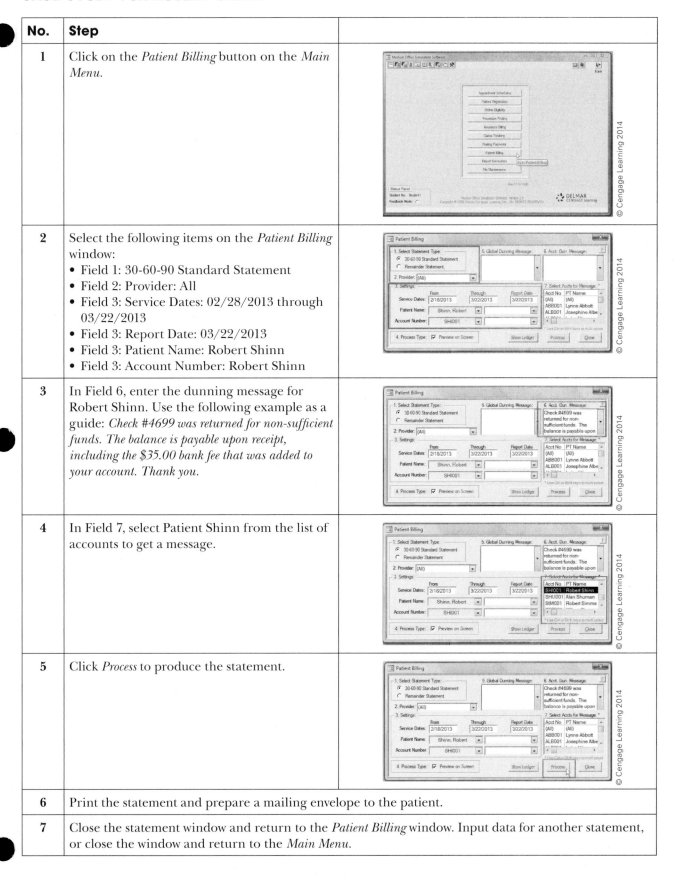
2	Select the following items on the *Patient Billing* window: • Field 1: 30-60-90 Standard Statement • Field 2: Provider: All • Field 3: Service Dates: 02/28/2013 through 03/22/2013 • Field 3: Report Date: 03/22/2013 • Field 3: Patient Name: Robert Shinn • Field 3: Account Number: Robert Shinn	
3	In Field 6, enter the dunning message for Robert Shinn. Use the following example as a guide: *Check #4699 was returned for non-sufficient funds. The balance is payable upon receipt, including the $35.00 bank fee that was added to your account. Thank you.*	
4	In Field 7, select Patient Shinn from the list of accounts to get a message.	
5	Click *Process* to produce the statement.	
6	Print the statement and prepare a mailing envelope to the patient.	
7	Close the statement window and return to the *Patient Billing* window. Input data for another statement, or close the window and return to the *Main Menu*.	

Name_____ **Date**_____ **Score**_____

● COMPETENCY ASSESSMENT

Procedure 20-5: Preparing Collection Letters Using Medical Office Simulation Software (MOSS)

Task: To transcribe (type) medical collection letters using MOSS based on office manager dictation.

Conditions: • Computer with MOSS installed

Standards: Perform each Task within 15 minutes with a minimum score of ___ points, as determined by your instructor.

Competency Assessment Information

Use the following information to complete this procedure. The Case Study for Evan LaGasse and all Source Documents are found directly following this Competency Assessment checklist.

Today's date is March 25, 2013. You are working in the Medical Transcription area. After reviewing account receivables, the office manager has dictated collection letters to be sent to the following patients: Evan LaGasse, Justin McNamara, and Eugene Sykes. The dictation can be found on the Source Documents.

Using the Correspondence feature in MOSS, transcribe (type) the documents, being sure to format the letters properly. Pay special attention to spelling, grammar, and punctuation. All transcribed documents will be placed on the office manager's desk for signature. The mailing envelope should also be prepared and attached to mail the letter in.

● **Time began:** _____ **Time ended:** _____ **Total time:** _____

No.	Step	Points	Check #1	Check #2	Check #3
1	After setting up the transcription equipment and inserting the tape, click on the *Billing* drop-down menu option in MOSS (along the top left) and click on *Patient Ledger.*				
2	Select the patient from the *Patient Account* list and click on *View.* This will display the patient's ledger. Hint: Click on the magnifying glass icon to drop down the list of patients.				
3	At the bottom left of the ledger screen, click on the *Correspondence* button.				
4	The *Output To* dialog box will open. Select a location to save your letter and name it as follows: patientlastname_collection letter_yourlastname. Click *OK* to save the letter.				
5	After a short pause, the letterhead for Douglasville Medicine Associates opens. Change the date of the letter to the desired date and put your own last name in the *Student No.* field.				
6	Include a subject line with the date(s) of service and balance due amount before the salutation, as indicated in the dictation. Next, with the cursor, click at *Type Message Here* and delete that line. Start the body of the letter at that location.				

No.	Step	Points	Check #1	Check #2	Check #3
7	Transcribe (type) the office manager's dictation as shown on the source document. Be sure to format the letter, use punctuation, and use proper grammar.				
8	When complete, save the document by clicking on the *Save* button on the word processor.				
9	Print the letter so the office manager may sign it and turn in a copy to your instructor. Prepare mailing envelopes for all recipients.				
10	Close the word processor and return to the Main Menu in MOSS.				
Student's Total Points					
Points Possible					
Final Score (Student's Total Points/Possible Points)					

Instructor's/Evaluator's Comments and Suggestions:

_____

_____

_____

_____

_____

CHECK #1	
Evaluator's Signature:	Date:

CHECK #2	
Evaluator's Signature:	Date:

CHECK #3	
Evaluator's Signature:	Date:

ABHES Competencies: MA.A.1.7.b(2) Apply computer application skills using variety of different electronic programs including both practice management software and EMR software; MA.A.1.8.b Prepare and maintain medical records

CAAHEP Competencies: V.P.5 Execute data management using electronic healthcare records such as the EMR; V.P.6 Use office hardware and software to maintain office systems

CASE STUDY FOR EVAN LAGASSE

No.	Step	
1	After setting up the transcription equipment and inserting the tape, click on the *Billing* drop-down menu option in MOSS (along the top left) and click on *Patient Ledger*.	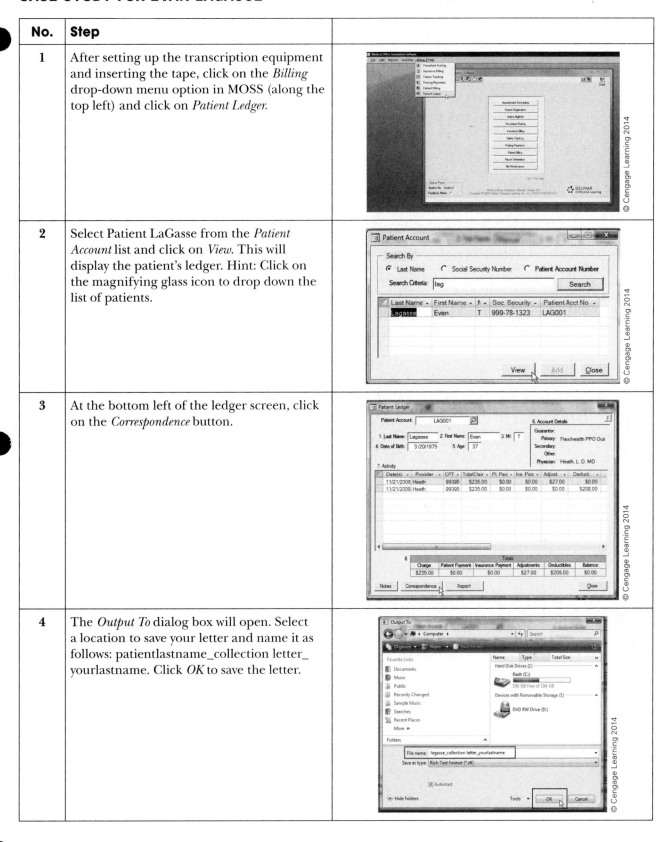
2	Select Patient LaGasse from the *Patient Account* list and click on *View*. This will display the patient's ledger. Hint: Click on the magnifying glass icon to drop down the list of patients.	
3	At the bottom left of the ledger screen, click on the *Correspondence* button.	
4	The *Output To* dialog box will open. Select a location to save your letter and name it as follows: patientlastname_collection letter_yourlastname. Click *OK* to save the letter.	

© Cengage Learning 2014

No.	Step
5	After a short pause, the letterhead for Douglasville Medicine Associates opens. Change the date of the letter to the desired date and put your own last name in the *Student No.* field.
6	Include a subject line with the date(s) of service and balance due amount before the salutation, as indicated in the dictation. Next, with the cursor, click at *Type Message Here* and delete that line. Start the body of the letter at that location.
7	Transcribe (type) the office manager's dictation as shown on the source document. Be sure to format the letter, use punctuation, and use proper grammar.
8	When complete, save the document by clicking on the *Save* button on the word processor.
9	Print the letter so the office manager may sign it and turn in a copy to your instructor. Prepare a mailing envelope.
10	Close the word processor and return to the Main Menu in MOSS.

For step 6, the source document letter shows:

Douglasville Medicine Associates
5076 Brand Blvd., Suite 401
Douglasville, NY 01234
Ph: (123) 456-7890
Fax: (123) 456-7891
Email: admin@dfma.com
Website: www.dfma.com

EVAN LAGASSE
208 Jackman Lane
Compton, NY 01255

Date: 03/25/2013
Account No: LAG001
Student No: Your Name

SUBJECT: SERVICE DATE 11/21/2008 - BALANCE DUE 208.00

Dear Mr. Lagasse:

© Cengage Learning 2014

SOURCE DOCUMENTS FOR PROCEDURE 20-5: DICTATION

Patient: Evan Lagasse

Dictation: Jackie Simmons, CMA, Office Manager

Dictated Correspondence:

this letter is to . . . evan lagasse . . . l-a-g-a-s-s-e . . . please get his address from the computer system database . . . subject line . . . service dates november twenty first two thousand and eight . . . balance due is two hundred and eight dollars . . . dear mister lagasse . . . i am writing you today since our repeated requests for payment have been ignored . . . according to our records your balance . . . remains unpaid to our practice. . . . we have not received . . . a response . . . despite attempts to reach you . . . to set up a payment plan . . . and my instructions to my staff . . . to make every effort available . . . to you...to pay your . . . correction . . . say . . . to satisfy any misunderstanding you may have . . . concerning your balance . . . new paragraph . . . i am deliberately withholding . . . any action on your account for . . . the next ten days . . . if we do not receive any response . . . from you . . . i will be forced to turn your account over to our collection agency . . . northern recovery services incorporated . . . new paragraph . . . we understand that many of our patients . . . experience financial . . . difficulties . . . if this is . . . the case . . . please let us know so we can assist you. . . . if you would like to discuss your account please do not . . . hesitate to contact me at the office . . . sincerely yours . . . jackie simmons . . . c-m-a . . . office manager . . .

Patient: Justin McNamara

Dictation: Jackie Simmons, CMA, Office Manager

Dictated Correspondence:

this letter is to . . . evan lagasse . . . l-a-g-a-s-s-e . . . please get his address from the computer system database . . . subject line . . . service dates . . . december eighteenth . . . two thousand and eight . . . balance due sixty four dollars . . . dear mister mcnamara . . . capital m . . . c-n-a-m-a-r-a . . . as you are aware . . . you have a past due balance . . . of . . . of six four dollars . . . the amount due was an amount . . . applied to your deductible . . . by . . . your insurance . . . company . . . new paragraph . . . to date . . . we have not received payment . . . and . . . have not heard from you regarding payment arrangements . . . please send payment . . . or contact us . . . within ten days . . . to avoid assigning your account to a collection agency . . . we want to help you fulfill your commitment . . . without causing undue hardship . . . and are available to discuss . . . your account . . . i can be reached at the office . . . between eight a-m and . . . five p-m daily . . . new paragraph . . . your prompt attention is appreciated . . . sincerely . . . yours . . . jackie simmons . . . c-m-a . . . office manager . . .

Patient: Eugene Sykes

Dictation: Jackie Simmons, CMA, Office Manager

Dictated Correspondence:

this letter is to . . . eugene . . . sykes . . . s-y-k-e-s . . . his address is in the computer system database . . . subject line . . . service dates . . . october sixteenth two thousand and nine . . . and . . . november second two thousand and nine . . . dear mister sykes . . . on several dates over the past year . . . we called your attention to your account balance . . . in the amount of . . . three hundred dollars . . . new paragraph . . . according to our records . . . we have not received a response from you . . . as you know . . . at the time you received services . . . your insurance coverage had lapsed . . . and resulted in . . . none . . . of the service charges . . . being paid . . . new paragraph . . . we extended credit to you on your account in good faith and expected payment under our normal terms . . . which we feel are most reasonable . . . given the amount of time . . . that has passed . . . new paragraph . . . so that no further action . . . on our part . . . will be necessary we shall expect . . . payment within five days of receipt of this letter . . . or the courtesy of reply to our letter as to why payment is being withheld . . . if we do not receive . . . any response from you . . . i will be forced to turn your account over to our collection agency . . . northern recovery services incorporated . . . thank you for your prompt attention . . . to this matter . . . sincerely . . . yours . . . jackie simmons . . . c-m-a . . . office manager . . .

Name_____ **Date**_____ **Score**_____

● COMPETENCY ASSESSMENT

Procedure 20-6: Posting Non-Sufficient Fund (NSF) Checks Using Medical Office Simulation Software (MOSS)

Task: To post and charge back NSF checks to patient accounts, including bank fees.

Conditions: • Computer with MOSS installed

Standards: Perform each Task within 10 minutes with a minimum score of ___ points, as determined by your instructor.

Competency Assessment Information

Use the following information to complete this procedure. The Case Study for Robert Simms is found directly following this Competency Assessment checklist.

You are working in the Patient Accounts office on March 21, 2013. Post charges for NSF to patient accounts as indicated below, using MOSS:

1. Case Study – The bank has notified the clinic that check number 162 in the amount of $326.00 has been returned for non-sufficient funds. The check was written by Robert Simms. There is an additional $35.00 fee charged by the bank for the return. Post the NSF and charge back the original amount of the check and the bank fee to the patient's account.
2. The bank has notified the clinic that check number 4699 in the amount of $10.00 has been returned for non-sufficient funds. The check was written by Karl Shinn (for patient Robert Shinn). There is an additional $35.00 fee charged by the bank for the return. Post the NSF and charge back the original amount of the check and the bank fee to the patient's account.

Time began: _____ **Time ended:** _____ **Total time:** _____

No.	Step	Points	Check #1	Check #2	Check #3
1	Click on the *Posting Payments* button on the *Main Menu.*				
2	Select the patient and then click the *Apply Payment* button.				
3	Select the line item for service date to be charged back and then click on *Select/Edit.*				
4	Change the date to the date of posting and then drop down the box for Field 10, *Adjustments* and select *Adjustment Debit.*				
5	In Field 11, enter the amount to be charged back to the account. Include the original amount and add any additional fees, if applicable.				
6	Write a note in Field 14 regarding the adjustment so that the reason for the charge back is documented for the line item.				

No.	Step	Points	Check #1	Check #2	Check #3
7	Click *Post* to apply the charges.				
8	Click *Close* and return to the *Main Menu*.				
Student's Total Points					
Points Possible					
Final Score (Student's Total Points/Possible Points)					

Instructor's/Evaluator's Comments and Suggestions:

_____

_____

_____

_____

_____

_____

CHECK #1	
Evaluator's Signature:	Date:

CHECK #2	
Evaluator's Signature:	Date:

CHECK #3	
Evaluator's Signature:	Date:

ABHES Competencies: MA.A.1.7.b(2) Apply computer application skills using variety of different electronic programs including both practice management software and EMR software; MA.A.1.8.b Prepare and maintain medical records

CAAHEP Competencies: V.P.5 Execute data management using electronic healthcare records such as the EMR; V.P.6 Use office hardware and software to maintain office systems

CASE STUDY FOR ROBERT SIMMS

No.	Step	
1	Click on the *Posting Payments* button on the *Main Menu*.	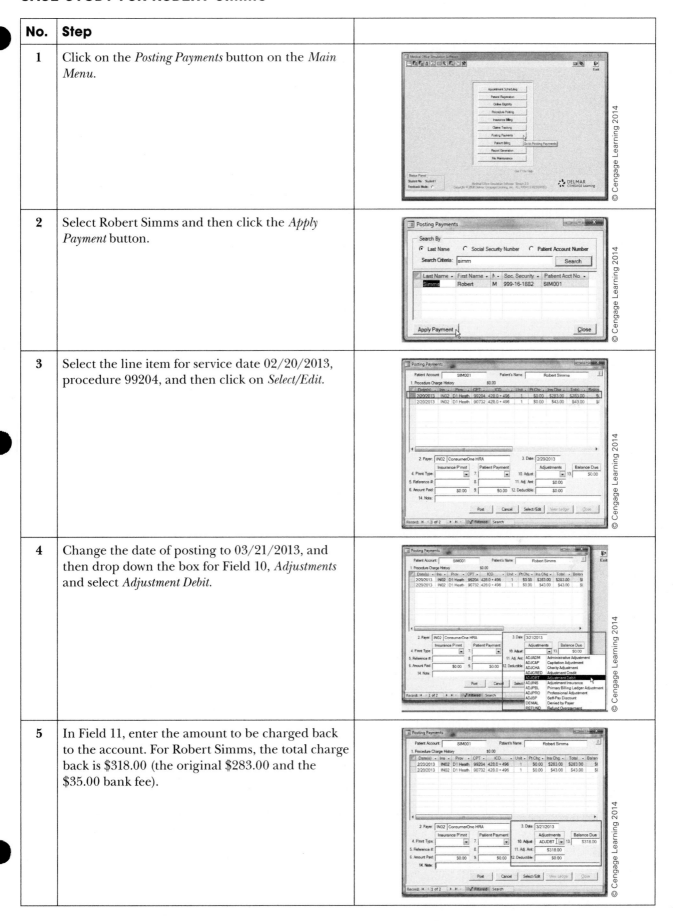
2	Select Robert Simms and then click the *Apply Payment* button.	
3	Select the line item for service date 02/20/2013, procedure 99204, and then click on *Select/Edit*.	
4	Change the date of posting to 03/21/2013, and then drop down the box for Field 10, *Adjustments* and select *Adjustment Debit*.	
5	In Field 11, enter the amount to be charged back to the account. For Robert Simms, the total charge back is $318.00 (the original $283.00 and the $35.00 bank fee).	

© Cengage Learning 2014

No.	Step	
6	Write a note in Field 14 regarding the adjustment: "NSF CHECK #162 for $283.00 plus $35.00 bank fee charged back."	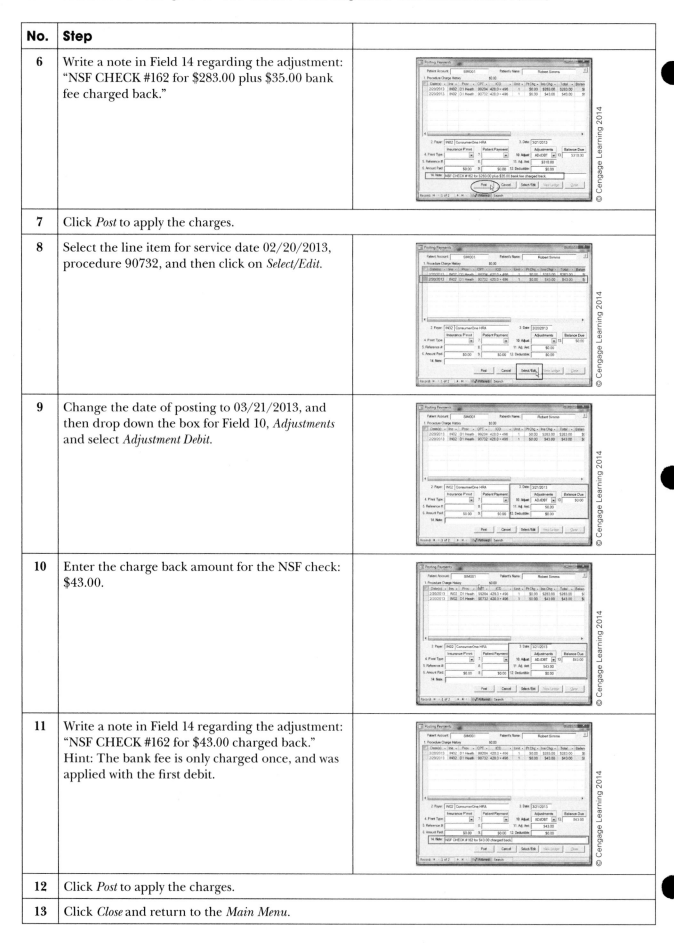
7	Click *Post* to apply the charges.	
8	Select the line item for service date 02/20/2013, procedure 90732, and then click on *Select/Edit*.	
9	Change the date of posting to 03/21/2013, and then drop down the box for Field 10, *Adjustments* and select *Adjustment Debit*.	
10	Enter the charge back amount for the NSF check: $43.00.	
11	Write a note in Field 14 regarding the adjustment: "NSF CHECK #162 for $43.00 charged back." Hint: The bank fee is only charged once, and was applied with the first debit.	
12	Click *Post* to apply the charges.	
13	Click *Close* and return to the *Main Menu*.	

© Cengage Learning 2014

Name_____ **Date**_____ **Score**_____

● COMPETENCY ASSESSMENT

Procedure 20-7: Post/Record Collection Agency Adjustments in a Manual System

Task: To keep track of financial adjustments.

Conditions:
- Manual bookkeeping system
- Patient's account
- Black or blue and red pens for use in manual bookkeeping system

Standards: Perform the Task within 15 minutes with a minimum score of ___ points, as determined by your instructor.

Time began: _____ **Time ended:** _____ **Total time:** _____

No.	Step	Points	Check #1	Check #2	Check #3
1	With the daily schedule of services/charges in front of you (the manual daily sheet), enter amount received from the collection agency on a patient's account and a note such as "Payment from ABC Collection Agency" in the explanation section.				
2	Record the amount received and the explanation in the patient's account as well. The amount received is *subtracted* from the account balance. The balance amount of the account is placed in the "adjustment" column. If there is no adjustment column, put the amount in the charge column with parentheses around it or circle the amount in red. These data are copied to the patient's account in the write-it-once system.				
3	Subtract the amount paid by the collection agency from the total charges to create the new balance.				
4	Write off this balance, indicating a zero balance on the patient's account. In the daily sheet, the difference between the amount collected and the amount paid by the collection agency (plus the agency's fee) is entered as a negative adjustment.				
Student's Total Points					
Points Possible					
Final Score (Student's Total Points/Possible Points)					

Instructor's/Evaluator's Comments and Suggestions:

_____

_____

_____

_____

_____

_____

CHECK #1	
Evaluator's Signature:	Date:

CHECK #2	
Evaluator's Signature:	Date:

CHECK #3	
Evaluator's Signature:	Date:

ABHES Competencies: MA.A.1.8.q Post collection agency payments; MA.A.1.8.j Perform accounts payable procedures; MA.A.1.8.k Perform accounts receivable procedures

CAAHEP Competencies: VI.P.2.a Post entries on a day sheet; VI.P.2.h Post collection agency payments

Name_____   **Date**_____   **Score**_____

● COMPETENCY ASSESSMENT

Procedure 20-8:   Post/Record Collection Agency Adjustments Using Medical Office Simulation Software (MOSS)

Task: To post payments collected by a collection agency to patient accounts and adjust commission fees and uncollectable amounts.

Conditions: • Computer with MOSS installed

Standards: Perform each Task within 15 minutes with a minimum score of ___ points, as determined by your instructor.

Competency Assessment Information

Use the following information to complete this procedure. The Case Study for Evan Lagasse and Source Document are found directly following this Competency Assessment checklist.

Today's date is June 3, 2013. You are working in Patient Accounts. The collection agency, Northern Recovery Services Inc., retains 22% of recovered monies and has sent a check to the office for payments collected on accounts that have been assigned to their service. Post the payments as indicated below:

1. Case Study – Review the Monthly Collection Report from Northern Recovery Services Inc. on the Source Document. Post the payment for Account LAG001, Lagasse, as shown on the report. Adjust the agency's commission fee and remaining balance. In the Note Field, document the payment as from Northern Recovery Services and the date of statement (05/31/2013) to flag the account.
2. Review the Monthly Collection Report from Northern Recovery Services Inc. on the Source Document. Post the payment for Account MCN001, McNamara, as shown on the report. Adjust the agency's commission fee and remaining balance. In the Note Field, document the payment as from Northern Recovery Services and the date of statement (05/31/2013) to flag the account.
3. Review the Monthly Collection Report from Northern Recovery Services Inc. on the Source Document. Post the payments for Account SYK001, Sykes, as shown on the report. Adjust the agency's commission fee and remaining balance. In the Note Field, document the payment as from Northern Recovery Services and the date of statement (05/31/2013) to flag the account.

Time began: _____   **Time ended:** _____   **Total time:** _____

No.	Step	Points	Check #1	Check #2	Check #3
1	Click on *Posting Payments* from the *Main Menu*.				
2	Select the patient from the *Posting Payments* patient selection window.				
3	Select the line item for the service for which a payment will be posted.				
4	Change the date of posting to the date the payment is being applied.				
5	In Field 7, drop down the box and select *Other* as the payment option.				
6	Input the check number and payment amount in Fields 8 and 9. Hint: See the Monthly Collection Report for the check number.				

No.	Step	Points	Check #1	Check #2	Check #3
7	In Field 10, enter the adjustment amount, which includes the agency's commission and, if applicable, remaining balances.				
8	In the Note, Field 14, enter the collection agency's business name and the date of the statement.				
9	Click on the *Post* button to apply the payment and adjustment.				
10	Close the posting window and select another patient, or return to the *Main Menu*.				
Student's Total Points					
Points Possible					
Final Score (Student's Total Points/Possible Points)					

Instructor's/Evaluator's Comments and Suggestions:

_____

_____

_____

_____

_____

_____

CHECK #1 Evaluator's Signature:	Date:

CHECK #2 Evaluator's Signature:	Date:

CHECK #3 Evaluator's Signature:	Date:

ABHES Competencies: MA.A.1.7.b(2) Apply computer application skills using variety of different electronic programs including both practice management software and EMR software; MA.A.1.8.b Prepare and maintain medical records

CAAHEP Competencies: V.P.5 Execute data management using electronic healthcare records such as the EMR; V.P.6 Use office hardware and software to maintain office systems

CASE STUDY FOR EVAN LAGASSE

No.	Step	
1	Click on *Posting Payments* from the *Main Menu*.	
2	Select Patient Lagasse from the *Posting Payments* patient selection window.	
3	Select the line item for the service for which a payment will be posted.	
4	Change the date of posting to 06/03/2013.	
5	In Field 7, drop down the box and select *Other* as the payment option.	

No.	Step	
6	Input the check number and payment amount in Fields 8 and 9. Hint: See the Monthly Collection Report for the check number.	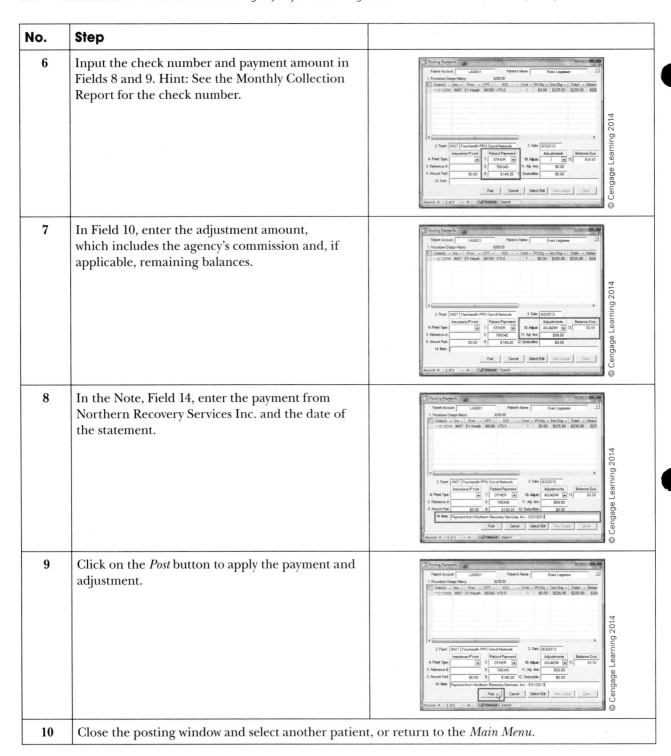
7	In Field 10, enter the adjustment amount, which includes the agency's commission and, if applicable, remaining balances.	
8	In the Note, Field 14, enter the payment from Northern Recovery Services Inc. and the date of the statement.	
9	Click on the *Post* button to apply the payment and adjustment.	
10	Close the posting window and select another patient, or return to the *Main Menu*.	

© Cengage Learning 2014

SOURCE DOCUMENT FOR PROCEDURE 20-8: MONTHLY COLLECTION REPORT

MONTHLY COLLECTION REPORT – 05/31/2013

PREPARED BY: NORTHERN RECOVERY SERVICES, INC.
6800 INDUSTRY WAY, SUITE 100, DOUGLASVILLE, NY 01235   (123) 457-9000

CLIENT
DOUGLASVILLE MEDICINE ASSOCIATES – ACCOUNT 89110   5/31/2013
5076 BRAND BLVD., SUITE 401, DOUGLASVILLE, NY 01234

PATIENT	DOS	BALANCE DUE	DATE PAID	PAID TO AGENCY	AGENCY COMMISSION	REMAINING BALANCE	PAYMENT PLAN?	PAID TO CLIENT
LAGASSE, E LAG001	11/21/2008	$208.00	5/02/2013	$190.00	$ 41.80	$18.00	NO	$148.20
MCNAMARA, J MCN001	12/18/2008	$ 64.00	5/01/2013	$ 64.00	$ 14.08	$0.00	NO	$ 49.92
SYKES, E SYK001	11/02/2009	$180.00	5/17/2013	$170.00	$ 37.40	$10.00	NO	$132.60
SYKES, E SYK001	10/16/2009	$111.00	5/29/2013	$ 101.00	$ 22.22	$10.00	NO	$ 78.78
SYKES, E SYK001	10/16/2009	$ 11.00	5/29/2013	$ 11.00	$ 2.42	$0.00	NO	$ 8.58
SYKES, E SYK001	10/16/2009	$ 18.00	5/29/2013	$ 18.00	$ 3.96	$0.00	NO	$ 14.04
							TOTAL PAID:	$ 353.34
							Check number:	789345

© Cengage Learning 2014

Name_____ **Date**_____ **Score**_____

● COMPETENCY ASSESSMENT

Procedure 21-1:   Preparing Accounts Receivable Trial Balance in a Manual System

Task: A trial balance will determine if there is any problem between the daily journal and the ledger or patient accounts.

Conditions: • Patient accounts
                • Calculator

Standards: Perform the Task within 20 minutes with a minimum score of ___ points, as determined by your instructor.

Time began: _____   **Time ended:** _____   **Total time:** _____

No.	Step	Points	Check #1	Check #2	Check #3
1	Pull all patient accounts that have a balance due.				
2	Enter the balance of those accounts into the calculator.				
3	Add the balances and total.				
4	Create an accounts receivable total: a. Enter the accounts receivable total from the first of the month into the calculator. b. Add total charges for this month and subtotal. c. Total the amount of all payments received this month. d. Subtract the total of payments from subtotal of "b" above and subtotal. e. Total the amount of the month's adjustments and subtract from the subtotal in "d" above. f. This total is the accounts receivable amount.				
Student's Total Points					
Points Possible					
Final Score (Student's Total Points/Possible Points)					

Instructor's/Evaluator's Comments and Suggestions:

_____

_____

_____

_____

_____

_____

_____

CHECK #1	
Evaluator's Signature:	Date:

CHECK #2	
Evaluator's Signature:	Date:

CHECK #3	
Evaluator's Signature:	Date:

ABHES Competencies: MA.A.1.8.j Perform accounts payable procedures; MA.A.1.8.k Perform accounts receivable procedures

Work Documentation Form(s)

Total of Patient Ledgers that have balances: _____

Accounts receivable total:

    A. Monthly accounts receivable total: _____

    B. Add total of this month's charges: +_____

                          Subtotal: _____

    C. Subtract total payments: −_____

                          Subtotal: _____

    D. Total of the month's adjustments: _____

        Subtract D from C for TOTAL: _____

Name_____ **Date**_____ **Score**_____

COMPETENCY ASSESSMENT

Procedure 21-2: Preparing Accounts Receivable Trial Balance Using Medical Office Simulation Software (MOSS)

Task: To generate a trial balance using a monthly summary report showing all transactions for a given month.

Conditions:
- Computer with MOSS installed

Standards: Perform the Task within 10 minutes with a minimum score of ___ points, as determined by your instructor.

Competency Assessment Information

Use the following information to complete this procedure. The Case Study is found directly following this Competency Assessment checklist.

1. Case Study-Generate a monthly summary report using MOSS for the period 02/01/2013 through 02/28/2013.

Time began: _____ **Time ended:** _____ **Total time:** _____

No.	Step	Points	Check #1	Check #2	Check #3
1	Click on the *Report Generation* button on the *Main Menu.*				
2	Select Option 4, *Monthly Summary.*				
3	Enter the *Start Date.*				
4	Enter the *End Date*, and then click *OK.*				
5	Print the *Monthly Summary* report.				
6	Close the report and *Reports Panel*, and return to the *Main Menu.*				
Student's Total Points					
Points Possible					
Final Score (Student's Total Points/Possible Points)					

Instructor's/Evaluator's Comments and Suggestions:

_____

_____

_____

_____

_____

_____

CHECK #1	
Evaluator's Signature:	Date:

CHECK #2	
Evaluator's Signature:	Date:

CHECK #3	
Evaluator's Signature:	Date:

ABHES Competencies: MA.A.1.7.b(2) Apply computer application skills using variety of different electronic programs including both practice management software and EMR software; MA.A.1.8.b Prepare and maintain medical records

CAAHEP Competencies: V.P.5 Execute data management using electronic healthcare records such as the EMR; V.P.6 Use office hardware and software to maintain office systems

CASE STUDY FOR PREPARING AN ACCOUNTS RECEIVABLE TRIAL BALANCE

No.	Step	
1	Click on the *Report Generation* button on the *Main Menu*.	
2	Select Option 4, *Monthly Summary*.	
3	Enter the *Start Date* of 02/01/2013.	
4	Enter the *End Date* of 02/28/2013, and then click *OK*.	
5	Print the *Monthly Summary* report.	
6	Close the report and *Reports Panel*, and return to the *Main Menu*.	

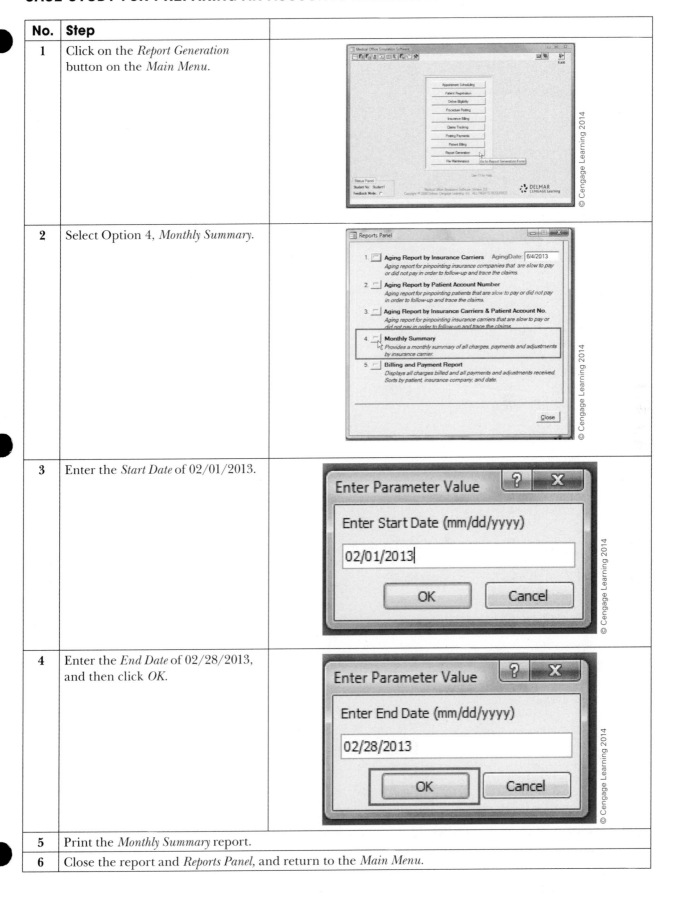

© Cengage Learning 2014

Name _____ **Date** _____ **Score** _____

COMPETENCY ASSESSMENT

Procedure 22-1: Medical Asepsis Hand Wash (Hand Hygiene)

Task: To reduce pathogens on the hands and wrists, thereby decreasing direct and indirect transmission of infectious microorganisms. Average duration is 1 minute before beginning to work with patients, 15 seconds (CDC Hand Hygiene recommendation) following each patient contact.

Conditions:
- Sink (preferably with foot-operated controls)
- Soap (preferably liquid soap in a foot-operated container; bar soap is discouraged)
- Water-based antibacterial lotion
- Disposable paper towels
- Nail stick or brush

Standards: Perform the Task within 5 minutes with a minimum score of ___ points, as determined by your instructor.

Time began: _____ **Time ended:** _____ **Total time:** _____

No.	Step	Points	Check #1	Check #2	Check #3
1	Remove all jewelry (plain wedding band is the only acceptable jewelry). Push watch up on arm or remove.				
2	Ensure that nails are clipped short.				
3	Roll sleeves to above the elbow.				
4	Prepare disposable paper towel (if using a pull-down dispenser, prepare the amount of paper toweling needed for drying hands after wash; if using folded towels, have accessible).				
5	Never allow clothing to touch the sink; never touch the inside of the sink with your hands.				
6	Turn on the faucet with a dry paper towel. Discard the paper towel after adjusting the water temperature to lukewarm.				
7	Wet hands and apply soap in a circular motion and apply friction to rub into a lather.				
8	Use an orange stick or a brush at the first hand washing of each day.				
9	Rinse hands with hands pointed down and lower than elbows.				
10	Repeat soap application and lather; interlace fingers well; wash with vigorous, circular motions all parts of hands including wrists; wash for at least one minute or longer depending on degree of contamination.				
11	Rinse well, keeping hands pointed downward.				
12	Repeat hand washing for the first hand washing of the day or if necessary for contaminated or visibly soiled hands. Lather wrists using a circular motion and friction. Rinse arms and hands.				

No.	Step	Points	Check #1	Check #2	Check #3
13	Dry hands and wrists with disposable paper towel; do not touch towel dispenser after hand washing; blot instead of rubbing with towel; if sink is not foot operated, use a clean disposable towel to turn off the water faucet.				
14	Discard paper towel in waste container. Do not leave contaminated towels for repeated use.				
Student's Total Points					
Points Possible					
Final Score (Student's Total Points/Possible Points)					

Instructor's/Evaluator's Comments and Suggestions:

_____

_____

_____

_____

_____

_____

_____

CHECK #1 Evaluator's Signature:	Date:

CHECK #2 Evaluator's Signature:	Date:

CHECK #3 Evaluator's Signature:	Date:

ABHES Competency: MA.A.1.9.i Use standard precautions

CAAHEP Competency: III.P.4 Perform handwashing

Name_____ **Date**_____ **Score**_____

● COMPETENCY ASSESSMENT

Procedure 22-2: Correct Use of Alcohol-Based Hand Rubs (ABHR)

Task: To avoid transmission of pathogens via the hands of health care personnel.

Conditions: • Alcohol-based hand rub containing 60% to 90% alcohol

Standards: Perform the Task within 3 minutes with a minimum score of ____ points, as determined by your instructor.

Time began: _____ **Time ended:** _____ **Total time:** _____

No.	Step	Points	Check #1	Check #2	Check #3
1	Assure there is no gross contamination of hands.				
2	Dispense 2–3 mL of the alcohol-based hand rub into the palm of the hand.				
3	The ABHR must be applied in the following manner: • Rub palms together. • Place the right palm over the dorsal aspect of the left hand and vice versa. • Face palm to palm with fingers interlaced. • Place backs of fingers to opposing palms with fingers interlaced. • Employ rotational rubbing of left thumb clasped in right palm and vice versa. • Continue rotation rubbing, backwards and forwards, with clasped fingers of right hand on the left palm and vice versa.				
4	Hands should be rubbed together for at least 30 seconds until the hands are dry.				
Student's Total Points					
Points Possible					
Final Score (Student's Total Points/Possible Points)					

Instructor's/Evaluator's Comments and Suggestions:

_____

_____

_____

_____

_____

_____

_____

CHECK #1	
Evaluator's Signature:	Date:

CHECK #2	
Evaluator's Signature:	Date:

CHECK #3	
Evaluator's Signature:	Date:

ABHES Competencies: MA.A.1.9.b Apply principles of aseptic techniques and infection control; MA.A.1.9.i Use standard precautions

CAAHEP Competency: III.P.4 Perform handwashing

Name _____ **Date** _____ **Score** _____

● COMPETENCY ASSESSMENT

Procedure 22-3:   Removing Contaminated Gloves

Task: To carefully remove and dispose of contaminated gloves to contain exposure.

Conditions: • Biohazard waste container

Standards: Perform the Task within 3 minutes with a minimum score of ___ points, as determined by your
                 instructor.

Time began: _____   **Time ended:** _____   **Total time:** _____

No.	Step	Points	Check #1	Check #2	Check #3
1	Grasp the palm of the used left glove with the right hand to begin removing the first glove. Hands are held away from the body and pointed downward.				
2	Turn the used left glove inside out and hold it in the right gloved hand. Be careful not to touch your bare left hand on the contaminated right glove.				
3	Holding the glove that has been removed with the hand that still has a glove on, insert two fingers of the ungloved hand between your arm and the inside of the dirty glove.				
4	Turn the right dirty glove inside out over the other. One glove is inside the other.				
5	Dispose of the inverted gloves into a biological waste receptacle.				
6	Wash hands thoroughly.				
Student's Total Points					
Points Possible					
Final Score (Student's Total Points/Possible Points)					

Instructor's/Evaluator's Comments and Suggestions:

_____

_____

_____

_____

_____

_____

_____

CHECK #1	
Evaluator's Signature:	Date:

CHECK #2	
Evaluator's Signature:	Date:

CHECK #3	
Evaluator's Signature:	Date:

ABHES Competencies: MA.A.1.9.b Apply principles of aseptic techniques and infection control; MA.A.1.9.i Use standard precautions

CAAHEP Competency: III.P.2 Practice standard precautions

Name_____   **Date**_____   **Score**_____

⬤ COMPETENCY ASSESSMENT

Procedure 22-4: Transmission-Based Precautions: Donning a Gown, Mask, Gloves, and Cap (Isolation Technique)

Task: To provide barriers for the medical assistant to be protected from airborne, contact, or droplet infectious diseases.

Conditions:
- Disposable gowns
- Disposable caps if needed
- Disposable masks
- Gloves (nonsterile and sterile)
- Room with sink and running water
- Paper towels
- Other supplies relative to the patient's condition

Standards: Perform the Task within 20 minutes with a minimum score of ___ points, as determined by your instructor.

Time began: _____   **Time ended:** _____   **Total time:** _____

No.	Step	Points	Check #1	Check #2	Check #3
1	Review provider orders and agency protocols relative to the type of isolation precautions.				
2	Place appropriate isolation supplies outside the patient's room and note type of isolation sign on the door.				
3	Remove jewelry, laboratory coat, and other items not necessary in providing patient care.				
4	Wash hands and don disposable clothing: • Apply cap to cover hair and ears completely. • Apply gown to cover outer garments completely. Hold gown in front of body and place arms through sleeves. Pull sleeves down to wrist. Tie gown securely at neck and waist. • Don nonsterile gloves and pull gloves over the cuff to cover completely. • Apply mask by placing the top of the mask over the bridge of your nose (top part of mask has a metal strip) and pinch the metal strip to fit snugly against the skin of the nose.				
5	Enter patient's room with all gathered supplies.				
6	Assess vital signs and perform other functions (ECG, phlebotomy) of care to meet the needs of the patient. Record assessment data on a piece of paper, avoiding contact with any articles in the patient room.				
7	Dispose of soiled articles in the impermeable biohazard bags, which should be labeled correctly according to contents. If soiled, reusable equipment is removed from the room; label bag accordingly.				

No.	Step	Points	Check #1	Check #2	Check #3
Exiting the Isolation Room: Removing Gown, Gloves, Mask, and Cap					
1	Remove contaminated gloves. Wash hands and then untie waist tie of gown.				
2	Remove mask by untying bottom ties first, then top ties. Holding mask by ties, place in contaminated waste.				
3	Untie neckties of gown. Wash hands.				
4	Slip fingers of one hand inside cuff of the other hand. Pull the gown over the hand, being careful not to touch the outside of the gown.				
5	Using the hand covered by the gown, pull down the gown over the other hand.				
6	Pull gown off your arms. Hold gown away from yourself and roll into a ball with the contaminated side inside.				
7	Dispose of gown in biohazard container.				
8	Wash hands thoroughly.				
9	Document procedures performed on patient in patient record or electronic medical record.				
Student's Total Points					
Points Possible					
Final Score (Student's Total Points/Possible Points)					

Instructor's/Evaluator's Comments and Suggestions:

_____

_____

_____

_____

_____

CHECK #1	
Evaluator's Signature:	Date:

CHECK #2	
Evaluator's Signature:	Date:

CHECK #3	
Evaluator's Signature:	Date:

ABHES Competencies: MA.A.1.9.b Apply principles of aseptic techniques and infection control; MA.A.1.9.i Use standard precautions

CAAHEP Competencies: III.P.2 Practice standard precautions; III.P.4 Perform hand washing; IV.P.8 Document patient care

Name _____ **Date** _____ **Score** _____

● COMPETENCY ASSESSMENT

Procedure 22-5:   Sanitization of Instruments

Task: To properly clean contaminated instruments to remove tissue and debris.

Conditions: • Sink (or ultrasonic cleaner; follow manufacturer's instructions)
                 • Sanitizing agent (low-sudsing detergent, approved chemical disinfectant, or blood solvent)
                 • Brush
                 • Disposable paper towels
                 • Plastic apron
                 • Disposable gloves, heavy-duty if cleaning sharps
                 • Goggles
                 • Biohazard waste container

Standards: Perform the Task within 15 minutes with a minimum score of ___ points, as determined by your instructor.

Time began: _____   Time ended: _____   Total time: _____

No.	Step	Points	Check #1	Check #2	Check #3
1	Wear heavy duty gloves, goggles, and apron.				
2	As soon as possible after the procedure in which an instrument is contaminated, rinse the instrument in water and disinfectant solution; rinse again under running water.				
3	If contaminated instrument must be carried from one place to another for sanitization, place the instrument in a basin labeled "Biohazard."				
4	Scrub each instrument well with detergent and water; scrub under running water, and be sure to scrub inside any edges, serrations, and all surfaces.				
5	Rinse well with hot water.				
6	After they are rinsed, place instruments on muslin or disposable paper towels until all instruments have been scrubbed and rinsed.				
7	Dry instruments with muslin or disposable paper towels.				
8	Remove gloves and wash hands.				
Student's Total Points					
Points Possible					
Final Score (Student's Total Points/Possible Points)					

Instructor's/Evaluator's Comments and Suggestions:

_____
_____
_____
_____
_____
_____
_____

CHECK #1 Evaluator's Signature:	Date:

CHECK #2 Evaluator's Signature:	Date:

CHECK #3 Evaluator's Signature:	Date:

ABHES Competencies: MA.A.1.9.b Apply principles of aseptic techniques and infection control; MA.A.1.9.i Use standard precautions

CAAHEP Competencies: III.P.2 Practice standard precautions; III.P.4 Perform handwashing; III.P.5 Prepare items for autoclaving

Name _____ **Date** _____ **Score** _____

● COMPETENCY ASSESSMENT

Procedure 23-1: Taking a Medical History for a Paper Medical Record

Task: To obtain a medical history from a patient new to the ambulatory care setting.

Conditions:
- Patient history forms
- Clipboard
- Pen

Standards: Perform the Task within 25 minutes with a minimum score of ___ points, as determined by your instructor.

Time began: _____   **Time ended:** _____   **Total time:** _____

No.	Step	Points	Check #1	Check #2	Check #3
1	*Introduce yourself to the new patient. Confirm identity of the patient* and escort to the examination room or private area.				
2	Make sure the environment is private and there are few distractions.				
3	*Make eye contact and use positive body language.*				
4	Explain the purpose and importance of obtaining the patient information, *speaking at the patient's level of understanding*. Ask the questions on the form, trying to get as much information as possible without letting the patient wander from the subject.				
5	Ask each question clearly. *Be sure patient understands all questions.* Ask about allergies.				
6	Repeat patient answers when needed to confirm. Be specific when documenting answers. Do not just write "yes" for tobacco use. List "2 packs per day." Be specific.				
7	Write legibly using dark ink (blue or black).				
8	Recheck the medical history form to be sure all parts are complete. *Pay attention to detail.* Note any additional information provided by patient. Make sure numbers, dates, spelling, and other information are accurate and legible.				
9	Prepare the patient for the review of systems and physical examination if this is indicated.				
10	Document the procedure.				
Student's Total Points					
Points Possible					
Final Score (Student's Total Points/Possible Points)					

Instructor's/Evaluator's Comments and Suggestions:

_____

_____

_____

_____

_____

_____

CHECK #1	
Evaluator's Signature:	Date:

CHECK #2	
Evaluator's Signature:	Date:

CHECK #3	
Evaluator's Signature:	Date:

ABHES Competencies: MA.A.1.4.a Document accurately; MA.A.1.8.aa Are attentive, listen, and learn; MA.A.1.8.ff Interview effectively; MA.A.1.8.ii Recognize and respond to verbal and nonverbal communication; MA.A.1.8.kk Adapt to individual needs; MA.A.1.9.a Obtain chief complaint, recording patient history

CAAHEP Competencies: I.P.6 Perform patient screening using established protocols; I.A.1 Apply critical thinking skills in performing patient assessment and care; IV.C.6 Differentiate between subjective and objective information; IV.P.1 Use reflection, restatement and clarification techniques to obtain a patient history; IV.P.2 Report relevant information to others succinctly and accurately; IV.P.3 Use medical terminology, pronouncing medical terms correctly, to communicate information, patient history, data and observations; IV.A.10 Demonstrate respect for individual diversity, incorporating awareness of one's own biases in areas including gender, race, religion, age and economic status; IX.P.7 Document accurately in the patient record; IX.A.1 Demonstrate sensitivity to patient rights

Work Documentation Form(s)

CONFIDENTIAL HEALTH HISTORY

Name: _____ Date: _____
Birthdate: _____ Age: _____ Date of last physical examination:_____
Occupation: _____
Reason for visit today: _____

MEDICATIONS List all medications you are currently taking	**ALLERGIES** List all allergies

SYMPTOMS Check {✓} symptoms you currently have had in the past year.

GENERAL	GASTROINTESTINAL	EYE, EAR, NOSE, THROAT	MEN only
☐ Chills	☐ Appetite poor	☐ Bleeding gums	☐ Breast lump
☐ Depression	☐ Bloating	☐ Blurred vision	☐ Erection difficulties
☐ Dizziness	☐ Bowel changes	☐ Crossed eyes	☐ Lump in testicles
☐ Fainting	☐ Constipation	☐ Difficulty swallowing	☐ Penis discharge
☐ Fever	☐ Diarrhea	☐ Double vision	☐ Sore on penis
☐ Forgetfulness	☐ Excessive hunger	☐ Earache	☐ Other
☐ Headache	☐ Excessive thirst	☐ Ear discharge	**WOMEN only**
☐ Loss of sleep	☐ Gas	☐ Hay fever	☐ Abnormal Pap Smear
☐ Loss of weight	☐ Hemorrhoids	☐ Hoarseness	☐ Bleeding between periods
☐ Nervousness	☐ Indigestion	☐ Loss of hearing	☐ Breast lump
☐ Numbness	☐ Nausea	☐ Nosebleeds	☐ Extreme menstrual pain
☐ Sweats	☐ Rectal bleeding	☐ Persistent cough	☐ Hot flashes
MUSCLE/JOINT/BONE	☐ Stomach pain	☐ Ringing in ears	☐ Nipple discharge
Pain, weakness, numbness in:	☐ Vomiting	☐ Sinus problems	☐ Painful intercourse
☐ Arms ☐ Hips	☐ Vomiting blood	☐ Vision – Flashes	☐ Vaginal discharge
☐ Back ☐ Legs	**CARDIOVASCULAR**	☐ Vision – Halos	☐ Other
☐ Feet ☐ Neck	☐ Chest pain	**SKIN**	
☐ Hands ☐ Shoulders	☐ High blood pressure	☐ Bruise easily	Date of last menstrual period_____
GENITO-URINARY	☐ Irregular heart beat	☐ Hives	Date of last Pap Smear_____
☐ Blood in urine	☐ Low blood pressure	☐ Itching	
☐ Frequent urination	☐ Poor circulation	☐ Change in moles	Have you had a mammogram?_____
☐ Lack of bladder control	☐ Rapid heart beat	☐ Rash	Are you pregnant?_____
☐ Painful urination	☐ Swelling of ankles	☐ Scars	Number of children_____
	☐ Varicose veins	☐ Sores that won't heal	

MEDICAL HISTORY Check {✓} the medical conditions you have or have had in the past.

☐ AIDS	☐ Chemical dependency	☐ Herpes	☐ Polio
☐ Alcoholism	☐ Chicken Pox	☐ High Cholesterol	☐ Prostate Problem
☐ Anemia	☐ Diabetes	☐ HIV Positive	☐ Psychiatric Care
☐ Anorexia	☐ Emphysema	☐ Kidney Disease	☐ Rheumatic Fever
☐ Appendicitis	☐ Epilepsy	☐ Liver Disease	☐ Scarlet Fever
☐ Arthritis	☐ Gall Bladder Disease	☐ Measles	☐ Stroke
☐ Asthma	☐ Glaucoma	☐ Migraine Headaches	☐ Suicide Attempt
☐ Bleeding Disorders	☐ Goiter	☐ Miscarriage	☐ Thyroid Problems
☐ Breast Lump	☐ Gonorrhea	☐ Mononucleosis	☐ Tonsilitis
☐ Bronchitis	☐ Gout	☐ Multiple Sclerosis	☐ Tuberculosis
☐ Bulimia	☐ Heart Disease	☐ Mumps	☐ Typhoid Fever
☐ Cancer	☐ Hepatitis	☐ Pacemaker	☐ Ulcers
☐ Cataracts	☐ Hernia	☐ Pneumonia	☐ Vaginal Infections
			☐ Venereal Disease

CONFIDENTIAL HEALTH HISTORY

Work Form 23-1 (*continued*)

HOSPITALIZATIONS

Year	Hospital	Reason for Hospitalization and Outcome

Have you ever had a blood transfusion?   ☐ Yes ☐ No

If yes, please give approximate dates: _____

OCCUPATIONAL CONCERNS Check {✓} if your work exposes you to the following:	HEALTH HABITS Check {✓} which substances you use and indicate how much you use per day/week.	PREGNANCY HISTORY		
		Year of Birth	**Sex of Birth**	**Complications if any**
☐ Stress	☐ Caffeine			
☐ Hazardous Substances	☐ Tobacco			
☐ Heavy Lifting	☐ Drugs			
☐ Other	☐ Alcohol			

SERIOUS ILLNESS/INJURIES	DATE	OUTCOME

FAMILY HISTORY Fill in health information about your family.

Relation	Age	State of Health	Age of Death	Cause of Death	Check {✓} if your blood relatives had any of the following	
					Disease	**Relationship to you**
Father					☐ Arthritis, Gout	
Mother					☐ Asthma, Hay Fever	
Brothers					☐ Cancer	
					☐ Chemical Dependency	
					☐ Diabetes	
					☐ Heart Disease, Strokes	
Sisters					☐ High Blood Pressure	
					☐ Kidney Disease	
					☐ Tuberculosis	
					☐ Other	

I certify that the above information is correct to the best of my knowledge. I will not hold my doctor or any members of his/her staff responsible for any errors or omissions that I may have made in the completion of this form.

_____   _____
            Signature   Date

_____   _____
            Reviewed By   Date

Name_____ **Date**_____ **Score**_____

● COMPETENCY ASSESSMENT

Procedure 24-1:   Measuring an Oral Temperature Using an Electronic Thermometer

Task: To obtain an oral temperature.

Conditions: • Electronic thermometer
               • Probe covers
               • Biohazard waste container

Standards: Perform the Task within 3 minutes with a minimum score of ___ points, as determined by your instructor.

Time began: _____   **Time ended:** _____   **Total time:** _____

No.	Step	Points	Check #1	Check #2	Check #3
1	Wash hands and follow Standard Precautions.				
2	*Paying attention to detail,* assemble equipment.				
3	*Introduce yourself to the patient. Identity patient.*				
4	Position the patient in a comfortable position.				
5	Inquire if the patient has ingested hot or cold drinks or food or has been smoking within the previous half hour.				
6	*Being courteous and respectful to the patient, explain the procedure, speaking at the patient's level of understanding.*				
7	Select the correct probe for an oral temperature.				
8	Cover with the correct probe cover.				
9	Insert the probe on either side of the frenulum.				
10	Instruct patient to close mouth without placing teeth on thermometer.				
11	Leave in place until the beep is heard.				
12	Remove the thermometer probe after appropriate time has elapsed.				
13	Read the results on the digital display window.				
14	Discard probe cover in biohazard waste container.				
15	Replace the electronic thermometer in the base holder, if required for recharging.				
16	Wash hands.				
17	Record temperature in patient's chart or electronic medical record.				
Student's Total Points					
Points Possible					
Final Score (Student's Total Points/Possible Points)					

Instructor's/Evaluator's Comments and Suggestions:

_____

_____

_____

_____

_____

_____

_____

CHECK #1	
Evaluator's Signature:	Date:

CHECK #2	
Evaluator's Signature:	Date:

CHECK #3	
Evaluator's Signature:	Date:

Work Documentation Form(s)

*Progress Note Template can be downloaded from the Premium Website

ABHES Competencies: MA.A.1.9.b Apply principles of aseptic techniques and infection control; MA.A.1.9.c Take vital signs; MA.A.1.9.i Use standard precautions

CAAHEP Competencies: I.P.1 Obtain vital signs; III.P.2 Practice standard precautions; III.P.4 Perform handwashing; IX.P.7 Document accurately in the patient record

Name_____ **Date**_____ **Score**_____

● **COMPETENCY ASSESSMENT**

Procedure 24-2:   Measuring an Aural Temperature Using a Tympanic Thermometer

Task: To obtain an aural temperature using a tympanic thermometer.

Conditions: • Tympanic thermometer
                • Probe covers or ear speculum
                • Waste container

Standards: Perform the Task within 3 minutes with a minimum score of ___ points, as determined by your instructor.

Time began: _____   **Time ended:** _____   **Total time:** _____

No.	Step	Points	Check #1	Check #2	Check #3
1	Wash hands following Standard Precautions.				
2	*Paying attention to detail,* assemble equipment.				
3	*Introduce yourself to the patient. Identify the patient.*				
4	*Explain procedure, speaking at the patient's level of understanding.*				
5	Place cover on thermometer.				
6	Set thermometer to start.				
7	Gently straighten ear canal up and back for adults and place probe into ear canal to seal the area and activate the system.				
8	Wait until the temperature is displayed on the screen.				
9	Remove from the ear.				
10	Discard cover into waste container by pressing the release button.				
11	Replace thermometer.				
12	Wash hands.				
13	Record temperature in patient's chart or electronic medical record, indicating tympanic measurement (Tym).				
Student's Total Points					
Points Possible					
Final Score (Student's Total Points/Possible Points)					

Instructor's/Evaluator's Comments and Suggestions:

_____

_____

_____

_____

_____

_____

_____

CHECK #1	
Evaluator's Signature:	Date:

CHECK #2	
Evaluator's Signature:	Date:

CHECK #3	
Evaluator's Signature:	Date:

Work Documentation Form(s)

*Progress Note Template can be downloaded from the Premium Website

ABHES Competencies: MA.A.1.9.b Apply principles of aseptic techniques and infection control; MA.A.1.9.c Take vital signs; MA.A.1.9.i Use standard precautions

CAAHEP Competencies: I.P.1 Obtain vital signs; III.P.2 Practice standard precautions; III.P.4 Perform handwashing; IX.P.7 Document accurately in the patient record

Name_____ **Date**_____ **Score**_____

● COMPETENCY ASSESSMENT

Procedure 24-3:   Measuring a Temperature Using a Temporal Artery (TA) Thermometer

Task: To obtain a temporal artery temperature using a temporal artery (TA) thermometer.

Conditions: • Temporal artery thermometer
                 • Probe cover, cap or sheath
                 • Alcohol wipes

Standards: Perform the Task within 3 minutes with a minimum score of ___ points, as determined by your instructor.

Time began: _____   **Time ended:** _____   **Total time:** _____

No.	Step	Points	Check #1	Check #2	Check #3
1	Wash hands and follow Standard Precautions.				
2	*Paying attention to detail,* assemble equipment. Clean probe with alcohol or attach a probe.				
3	*Introduce yourself to the patient. Identify the patient.*				
4	*Explain the procedure, speaking at the patient's level of understanding.*				
5	Remove perspiration from forehead, remove hat, push back hair from forehead.				
6	Hold the probe in the center of patient's forehead flush against the skin.				
7	Press the scan button and hold while sliding the thermometer slowly across the forehead to the temple area of the hair line. There will be a tapping or clicking sound that will stop when the temperature has been reached.				
8	Release the button and remove the thermometer from the forehead.				
9	Read the display for temperature measurement.				
10	Turn upside down and wipe probe with alcohol wipe. Let dry. Return to holder.				
11	Wash hands.				
12	Record temperature in patient's chart or electronic medical record, indicating TA temperature.				
Student's Total Points					
Points Possible					
Final Score (Student's Total Points/Possible Points)					

Instructor's/Evaluator's Comments and Suggestions:

_____

_____

_____

_____

_____

_____

_____

CHECK #1	
Evaluator's Signature:	Date:

CHECK #2	
Evaluator's Signature:	Date:

CHECK #3	
Evaluator's Signature:	Date:

Work Documentation Form(s)

*Progress Note Template can be downloaded from the Premium Website

ABHES Competencies: MA.A.1.9.b Apply principles of aseptic techniques and infection control; MA.A.1.9.c Take vital signs; MA.A.1.9.i Use standard precautions

CAAHEP Competencies: I.P.1 Obtain vital signs; III.P.2 Practice standard precautions; III.P.4 Perform handwashing; IX.P.7 Document accurately in the patient record

Name_____ Date_____ Score_____

● **COMPETENCY ASSESSMENT**

Procedure 24-4:   Measuring a Rectal Temperature Using a Digital Thermometer

Task: To obtain a rectal temperature using a digital thermometer.

Conditions: • Digital thermometer with red probe (rectal)
                 • Probe cover
                 • Lubricating jelly on a 4 × 4 gauze or in a packet
                 • Gloves
                 • Biohazard waste container

Standards: Perform the Task within 3 minutes with a minimum score of ___ points, as determined by your instructor.

Time began: _____ **Time ended:** _____ **Total time:** _____

No.	Step	Points	Check #1	Check #2	Check #3
1	Wash hands and don gloves following Standard Precautions.				
2	*Paying attention to detail,* assemble equipment.				
3	*Introduce yourself to the patient. Identify patient.*				
4	*Explain procedure to patient, speaking at the patient's level of understanding.*				
5	Remove patient's clothing from the waist down, *protecting patient's personal boundaries;* drape as necessary.				
6	Position patient in Sims' position.				
7	Place probe cover on red probe (rectal).				
8	Lubricate with lubricating jelly.				
9	Spread buttocks and gently insert thermometer into the rectum past the sphincter (1½ inches for an adult).				
10	Hold buttocks together while holding the thermometer. Do not let go of the thermometer.				
11	Hold in place until the beep is heard.				
12	Read the results on the digital display window.				
13	Remove from the rectum.				
14	Discard probe cover into biohazard waste container by pushing the release button.				
15	Replace thermometer on holder base.				
16	Remove gloves, discard in biohazard waste container, and wash hands.				
17	Offer tissue to patient to wipe anus. Assist patient in dressing and position as necessary, *attending to any special needs of the patient.*				
18	Accurately temperature in patient's chart or electronic medical record, indicating a rectal temperature (R).				
Student's Total Points					
Points Possible					
Final Score (Student's Total Points/Possible Points)					

Instructor's/Evaluator's Comments and Suggestions:

_____

_____

_____

_____

_____

_____

_____

CHECK #1	
Evaluator's Signature:	Date:

CHECK #2	
Evaluator's Signature:	Date:

CHECK #3	
Evaluator's Signature:	Date:

Work Documentation Form(s)

*Progress Note Template can be downloaded from the Premium Website

ABHES Competencies: MA.A.1.9.b Apply principles of aseptic techniques and infection control; MA.A.1.9.c Take vital signs; MA.A.1.9.i Use standard precautions

CAAHEP Competencies: I.P.1 Obtain vital signs; III.P.2 Practice standard precautions; III.P.4 Perform handwashing; IX.P.7 Document accurately in the patient record

Name_____ **Date**_____ **Score**_____

● **COMPETENCY ASSESSMENT**

Procedure 24-5: Measuring an Axillary Temperature

Task: To obtain an axillary temperature using a digital thermometer.

Conditions:
- Digital thermometer
- Sheath
- Towelettes
- Paper towels

Standards: Perform the Task within 3 minutes with a minimum score of ___ points, as determined by your instructor.

Time began: _____ **Time ended:** _____ **Total time:** _____

No.	Step	Points	Check #1	Check #2	Check #3
1	Wash hands following Standard Precautions.				
2	*Paying attention to detail,* assemble equipment; place sheath on thermometer.				
3	*Introduce yourself to the patient. Identify patient.*				
4	*Explain procedure, speaking at the patient's level of understanding.*				
5	Ask patient to remove clothing to provide access to axilla.				
6	Cover patient with gown as necessary to maintain patient modesty and warmth.				
7	Wipe axillary area with dry towel or towelette to remove moisture.				
8	Place thermometer in axilla.				
9	Ask patient to fold arm against chest or abdomen.				
10	Hold in place until the beep is heard.				
11	Carefully remove from the axillary area.				
12	Eject probe cover and appropriately discard.				
13	Read temperature in the digital window.				
14	Replace thermometer on holder base.				
15	Wash hands.				
16	Accurately record temperature in patient's chart or electronic medical record, indicating axillary temperature (A).				
Student's Total Points					
Points Possible					
Final Score (Student's Total Points/Possible Points)					

Instructor's/Evaluator's Comments and Suggestions:

_____

_____

_____

_____

_____

_____

_____

CHECK #1	
Evaluator's Signature:	Date:

CHECK #2	
Evaluator's Signature:	Date:

CHECK #3	
Evaluator's Signature:	Date:

Work Documentation Form(s)

*Progress Note Template can be downloaded from the Premium Website

ABHES Competencies: MA.A.1.9.b Apply principles of aseptic techniques and infection control; MA.A.1.9.c Take vital signs; MA.A.1.9.i Use standard precautions

CAAHEP Competencies: I.P.1 Obtain vital signs; III.P.2 Practice standard precautions; III.P.4 Perform handwashing; IX.P.7 Document accurately in the patient record

Name_____ Date_____ Score_____

● **COMPETENCY ASSESSMENT**

Procedure 24-6: Measuring an Oral Temperature Using a Disposable Oral Strip Thermometer

Task: To obtain an oral temperature.

Conditions: • Oral strip thermometer
                   • Gloves
                   • Biohazard waste container

Standards: Perform the Task within 3 minutes with a minimum score of ___ points, as determined by your
                   instructor.

Time began: _____   **Time ended:** _____   **Total time:** _____

No.	Step	Points	Check #1	Check #2	Check #3
1	Wash hands following Standard Precautions.				
2	*Paying attention to detail,* assemble equipment.				
3	*Introduce yourself to the patient. Identify patient.*				
4	Position the patient in a comfortable position.				
5	Determine if the patient has ingested hot or cold drinks or food or has smoked within the previous half hour.				
6	*Explain the procedure, speaking at the patient's level of understanding.*				
7	Apply gloves.				
8	Insert disposable oral strip thermometer under the tongue to the side of the mouth.				
9	Instruct patient to close mouth tightly.				
10	Leave in place for 60 seconds or according to manufacturer's instructions.				
11	Remove thermometer after the appropriate time has elapsed.				
12	Wait 10 seconds to read the dots.				
13	Read temperature by locating the last dot that has changed color.				
14	Discard strip in biohazard waste container.				
15	Remove gloves and discard in biohazard waste container.				
16	Wash hands.				
17	Accurately record temperature in patient's chart or electronic medical record.				
Student's Total Points					
Points Possible					
Final Score (Student's Total Points/Possible Points)					

Instructor's/Evaluator's Comments and Suggestions:

_____

_____

_____

_____

_____

_____

_____

CHECK #1	
Evaluator's Signature:	Date:

CHECK #2	
Evaluator's Signature:	Date:

CHECK #3	
Evaluator's Signature:	Date:

Work Documentation Form(s)

*Progress Note Template can be downloaded from the Premium Website

ABHES Competencies: MA.A.1.9.b Apply principles of aseptic techniques and infection control; MA.A.1.9.c Take vital signs; MA.A.1.9.i Use standard precautions

CAAHEP Competencies: I.P.1 Obtain vital signs; III.P.2 Practice standard precautions; III.P.4 Perform handwashing; IX.P.7 Document accurately in the patient record

Name _____ **Date** _____ **Score** _____

● COMPETENCY ASSESSMENT

Procedure 24-7:   Measuring a Radial Pulse

Task: To obtain a radial pulse rate.

Conditions: • Watch with second hand

Standards: Perform the Task within 3 minutes with a minimum score of ___ points, as determined by your instructor.

Time began: _____   **Time ended:** _____   **Total time:** _____

No.	Step	Points	Check #1	Check #2	Check #3
1	Wash hands.				
2	*Introduce yourself to the patient. Identify patient.*				
3	*Explain procedure, speaking at the patient's level of understanding.*				
4	Position patient with the wrist resting either on a table or on lap.				
5	Locate the radial pulse using the pads of your first three fingers. Do not use your thumb; it has its own pulse.				
6	Gently compress the radial artery enough to feel the pulse.				
7	Count the pulsations for 1 full minute using a watch with a second hand or digital readout. Counting for a full minute allows for the most accuracy. However, with practice, counting for 30 seconds and multiplying the pulsations by two or counting for 15 seconds and multiplying by four to obtain the beats per minute is allowed as long as the pulse is regular.				
8	Note any irregularities in rhythm, volume, and condition of artery.				
9	Wash hands.				
10	Accurately record pulse in patient chart or electronic medical record after the temperature, noting any irregularities.				
	Student's Total Points				
	Points Possible				
	Final Score (Student's Total Points/Possible Points)				

Instructor's/Evaluator's Comments and Suggestions:

CHECK #1	
Evaluator's Signature:	Date:

CHECK #2	
Evaluator's Signature:	Date:

CHECK #3	
Evaluator's Signature:	Date:

Work Documentation Form(s)

*Progress Note Template can be downloaded from the Premium Website

ABHES Competencies: MA.A.1.9.c Take vital signs; MA.A.1.9.i Use standard precautions

CAAHEP Competencies: I.P.1 Obtain vital signs; III.P.2 Practice standard precautions; III.P.4 Perform handwashing; IX.P.7 Document accurately in the patient record

Name _____ **Date** _____ **Score** _____

● **COMPETENCY ASSESSMENT**

Procedure 24-8: Taking an Apical Pulse

Task: To obtain an apical pulse rate.

Conditions:
- Stethoscope
- Watch with second hand
- Alcohol wipes

Standards: Perform the Task within 3 minutes with a minimum score of ___ points, as determined by your instructor.

Time began: _____ **Time ended:** _____ **Total time:** _____

No.	Step	Points	Check #1	Check #2	Check #3
1	Wash hands.				
2	*Paying attention to detail,* assemble equipment.				
3	Wipe earpiece with alcohol wipes.				
4	*Introduce yourself to the patient. Identify patient.*				
5	*Explain procedure, speaking at the patient's level of understanding.*				
6	Assist patient in disrobing, removing clothing from the waist up, *while protecting patient's personal boundaries.*				
7	Provide a gown or drape for patient modesty and warmth.				
8	Position the patient in a supine position.				
9	Locate the fifth intercostal space, midclavicular, left of sternum.				
10	Place stethoscope on the site and listen for the lub-dub sound of the heart.				
11	Count the pulse for 1 minute; each lub-dub equals one pulse. Note any additional heart sounds or arrythmias.				
12	Assist the patient to sit up and dress, *attending to any special needs of the patient.*				
13	Wash hands.				
14	Wipe earpieces, diaphragm, and tubing of stethoscope.				
15	Accurately pulse in patient chart or electronic medical record with the designation of apical pulse (AP) to denote method of obtaining the pulse and note any arrhythmias.				
Student's Total Points					
Points Possible					
Final Score (Student's Total Points/Possible Points)					

Instructor's/Evaluator's Comments and Suggestions:

_____

_____

_____

_____

_____

_____

_____

CHECK #1	
Evaluator's Signature:	Date:

CHECK #2	
Evaluator's Signature:	Date:

CHECK #3	
Evaluator's Signature:	Date:

Work Documentation Form(s)

*Progress Note Template can be downloaded from the Premium Website

ABHES Competencies: MA.A.1.9.c Take vital signs; MA.A.1.9.i Use standard precautions

CAAHEP Competencies: I.P.1 Obtain vital signs; III.P.2 Practice standard precautions; III.P.4 Perform handwashing; IX.P.7 Document accurately in the patient record

Name_____ **Date**_____ **Score**_____

● **COMPETENCY ASSESSMENT**

Procedure 24-9: Measuring the Respiration Rate

Task: To obtain an accurate respiratory rate.

Conditions: • Watch with second hand

Standards: Perform the Task within 3 minutes with a minimum score of ___ points, as determined by your instructor.

Time began: _____   **Time ended:** _____   **Total time:** _____

No.	Step	Points	Check #1	Check #2	Check #3
1	Wash hands.				
2	*Introduce yourself to the patient. Identify the patient.*				
3	Position patient in a comfortable position.				
4	Watch the rise and fall of the chest wall for 1 minute, or while holding the patient's arm, place it across the chest and feel for the rise and fall of the chest wall. Alternatively, place a hand on the patient's shoulder and feel and watch for the rise and fall of the chest wall. With practice, counting respirations for 30 seconds and multiplying by 2 or counting for 15 seconds and multiplying by 4 is allowable as long as the respiratory rate is regular.				
5	Note depth, rhythm, and breath sounds while counting.				
6	Wash hands.				
7	Accurately record respiration rate in patient's chart or electronic medical record, noting any irregularities and sounds.				
Student's Total Points					
Points Possible					
Final Score (Student's Total Points/Possible Points)					

Instructor's/Evaluator's Comments and Suggestions:

_____

_____

_____

_____

_____

_____

_____

CHECK #1	
Evaluator's Signature:	Date:

CHECK #2	
Evaluator's Signature:	Date:

CHECK #3	
Evaluator's Signature:	Date:

Work Documentation Form(s)

*Progress Note Template can be downloaded from the Premium Website

ABHES Competencies: MA.A.1.9.c Take vital signs; MA.A.1.9.i Use standard precautions

CAAHEP Competencies: I.P.1 Obtain vital signs; III.P.2 Practice standard precautions; III.P.4 Perform handwashing; IX.P.7 Document accurately in the patient record

Name_____ **Date**_____ **Score**_____

⬤ **COMPETENCY ASSESSMENT**

Procedure 24-10: Measuring Blood Pressure

Task: To measure blood pressure.

Conditions:
- Stethoscope
- Sphygmomanometer
- Alcohol wipes

Standards: Perform the Task within 3 minutes with a minimum score of ___ points, as determined by your instructor.

Time began: _____   **Time ended:** _____   **Total time:** _____

No.	Step	Points	Check #1	Check #2	Check #3
1	Wash hands.				
2	*Paying attention to detail,* assemble equipment, making sure that cuff size is correct.				
3	Clean earpieces of stethoscope with alcohol wipe.				
4	*Introduce yourself to the patient. Identify patient.*				
5	*Explain procedure, speaking at the patient's level of understanding.*				
6	Position patient comfortably; feet flat on the floor, arm resting at heart level on the lap or a table.				
7	Bare the right upper arm. If clothing is restrictive, have the patient remove it.				
8	Position the patient so that the brachial artery is at the level of the heart and the arm is supported so that there is not additional muscular tension.				
9	Palpate the brachial artery.				
10	Securely center the bladder of the cuff over the brachial artery above the bend of the elbow.				
11	Locate and palpate the radial pulse and smoothly inflate cuff until the pulse is no longer felt; note the number.				
12	Quickly deflate the cuff and allow the arm to rest for one minute. Calculate peak inflation level. Make sure cuff is completely deflated.				
13	Position stethoscope over the brachial artery and hold in position with the fingers only.				
14	Inflate cuff smoothly and quickly to the peak inflation level plus 30 mm Hg.				
15	Deflate the cuff at a rate of 2 to 4 mm Hg per heartbeat.				
16	Listen for Korotkoff Phase I; note when it appears.				
17	Continue deflation, noting the Korotkoff phases.				
18	Note when all sounds disappear, Korotkoff Phase V.				

No.	Step	Points	Check #1	Check #2	Check #3
19	Continue deflating the cuff at the same rate for at least 10 mm Hg after sounds have disappeared.				
20	Deflate the cuff quickly.				
21	Remove the cuff.				
22	Clean the earpieces and diaphragm of the stethoscope with alcohol wipes.				
23	Wash hands.				
24	Accurately record blood pressure in patient's chart or electronic medical record.				
Student's Total Points					
Points Possible					
Final Score (Student's Total Points/Possible Points)					

Instructor's/Evaluator's Comments and Suggestions:

CHECK #1 Evaluator's Signature:	Date:

CHECK #2 Evaluator's Signature:	Date:

CHECK #3 Evaluator's Signature:	Date:

Work Documentation Form(s)

*Progress Note Template can be downloaded from the Premium Website

ABHES Competencies: MA.A.1.9.c Take vital signs; MA.A.1.9.i Use standard precautions

CAAHEP Competencies: I.P.1 Obtain vital signs; III.P.2 Practice standard precautions; III.P.4 Perform handwashing; IX.P.7 Document accurately in the patient record

Name_____ **Date**_____ **Score**_____

COMPETENCY ASSESSMENT

Procedure 24-11: Measuring Height

Task: To obtain the height of a patient.

Conditions:
- Scale with measuring bar
- Paper towel

Standards: Perform the Task within 3 minutes with a minimum score of ___ points, as determined by your instructor.

Time began: _____   **Time ended:** _____   **Total time:** _____

No.	Step	Points	Check #1	Check #2	Check #3
1	Wash hands.				
2	*Introduce yourself to the patient. Identify patient.*				
3	*Explain the procedure, speaking at the patient's level of understanding,* to ensure understanding, cooperation, and consent.				
4	*Considering any special needs of the patient,* instruct patient to remove shoes and stand on paper towel on scale with back against scale, looking straight ahead.				
5	Assist patient onto scale.				
6	Lower measuring bar until firmly resting on the top of the patient's head.				
7	Assist patient's stepping off the scale. Allow patient to sit and help with shoes if necessary.				
8	*Paying attention to detail,* read line where measurement falls.				
9	Lower measuring bar to its original position.				
10	Wash hands.				
11	Accurately record height in patient's chart or electronic medical record.				
Student's Total Points					
Points Possible					
Final Score (Student's Total Points/Possible Points)					

Instructor's/Evaluator's Comments and Suggestions:

_____

_____

_____

_____

_____

_____

_____

CHECK #1	
Evaluator's Signature:	Date:

CHECK #2	
Evaluator's Signature:	Date:

CHECK #3	
Evaluator's Signature:	Date:

Work Documentation Form(s)

*Progress Note Template can be downloaded from the Premium Website

ABHES Competencies: MA.A.1.9.c Take vital signs; MA.A.1.9.i Use standard precautions

CAAHEP Competencies: I.P.1 Obtain vital signs; III.P.2 Practice standard precautions; III.P.4 Perform handwashing; IX.P.7 Document accurately in the patient record

Name_____ **Date**_____ **Score**_____

● COMPETENCY ASSESSMENT

Procedure 24-12:   Measuring Adult Weight

Task: To obtain the weight of the patient.

Conditions: • Balance beam scale or digital scale
             • Paper towels

Standards: Perform the Task within 3 minutes with a minimum score of ___ points, as determined by your instructor.

Time began: _____   **Time ended:** _____   **Total time:** _____

No.	Step	Points	Check #1	Check #2	Check #3
1	Wash hands.				
2	*Introduce yourself. Identify patient.*				
3	*Explain the procedure, speaking at the patient's level of understanding,* to ensure understanding and cooperation.				
4	Place a paper towel on the scale.				
5	Instruct the patient to place heavy objects on the area provided, including heavy objects that might be in pockets.				
6	Zero balance beam or digital scale.				
7	*Considering any special needs of the patient,* instruct the patient to remove shoes, jacket, and heavy sweater and step on the scale. Assist patient to the center of the scale.				
8	For balance beam scales, move the lower weight bar (measured in 50-pound increments) to the estimated number (the patient may be asked for approximate weight).				
9	Slowly slide the upper bar until the balance beam point is centered.				
10	Read the weight by adding the upper bar measurement to the lower bar measurement. If using a digital scale, simply read and remember the number.				
11	*Considering any special needs of the patient,* assist the patient in stepping off the scale.				
12	Provide a chair for the patient to sit and put on shoes. Return objects to the patient.				
13	If using a balance beam scale, return the weights to zero.				
14	Wash hands.				
15	Accurately record weight in patient's chart or electronic medical record.				
Student's Total Points					
Points Possible					
Final Score (Student's Total Points/Possible Points)					

Instructor's/Evaluator's Comments and Suggestions:

_____

_____

_____

_____

_____

_____

_____

CHECK #1	
Evaluator's Signature:	Date:

CHECK #2	
Evaluator's Signature:	Date:

CHECK #3	
Evaluator's Signature:	Date:

Work Documentation Form(s)

*Progress Note Template can be downloaded from the Premium Website

ABHES Competencies: MA.A.1.9.c Take vital signs; MA.A.1.9.i Use standard precautions

CAAHEP Competencies: I.P.1 Obtain vital signs; III.P.2 Practice standard precautions; III.P.4 Perform handwashing; IX.P.7 Document accurately in the patient record

Name _____ **Date** _____ **Score** _____

● **COMPETENCY ASSESSMENT**

Procedure 25-1: Assisting with a Complete Physical Examination

Task: To assist the provider with a complete physical examination.

Conditions: • Instruments utilized during physical exam.
              These might include the following:
    • Balance beam, digital, or electronic scale
    • Patient gown
    • Drape
    • Thermometer
    • Stethoscope
    • Alchohol wipes
    • Examination lights
    • Tuning fork
    • Otoscope and ophthalmoscope
    • Sphygmomanometer
    • Penlight
    • Tongue depressor
    • Percussion hammer
    • Tape measure
    • Cotton balls
    • Safety pin
    • Tissues
    • Emesis basin
    • Gauze sponges
    • Urine specimen container
    • Blood draw supplies
    • ECG machine
    • Speculum, pap slide, lubricant, swabs, gloves
    • Biohazard and regular waste containers
    • Other supplies as indicated

Standards: Perform the Task within 25 minutes with a minimum score of _____ points, as determined by
              your instructor.

Time began: _____   **Time ended:** _____   **Total time:** _____

No.	Step	Points	Check #1	Check #2	Check #3
1	Wash hands. Adhere to Standard Precautions.				
2	*Paying attention to detail,* assemble equipment.				
3	*Introduce yourself. Greet and identify patient. Explain procedure to the patient, speaking at the patient's level of understanding.*				
4	*Paying attention to detail,* place instruments in easily accessible sequence for provider use.				
5	*Using active listening skills,* review medical history with patient.				
6	Take patient vital signs, test visual acuity, and check hearing ability.				
7	Obtain a urine specimen.				
8	Obtain all required blood samples.				

No.	Step	Points	Check #1	Check #2	Check #3
9	Perform an electrocardiogram (ECG) if directed by the provider.				
10	Provide patient with appropriate gown and drape, and assist patient to disrobe completely while *protecting patient's personal boundaries.* Explain where the opening for the gown is to be placed.				
11	*Attending to any personal needs of the patient,* assist the patient in sitting at the end of the table; drape patient across lap and legs.				
12	Inform provider when patient is ready.				
13	When the provider arrives, *display a calm, professional, and caring manner,* remain by the patient, ready to assist the patient and provider.				
14	Position patient in a sitting or supine position for the head, throat, eye, ear, and neck examination.				
15	Lights may be turned off to allow pupils to dilate for retinal examination.				
16	*Paying attention to detail,* hand the provider instruments as required.				
17	The sitting position is maintained for auscultation of the chest and heart.				
18	Assist the patient into a supine position and drape for examination of the chest.				
19	Maintain a quiet atmosphere to enhance the ability of the provider in listening to heart and lung sounds.				
20	Position patient in supine position and drape for examinations of abdomen and extremities.				
21	Gynecologic examination may then be performed. Assist female patient into lithotomy position for gynecologic examination. Male genitals are examined.				
22	If a rectal examination is necessary, assist patient into Sims' position.				
23	Place patient in prone position for examination of posterior aspect of body.				
24	On completion of the exam, assist the patient to sitting position and allow patient to sit at the end of the table for a few moments.				
25	Ensure patient stability (check color of skin, pulse) before allowing the patient to stand.				
26	Assist patient with dressing; provide privacy.				
27	Accurately enter any notes or patient instructions on computer in patient's EMR per provider orders.				
28	Escort patient to provider's office for discussion of examination results.				
29	Don disposable gloves.				
30	Dispose of gown and drape in biohazard waste container if contaminated with blood or body fluids.				
31	Dispose of contaminated disposable materials in biohazard waste container.				

No.	Step	Points	Check #1	Check #2	Check #3
32	Remove table paper and dispose in biohazard waste container.				
33	Disinfect counters and examination table with a solution of 10% bleach. Clean, disinfect, or sterilize reusable instruments as appropriate.				
34	Remove gloves and discard in biohazard waste container.				
35	Wash hands.				
36	Replace table paper and equipment in preparation for the next patient.				
37	Document the procedure on computer in patient's chart or electronic medical record.				
Student's Total Points					
Points Possible					
Final Score (Student's Total Points/Possible Points)					

Instructor's/Evaluator's Comments and Suggestions:

_____

_____

_____

_____

_____

_____

CHECK #1	
Evaluator's Signature:	Date:

CHECK #2	
Evaluator's Signature:	Date:

CHECK #3	
Evaluator's Signature:	Date:

ABHES Competencies: MA.A.1.9.a Obtain chief complaint, recording patient history; MA.A.1.9.c Take vital signs; MA.A.1.9.i Use standard precautions; MA.A.1.9.k Prepare and maintain examination and treatment area; MA.A.1.9.l Prepare patient for examinations and treatments; MA.A.1.9.m Assist physician with routine and specialty examinations and treatments; MA.A.1.9.o Perform electrocardiograms and respiratory testing

CAAHEP Competencies: I.P.1 Obtain vital signs; I.P.5 Perform electrocardiography; I.P.10 Assist physician with patient care; I.A.1 Apply critical thinking skills in performing patient assessment and care; 1.A.2 Use language/verbal skills that enable patients' understanding; III.P.2 Practice Standard Precautions; III.P.4 Perform handwashing; III.A.2 Explain the rationale for performance of a procedure to a patient; IV.P.6 Prepare a patient for procedures and/or treatments; IV.P.8 Document patient care; IX.P.7 Document accurately in the patient record

Name_____   **Date**_____   **Score**_____

● **COMPETENCY ASSESSMENT**

Procedure 26-1:   Assisting with Routine Prenatal Visits

Task: To monitor the progress of the pregnancy.

Conditions:
- Scale
- Disposable gloves
- Patient gown
- Tape measure
- Sphygmomanometer
- Stethoscope
- Doppler fetoscope and coupling agent
- Urine specimen container
- Urinalysis testing supplies
- Biohazard waste container

Standards: Perform the Task within 10 minutes with a minimum score of ___ points, as determined by your instructor.

Time began: _____   **Time ended:** _____   **Total time:** _____

No.	Step	Points	Check #1	Check #2	Check #3
1	Wash hands and follow Standard Precautions.				
2	*Paying attention to detail,* assemble equipment.				
3	*Introduce yourself to the patient. Identify patient.*				
4	*Explain the procedure, speaking at the patient's level of understanding.*				
5	Instruct the patient in the correct method of obtaining a urine specimen.				
6	*Considering any special needs of the patient,* instruct and then assist the patient to remove shoes, jacket or sweater, and step on paper towels on the scale. Assist the patient to the center of the scale. Weigh patient. Accurately record findings.				
7	Measure blood pressure and accurately record findings.				
8	*Being courteous and respectful,* provide patient with gown and drape.				
9	*In a manner that protects the patient's personal boundaries,* have patient disrobe from waist down and put on a gown open in the front.				
10	Test the urine specimen while waiting for the provider.				
11	*Attending to any special needs,* assist patient onto examination table and drape her.				

No.	Step	Points	Check #1	Check #2	Check #3
12	Assist the provider as the examination is performed. • Hand the provider the tape measure to measure the height of the fundus. • Hand the provider the Doppler fetal pulse detector for measurement of the fetal heart rate. The medical assistant may spread the coupling agent onto the patient's abdomen.				
13	After the examination, assist the patient to sit for a few moments. Assess her color and pulse.				
14	Provide towel to patient to wipe off coupling agent.				
15	Provide any instructions or clarification of provider's orders, *speaking at the patient's level of understanding.*				
16	Apply gloves. Discard disposable supplies per OSHA guidelines. Disinfect equipment used.				
17	Remove gloves.				
18	Wash hands.				
19	Set up for the next patient.				
20	Accurately record all information in patient's chart or electronic medical record.				
Student's Total Points					
Points Possible					
Final Score (Student's Total Points/Possible Points)					

Instructor's/Evaluator's Comments and Suggestions:

_____

_____

_____

_____

_____

_____

_____

_____

CHECK #1	
Evaluator's Signature:	Date:

CHECK #2	
Evaluator's Signature:	Date:

CHECK #3	
Evaluator's Signature:	Date:

Work Documentation Form(s)

*Progress Note Template can be downloaded from the Premium Website

ABHES Competencies: MA.A.1.9.c Take vital signs; MA.A.1.9.i Use standard precautions; MA.A.1.9.k Prepare and maintain examination and treatment area; MA.A.1.9.l Prepare patient for examinations and treatments; MA.A.1.9.m Assist physician with routine and specialty examinations and treatments

CAAHEP Competencies: I.P.1 Obtain vital signs; I.P.10 Assist physician with patient care; I.A.1 Apply critical thinking skills in performing patient assessment and care; 1.A.2 Use language/verbal skills that enable patients' understanding; III.P.2 Practice Standard Precautions; III.P.4 Perform handwashing; III.A.1 Display sensitivity to patient rights and feelings in collecting specimens; III.A.2 Explain the rationale for performance of a procedure to a patient; IV.P.6 Prepare a patient for procedures and/or treatments; IV.P.8 Document patient care; IX.P.7 Document accurately in the patient record

Name_____ **Date**_____ **Score**_____

● COMPETENCY ASSESSMENT

Procedure 26-2: Assisting with Pelvic Examination and Pap Test (Conventional and ThinPrep® Methods)

Task: To assist the provider in collecting cervical cells for laboratory analysis for early detection of malignant cells of the cervix and to assess the health of the reproductive organs to detect diseases, leading to early diagnosis and treatment.

Conditions:
- Nonsterile gloves
- Vaginal speculum, disposable or nondisposable
- Warm water or warming light
- Light source
- Drape sheet
- Patient gown
- Tissues
- Vaginal lubricant
- Lab requisition
- Urine specimen container
- Urine testing supplies
- Biohazard specimen bag
- Biohazard waste container
- Adjustable stool for provider

Supplies for the Pap test according to the method used for ThinPrep® Pap:
- Cervical spatula
- Brush and broom
- ThinPrep® container with solution

For conventional Pap test:
- Microscope slides
- Fixative and/or specimen bottles
- Cervical spatula
- Cytology brush

Standards: Perform the Task within 25 minutes with a minimum score of ___ points, as determined by your instructor.

Time began: _____   **Time ended:** _____   **Total time:** _____

No.	Step	Points	Check #1	Check #2	Check #3
1	Wash hands and follow Standard Precautions.				
2	*Paying attention to detail,* assemble equipment.				
3	*Introduce yourself to the patient. Identify patient.*				
4	*Explain the procedure, speaking at the patient's level of understanding.*				
5	Request that patient empty her bladder. (Instruct patient to save urine specimen and provide specimen container if ordered by provider.)				
6	*Being courteous and respectful,* provide patient with gown and request her to completely undress, *being sure to protect patient's personal boundaries.*				

No.	Step	Points	Check #1	Check #2	Check #3
7	Instruct patient to sit at end of table when ready for pelvic examination. Drape patient for privacy. If performing conventional Pap test, label the frosted end of the slide with a marking pencil. Include patient's name on slide. Indicate site from where specimen is collected: c = cervix, v = vagina, e = endocervical.				
8	Assist patient into lithotomy position. Patient's knees should be relaxed and thighs rotated out as far as comfortable. Drape for privacy and warmth.				
9	Encourage patient to breathe slowly and deeply through the mouth during examination.				
10	Warm vaginal speculum with either warm water or under heat lamp or place on a heating pad.				
11	Hand speculum and spatula, cytology brush, and broom to the provider as needed.				
12	Apply gloves.				
13	For conventional Pap test, hold slides for provider to apply smear of exfoliated cells, one for vaginal smear (v), one for cervical smear (c), and one for endocervical smear (e), in that order. If spraying Pap fixative, spray it over the slide within 10 seconds at a distance of about 6 inches. Allow to dry for at least 10 minutes. If using Pap fixative in a bottle, place slide directly into bottle. If using ThinPrep®, swish the cytology broom vigorously in the ThinPrep® solution until the entire specimen has been deposited. Dispose of the brush into biohazard container.				
14	For ThinPrep® Pap testing, hand the speculum and cytology broom to the provider. Open the ThinPrep® solution container. When the cells have been obtained, take the broom and vigorously swish it into the container of solution until all the cells have been deposited. Replace the cap and label. Dispose of the broom into biohazard waste container.				
15	Place lubricant on provider's gloved fingers without touching the gloves, for bimanual and rectal examinations. The provider will insert the index and middle fingers into the vagina. The other hand is placed on the lower abdomen. The size, shape, and position of the uterus and ovaries are palpated.				
16	The provider will insert one gloved finger into the rectum to check the ovaries and the tone of the rectal and pelvic muscles. Hemorrhoids, rectal fissures, or other lesions may be palpated.				
17	Provide the patient tissues to wipe genitalia and rectum.				
18	After the examination, assist the patient to a sitting position, allowing her to rest a while. Check her pulse and skin color.				

No.	Step	Points	Check #1	Check #2	Check #3
19	Apply disposable gloves. Discard disposable supplies per OSHA guidelines. If stainless steel speculum was used, soak in cool water. Sanitize and sterilize as soon as convenient.				
20	Remove gloves and wash hands.				
21	Assist patient down and off the table if necessary, *attending to any special needs of the patient.*				
22	Assist the patient to dress; provide privacy. Escort the patient to provider's office for discussion of examination results.				
23	Prepare laboratory requisition (cytology request) form. Include provider name and address, date, source of specimen, patient's name and address, date of LMP, and hormone therapy, if any. Place slides in slide container or ThinPrep® container into biohazard specimen bag. Place requisition into outer pocket of bag and send to laboratory.				
24	Wash hands.				
25	Accurately document procedure in patient's chart or electronic medical record.				
Student's Total Points					
Points Possible					
Final Score (Student's Total Points/Possible Points)					

Instructor's/Evaluator's Comments and Suggestions:

_____

_____

_____

_____

_____

_____

_____

CHECK #1	
Evaluator's Signature:	Date:

CHECK #2	
Evaluator's Signature:	Date:

CHECK #3	
Evaluator's Signature:	Date:

Work Documentation Form(s)

*Progress Note Template and Laboratory Requisition Form can be downloaded from the Premium Website

ABHES Competencies: MA.A.1.9.c Take vital signs; MA.A.1.9.i Use standard precautions; MA.A.1.9.k Prepare and maintain examination and treatment area; MA.A.1.9.l Prepare patient for examinations and treatments; MA.A.1.9.m Assist physician with routine and specialty examinations and treatments

CAAHEP Competencies: I.P.1 Obtain vital signs; I.P.10 Assist physician with patient care; I.A.1 Apply critical thinking skills in performing patient assessment and care; 1.A.2 Use language/verbal skills that enable patients' understanding; III.P.2 Practice Standard Precautions; III.P.4 Perform handwashing; III.A.1 Display sensitivity to patient rights and feelings in collecting specimens; III.A.2 Explain the rationale for performance of a procedure to a patient; IV.P.6 Prepare a patient for procedures and/or treatments; IV.P.8 Document patient care; IX.P.7 Document accurately in the patient record

Name_____ **Date**_____ **Score**_____

● **COMPETENCY ASSESSMENT**

Procedure 26-3:   Assisting with Insertion of an Intrauterine Device (IUD)

Task: To assist the provider with the insertion of an intrauterine device.

Conditions: • Nonsterile gloves
                • Sterile gloves
                • Vaginal speculum
                • Light source and stool for provider
                • Drape and gown
                • Tissue
                • Lubricant
                • Prepackaged sterile IUD
                • Biohazard waste container
                • Local anesthetic
                • Syringe and needle
                • Antiseptic such as Betadine® solution or swabs
                • Emesis basin for used items such as speculum

Standards: Perform the Task within 25 minutes with a minimum score of ___ points, as determined by
                your instructor.

Time began: _____ **Time ended:** _____ **Total time:** _____

No.	Step	Points	Check #1	Check #2	Check #3
1	Wash hands and follow Standard Precautions.				
2	*Paying attention to detail,* assemble equipment.				
3	*Introduce yourself. Identify the patient.*				
4	Draw up local anesthetic into syringe as directed by provider.				
5	Request that the patient empty her bladder. Save urine for pregnancy test.				
6	*Being courteous and respectful,* ask patient to undress from the waist down and put on a gown, *being sure to protect the patient's personal boundaries.*				
7	*Explain procedure to patient, speaking at the patient's level of understanding. Allay the patient's fears regarding the procedure. Help her to feel safe and comfortable.*				
8	*Considering any special needs of the patient,* assist patient into lithotomy position. Drape for warmth and privacy.				
9	Administer medication to patient for pain as prescribed by provider.				
10	Hand speculum to provider.				
11	Provide nonsterile gloves to the practitioner for the initial pelvic examination.				
12	Encourage the patient to breathe slowly and deeply through her mouth during the procedure.				

No.	Step	Points	Check #1	Check #2	Check #3
13	The provider does a pelvic examination after donning nonsterile gloves.				
14	The provider checks for pelvic infection and position of the uterus.				
15	The provider swabs the cervix with an antiseptic and may inject a local anesthetic into the cervix.				
16	The provider puts the IUD into the insertion device. The arms of the IUD flatten (the top of the "T").				
17	The provider inserts the IUD with the insertion device through the cervix into the uterus.				
18	The insertion tube is withdrawn completely.				
19	Dispose of insertion device into biohazard waste container or emesis basin. The provider shortens the string on the IUD to 1–2 inches from the cervix and then removes speculum. Dispose of speculum into waste container or emesis basin.				
20	Place disposable speculum in biohazard waste container. Place nondisposable speculum into emesis basin.				
21	Provide the patient tissues to clean lubricant from exam area.				
22	Assist patient to sit for a few moments. Assess her pulse, skin color, and blood pressure if needed.				
23	Apply nonsterile gloves. Discard disposable supplies according to OSHA guidelines. If stainless steel speculum was used, soak in cool water. Sanitize and sterilize later when convenient.				
24	Remove gloves. Dispose in biohazard waste container. Wash hands.				
25	*Considering any special needs of the patient,* assist patient off table.				
26	Assist patient with dressing if needed; provide privacy.				
27	Explain to patient that she may experience light cramping and perhaps spotting for 1 to 2 days.				
28	Make an appointment in 4 to 6 weeks for the patient. Inform patient to make a yearly appointment thereafter for a check-up.				
29	Accurately document procedure in patient's chart or electronic medical record.				
Student's Total Points					
Points Possible					
Final Score (Student's Total Points/Possible Points)					

Instructor's/Evaluator's Comments and Suggestions:

_____
_____
_____
_____
_____
_____
_____

CHECK #1	
Evaluator's Signature:	Date:

CHECK #2	
Evaluator's Signature:	Date:

CHECK #3	
Evaluator's Signature:	Date:

Work Documentation Form(s)

*Progress Note Template can be downloaded from the Premium Website

ABHES Competencies: MA.A.1.9.c Take vital signs; MA.A.1.9.i Use standard precautions; MA.A.1.9.k Prepare and maintain examination and treatment area; MA.A.1.9.l Prepare patient for examinations and treatments; MA.A.1.9.m Assist physician with routine and specialty examinations and treatments

CAAHEP Competencies: I.P.1 Obtain vital signs; I.P.10 Assist physician with patient care; I.A.1 Apply critical thinking skills in performing patient assessment and care; 1.A.2 Use language/verbal skills that enable patients' understanding; III.P.2 Practice Standard Precautions; III.P.4 Perform handwashing; III.A.1 Display sensitivity to patient rights and feelings in collecting specimens; III.A.2 Explain the rationale for performance of a procedure to a patient; IV.P.6 Prepare a patient for procedures and/or treatments; IV.P.8 Document patient care; IX.P.7 Document accurately in the patient record

Name_____ **Date**_____ **Score**_____

● COMPETENCY ASSESSMENT

Procedure 26-4: Assisting with Insertion of a Hormonal Contraceptive (Implanon®)

Task: To assist the provider with the insertion of an implantable hormonal contraceptive such as Implanon®.

Conditions:
- Sterile gloves
- Sterile drape
- Skin marker
- Drape and gown
- Biohazard waste container
- Local anesthetic
- Syringe and needle
- Antiseptic such as Betadine® solution or swabs
- Sterile dressing materials

Standards: Perform the Task within 25 minutes with a minimum score of ___ points, as determined by your instructor.

Time began: _____ **Time ended:** _____ **Total time:** _____

No.	Step	Points	Check #1	Check #2	Check #3
1	Wash hands and follow Standard Precautions.				
2	*Paying attention to detail,* assemble equipment.				
3	*Introduce yourself. Identify patient.*				
4	Draw up local anesthetic into syringe as directed by provider.				
5	*Being courteous and respectful,* provide the patient with a gown and request that the patient undress from the waist down and put on a gown, *being sure to protect the patient's personal boundaries.*				
6	*Explain procedure to patient, speaking at the patient's level of understanding. Allay the patient's fears regarding the procedure. Help her to feel safe and comfortable.*				
7	*Considering any special needs of the patient,* assist the patient to recline on the exam table with her non-dominant arm flexed at the elbow and the wrist resting near the ear.				
8	Assist the provider with determination and marking the site for subdermal insertion.				
9	Assist the provider with cleaning the area with antiseptic and anesthetizing the area.				
10	Keep the patient informed during the procedure regarding what is happening and what is expected, *speaking at the patient's level of understanding.*				
11	Apply sterile gloves. Place a sterile dressing over the insertion site.				

No.	Step	Points	Check #1	Check #2	Check #3
12	Remove gloves. Dispose in biohazard waste container. Wash hands.				
13	Apply a pressure dressing to the site. Instruct the patient that it may be removed in 24 hours.				
14	***Considering any special needs of the patient,*** assist patient off table if she needs help.				
15	Assist the patient with dressing; provide privacy.				
16	Complete the user ID card and give it to the patient to keep. Apply the Patient Chart Label to the patient's chart.				
17	Make an appointment in 4 to 6 weeks for the patient. Inform patient to make a yearly appointment thereafter for a check-up.				
18	Accurately document procedure in patient's chart or electronic medical record.				
Student's Total Points					
Points Possible					
Final Score (Student's Total Points/Possible Points)					

Instructor's/Evaluator's Comments and Suggestions:

_____

_____

_____

_____

_____

_____

CHECK #1	
Evaluator's Signature:	Date:

CHECK #2	
Evaluator's Signature:	Date:

CHECK #3	
Evaluator's Signature:	Date:

Work Documentation Form(s)

*Progress Note Template can be downloaded from the Premium Website

ABHES Competencies: MA.A.1.9.b Apply principles of aseptic techniques and infection control; MA.A.1.9.c Take vital signs; MA.A.1.9.d Recognize and understand various treatment protocols; MA.A.1.9.e Recognize emergencies and treatments and minor office surgical procedures; MA.A.1.9.i Use standard precautions; MA.A.1.9.k Prepare and maintain examination and treatment area; MA.A.1.9.l Prepare patient for examinations and treatments; MA.A.1.9.m Assist physician with routine and specialty examinations and treatments; MA.A.1.9.p Advise patients of office policies and procedures

CAAHEP Competencies: I.P.10 Assist physician with patient care; I.A.1 Apply critical thinking skills in performing patient assessment and care; I.A.2 Use language/verbal skills that enable patients' understanding; III.P.2 Practice Standard Precautions; III.P.4 Perform handwashing; III.A.2 Explain the rationale for performance of a procedure to a patient; IV.P.6 Prepare a patient for procedures and/or treatments; IV.P.8 Document patient care; IV.A.7 Demonstrate recognition of the patient's level understanding in communication; IX.P.7 Document accurately in the patient record

Name _____ **Date** _____ **Score** _____

● COMPETENCY ASSESSMENT

Procedure 26-5:   Wet Prep/Wet Mount and Potassium Hydroxide (KOH) Prep

Task: To test a vaginal specimen to determine the cause of vaginitis. The wet prep/wet mount tests for yeast, bacteria, and trichomonas; the KOH prep tests for yeast.

Conditions: • Cotton-tipped applicator
   • Small test tube
   • Normal saline (0.5 mL or a few drops)
   • 10% potassium hydroxide (KOH; 0.5 mL or a few drops)
   • Two microscope slides and coverslips
   • Microscope
   • Vaginal speculum
   • Patient drape
   • Gloves
   • Other equipment as necessary for a vaginal examination

Standards: Perform the Task within 25 minutes with a minimum score of ____ points, as determined by your instructor.

Time began: _____   Time ended: _____   Total time: _____

No.	Step	Points	Check #1	Check #2	Check #3
1	Wash hands and follow Standard Precautions.				
2	*Paying attention to detail,* assemble equipment for vaginal examination.				
3	*Introduce yourself. Identify the patient.*				
4	*Being courteous and respectful,* provide patient with a gown and request that the patient undress from the waist down.				
5	*Explain the procedure, speaking at the patient's level of understanding. Allay the patient's fears regarding the procedure. Help her to feel safe and comfortable.*				
6	*Considering any special needs of the patient,* assist the patient into the lithotomy position.				
7	Prepare the patient for a pelvic examination as outlined in Procedure 26-2.				
8	Assist the provider with vaginal exam and obtaining the specimen for evaluation.				
9	Place several drops of normal saline into a small test tube.				
10	Don nonsterile gloves.				
11	Using the cotton-tipped applicator, the provider obtains a sampling of discharge from the vagina and hands it to the medical assistant.				
12	Rinse the swab vigorously in the test tube containing saline, pressing the cotton tip against the inside of the test tube to express all of the specimen.				

No.	Step	Points	Check #1	Check #2	Check #3
13	Dispose of the cotton-tipped applicator into a biohazard container.				
14	Apply a drop on a microscope slide and cover with a coverslip. Hand the slide to the provider for the microscopy examination.				
15	*Considering any special needs of the patient,* assist the patient back to a sitting position. Instruct her to dress and offer to assist if needed, *being sure to protect the patient's personal boundaries.*				
16	Escort patient to provider's office for discussion of examination results.				
17	In the laboratory, the provider will view the slide for yeast, bacteria, and trichomonas.				
18	After completion of the wet prep/wet mount, apply a few drips of KOH into the remaining solution in the test tube, place a drop on a fresh slide, and cover with a coverslip.				
19	The provider will perform a microscopic examination for yeast.				
20	Dispose of all slides and the test tube into a sharps container.				
21	Disinfect the laboratory area and equipment.				
22	Return to the patient and assist as needed, *attending to any special needs of the patient.*				
23	Remove gloves and dispose of properly. Wash hands.				
24	Accurately document procedure in patient's chart or electronic medical record. Input that a pelvic examination and wet prep were done, and that the provider examined the specimen. The provider will add his or her findings to the patient's electronic medical record. Be sure you sign the entry.				
Student's Total Points					
Points Possible					
Final Score (Student's Total Points/Possible Points)					

Instructor's/Evaluator's Comments and Suggestions:

_____

_____

_____

_____

_____

_____

CHECK #1	
Evaluator's Signature:	Date:

CHECK #2	
Evaluator's Signature:	Date:

CHECK #3	
Evaluator's Signature:	Date:

Work Documentation Form(s)

*Progress Note Template and Laboratory Requisition Form can be downloaded from the Premium Website

ABHES Competencies: MA.A.1.9.b Apply principles of aseptic techniques and infection control; MA.A.1.9.d Recognize and understand various treatment protocols; MA.A.1.9.e Recognize emergencies and treatments and minor office surgical procedures; MA.A.1.9.f Screen and follow up patient test results; MA.A.1.9.i Use standard precautions; MA.A.1.9.k Prepare and maintain examination and treatment area; MA.A.1.9.l Prepare patient for examinations and treatments; MA.A.1.9.m Assist physician with routine and specialty examinations and treatments; MA.A.1.9.p Advise patients of office policies and procedures

CAAHEP Competencies: I.P.10 Assist physician with patient care; I.A.1 Apply critical thinking skills in performing patient assessment and care; I.A.2 Use language/verbal skills that enable patients' understanding; III.P.2 Practice Standard Precautions; III.P.4 Perform handwashing; III.A.2 Explain the rationale for performance of a procedure to a patient; IV.P.6 Prepare a patient for procedures and/or treatments; IV.P.8 Document patient care; IV.A.7 Demonstrate recognition of the patient's level understanding in communication; IX.P.7 Document accurately in the patient record

Name _____ **Date** _____ **Score** _____

● COMPETENCY ASSESSMENT

Procedure 26-6: Amplified DNA ProbeTec Test for Chlamydia and Gonorrhea

Task: To test a vaginal specimen for diagnosis of chlamydia and gonorrhea and as a screening tool for the same for a pregnant woman.

Conditions:
- Amplified DNA ProbeTec Kit:
- Transport tube containing preservative
- Swabs (one large and one small Mini-Tip Culturette)
- Vaginal Speculum
- Patient drape
- Gloves
- Other equipment as necessary for a vaginal examination

Standards: Perform the Task within 25 minutes with a minimum score of ____ points, as determined by your instructor.

Time began: _____   **Time ended:** _____   **Total time:** _____

No.	Step	Points	Check #1	Check #2	Check #3
1	Prepare the patient for a pelvic examination as outlined in Procedure 26-2.				
2	Don nonsterile gloves.				
3	Assist the provider with vaginal exam and obtaining the specimen for evaluation.				
4	Hand the large swab to the provider, who will use it to clean the cervix.				
5	Discard the large swab into the biohazard waste container.				
6	Hand the small Mini-tip Culturette Swab to the provider, who will insert the swab into the cervical os and rotate it for 15 to 20 seconds.				
7	Immediately place the swab into the transport tube and recap.				
8	If using the ProbeTec Wet Transport Tube, break the tip of the swab off into the liquid before recapping.				
9	Remove gloves and dispose of them properly. Wash hands.				
10	*Paying attention detail,* attach requisition to specimen.				
11	Attend to your patient, *being sure to address any special needs.*				

No.	Step	Points	Check #1	Check #2	Check #3
12	Accurately record all information in patient's chart or electronic medical record. Document pelvic examination and wet prep were performed and that the provider examined the specimen. The provider will add his or her findings to the patient's electronic medical record. Be sure to sign the entry.				
	Student's Total Points				
	Points Possible				
	Final Score (Student's Total Points/Possible Points)				

Instructor's/Evaluator's Comments and Suggestions:

_____

_____

_____

_____

_____

CHECK #1	
Evaluator's Signature:	Date:

CHECK #2	
Evaluator's Signature:	Date:

CHECK #3	
Evaluator's Signature:	Date:

Work Documentation Form(s)

*Progress Note Template and Laboratory Requisition Form can be downloaded from the Premium Website

ABHES Competencies: MA.A.1.9.b Apply principles of aseptic techniques and infection control; MA.A.1.9.d Recognize and understand various treatment protocols; MA.A.1.9.e Recognize emergencies and treatments and minor office surgical procedures; MA.A.1.9.f Screen and follow up patient test results; MA.A.1.9.i Use standard precautions; MA.A.1.9.k Prepare and maintain examination and treatment area; MA.A.1.9.l Prepare patient for examinations and treatments; MA.A.1.9.m Assist physician with routine and specialty examinations and treatments; MA.A.1.9.p Advise patients of office policies and procedures

CAAHEP Competencies: I.P.10 Assist physician with patient care; I.A.1 Apply critical thinking skills in performing patient assessment and care; I.A.2 Use language/verbal skills that enable patients' understanding; III.P.2 Practice Standard Precautions; III.P.4 Perform handwashing; III.A.2 Explain the rationale for performance of a procedure to a patient; IV.P.6 Prepare a patient for procedures and/or treatments; IV.P.8 Document patient care; IV.A.7 Demonstrate recognition of the patient's level understanding in communication; IX.P.7 Document accurately in the patient record

Name_____ **Date**_____ **Score**_____

● **COMPETENCY ASSESSMENT**

Procedure 27-1:   Administration of a Vaccine

Task: To administer a vaccine.

Conditions:
- Vaccines as ordered by the provider
- Vaccine Information Statement (VIS)
- Medication card
- Appropriate syringe and needle
- Alcohol wipes
- Gloves (if office/clinic policy)
- Sharps container

Standards: Perform the Task within 15 minutes with a minimum score of _____ points, as determined by your instructor.

Time began: _____   **Time ended:** _____   **Total time:** _____

No.	Step	Points	Check #1	Check #2	Check #3
1	Review the provider's order. Write out a medication card.				
2	Follow the six "rights" of medication administration.				
3	Perform medical asepsis hand washing technique following OSHA guidelines.				
4	Work in a well-lit, quiet, clean area.				
5	*Paying attention to detail*, assemble the appropriate equipment.				
6	Give parents/guardians the Vaccine Information Statement (VIS) for the intended vaccine and *give them time to read the VIS and ask questions*.				
7	Be aware of the location of the emergency drugs (epinephrine and others).				
8	Carefully select the correct vial of vaccine. *Pay attention to detail.* Check the label three times and check the medication card.				
9	Check for the expiration date on the vial.				
10	Maintain sterile techniques throughout.				
11	Select the correct needle for the type of injection and the size of the patient.				
12	Shake the vial or reconstitute powder medication using all of the diluents according to the manufacturer's instructions.				

No.	Step	Points	Check #1	Check #2	Check #3
13	Invert the vial and withdraw the correct dose of the vaccine. Recheck the label on the vial and the medication card.				
14	Wash hands and, if office/clinic policy, put on nonsterile gloves.				
15	*Introduce yourself to the patient. Identity patient.*				
16	*Being courteous and respectful,* enlist the assistance of the parents to restrain the child.				
17	*Speaking at the patient's level of understanding, explain the procedure. Allay the patient's and parent's fears regarding the procedure. Help the patient to feel safe and comfortable.*				
18	Locate the appropriate site for administration. Cleanse the site with alcohol wipe and let dry.				
19	Inject the vaccine steadily at the appropriate angle.				
20	Withdraw the needle and syringe at the angle of insertion. Immediately dispose of needle and syringe in appropriate biohazard container.				
21	Apply gentle pressure to the injection site. Rub gently.				
22	Remove gloves, if required by office/clinic policy.				
23	Wash hands.				
24	Accurately record all information in patient's chart or electronic medical record and on the vaccine administration record. Include lot number, manufacturer, site, VIS date, and your name and initials.				
25	Update child's record of immunizations and remind parent or guardian to bring it to each visit.				
Student's Total Points					
Points Possible					
Final Score (Student's Total Points/Possible Points)					

Instructor's/Evaluator's Comments and Suggestions:

_____

_____

_____

_____

_____

_____

_____

CHECK #1	
Evaluator's Signature:	Date:

CHECK #2	
Evaluator's Signature:	Date:

CHECK #3	
Evaluator's Signature:	Date:

ABHES Competencies: MA.A.1.9.b Apply principles of aseptic techniques and infection control; MA.A.1.9.d Recognize and understand various treatment protocols; MA.A.1.9.g Maintain medication and immunization records; MA.A.1.9.i Use standard precautions; MA.A.1.9.j Prepare and administer oral and parenteral medications as directed by physician; MA.A.1.9.k Prepare and maintain examination and treatment area; MA.A.1.9.l Prepare patient for examinations and treatments; MA.A.1.9.m Assist physician with routine and specialty examinations and treatments; MA.A.1.9.p Advise patients of office policies and procedures

CAAHEP Competencies: I.P.9 Administer parenteral (excluding IV) medications; I.P.10 Assist physician with patient care; I.A.1 Apply critical thinking skills in performing patient assessment and care; I.A.2 Use language/verbal skills that enable patients' understanding; II.P.1 Prepare proper dosages of medication for administration; II.A.1 Verify ordered doses/dosages prior to administration; III.P.2 Practice Standard Precautions; III.P.4 Perform handwashing; III.A.2 Explain the rationale for performance of a procedure to a patient; IV.P.6 Prepare a patient for procedures and/or treatments; IV.P.8 Document patient care; IV.A.7 Demonstrate recognition of the patient's level understanding in communication; IX.P.7 Document accurately in the patient record

Work Documentation Form(s)

Vaccine Administration Record for Children and Teens

Patient name: _____

Birthdate: _____

Chart number: _____

Vaccine	Type of Vaccine[1] (generic abbreviation)	Date given (mo/day/yr)	Source (F,S,P)[2]	Site[3]	Vaccine		Vaccine Information Statement		Signature/ initials of vaccinator
					Lot #	Mfr.	Date on VIS[4]	Date given[4]	
Hepatitis B[5] (e.g., HepB, Hib-HepB, DTaP-HepB-IPV) Give IM.									
Diphtheria, Tetanus, Pertussis[5] (e.g., DTaP, DTaP-Hib, DTaP-HepB-IPV, DT, DTaP-Hib-IPV, Tdap, DTaP-IPV, Td) Give IM.									
Haemophilus influenzae **type b**[5] (e.g., Hib, Hib-HepB, DTaP-Hib-IPV, DTaP-Hib) Give IM.									
Polio[5] (e.g., IPV, DTaP-HepB-IPV, DTaP-Hib-IPV, DTaP-IPV) Give IPV SC or IM. Give all others IM.									
Pneumococcal (e.g., PCV, conjugate; PPV, polysaccharide) Give PCV IM. Give PPV SC or IM.									
Rotavirus (Rota) Give oral (po).									
Measles, Mumps, Rubella[5] (e.g., MMR, MMRV) Give SC.									
Varicella[5] (e.g., Var, MMRV) Give SC.									
Hepatitis A (HepA) Give IM.									
Meningococcal (e.g., MCV4; MPSV4) Give MCV4 IM and MPSV4 SC.									
Human papillomavirus (e.g., HPV) Give IM.									
Influenza[5] (e.g., TIV, inactivated; LAIV, live attenuated) Give TIV IM. Give LAIV IN.									
Other									

1. Record the generic abbreviation for the type of vaccine given (e.g., DTaP-Hib, PCV), *not* the trade name.
2. Record the source of the vaccine given as either F (Federally-supported), S (State-supported), or P (supported by Private insurance or other Private funds).
3. Record the site where vaccine was administered as either RA (Right Arm), LA (Left Arm), RT (Right Thigh), LT (Left Thigh), IN (Intranasal), or po (by mouth).
4. Record the publication date of each VIS as well as the date it is given to the patient.
5. For combination vaccines, fill in a row for each separate antigen in the combination.

Technical content reviewed by the Centers for Disease Control and Prevention, February 2008.

www.immunize.org/catg.d/p2022.pdf • Item #P2022 (2/08)

Distributed by the Immunization Action Coalition • (651) 647-9009 • www.immunize.org • www.vaccineinformation.org

From the Immunization Action Coalition, http://www.immunize.org

Name_____ **Date**_____ **Score**_____

● COMPETENCY ASSESSMENT

Procedure 27-2: Maintaining Immunization Records

Task: To establish and maintain a record of preventive immunizations against childhood diseases for the provider and parent or legal guardian.

Conditions:
- Vaccine Administration Record
- Vial of vaccine as ordered

Standards: Perform the Task within 15 minutes with a minimum score of _____ points, as determined by your instructor.

Time began: _____ **Time ended:** _____ **Total time:** _____

No.	Step	Points	Check #1	Check #2	Check #3
1	Give the parent or legal guardian the most recent copy of the Vaccine Information Statement (VIS). The statements explain risks and benefits of vaccines for each dose of vaccine given.				
2	After the administration of a scheduled vaccine for the child, accurately record all of the information in the patient's chart or electronic medical record and on the Vaccine Administration Record.				
3	Using the medicine card and the vaccine vial, fill out the Vaccine Administration Record according to which vaccine you administered. Note the headings, type of vaccine (use generic abbreviations, not the brand name), date given (month, day, year), dose, route, site, vaccine lot number and manufacturer, VIS; date on VIS, date given (VIS), and your initials as the individual who administered the vaccine.				
4	The immunization record is kept by the provider and the parent or legal guardian.				
Student's Total Points					
Points Possible					
Final Score (Student's Total Points/Possible Points)					

Instructor's/Evaluator's Comments and Suggestions:

_____

_____

_____

_____

_____

_____

_____

CHECK #1	
Evaluator's Signature:	Date:

CHECK #2	
Evaluator's Signature:	Date:

CHECK #3	
Evaluator's Signature:	Date:

ABHES Competencies: MA.A.1.9.d Recognize and understand various treatment protocols; MA.A.1.9.g Maintain medication and immunization records

CAAHEP Competencies: I.P.10 Assist physician with patient care; IV.P.8 Document patient care; IX.P.7 Document accurately in the patient record

Work Documentation Form(s)

Vaccine Administration Record for Children and Teens

Patient name: _____

Birthdate: _____

Chart number: _____

Vaccine	Type of Vaccine[1] (generic abbreviation)	Date given (mo/day/yr)	Source (F,S,P)[2]	Site[3]	Vaccine Lot #	Mfr.	Vaccine Information Statement Date on VIS[4]	Date given[4]	Signature/ initials of vaccinator
Hepatitis B[5] (e.g., HepB, Hib-HepB, DTaP-HepB-IPV) Give IM.									
Diphtheria, Tetanus, Pertussis[5] (e.g., DTaP, DTaP-Hib, DTaP-HepB-IPV, DT, DTaP-Hib-IPV, Tdap, DTaP-IPV, Td) Give IM.									
***Haemophilus influenzae* type b[5]** (e.g., Hib, Hib-HepB, DTaP-Hib-IPV, DTaP-Hib) Give IM.									
Polio[5] (e.g., IPV, DTaP-HepB-IPV, DTaP-Hib-IPV, DTaP-IPV) Give IPV SC or IM. Give all others IM.									
Pneumococcal (e.g., PCV, conjugate; PPV, polysaccharide) Give PCV IM. Give PPV SC or IM.									
Rotavirus (Rota) Give oral (po).									
Measles, Mumps, Rubella[5] (e.g., MMR, MMRV) Give SC.									
Varicella[5] (e.g., Var, MMRV) Give SC.									
Hepatitis A (HepA) Give IM.									
Meningococcal (e.g., MCV4; MPSV4) Give MCV4 IM and MPSV4 SC.									
Human papillomavirus (e.g., HPV) Give IM.									
Influenza[5] (e.g., TIV, inactivated; LAIV, live attenuated) Give TIV IM. Give LAIV IN.									
Other									

1. Record the generic abbreviation for the type of vaccine given (e.g., DTaP-Hib, PCV), *not* the trade name.
2. Record the source of the vaccine given as either F (Federally-supported), S (State-supported), or P (supported by Private insurance or other Private funds).
3. Record the site where vaccine was administered as either RA (Right Arm), LA (Left Arm), RT (Right Thigh), LT (Left Thigh), IN (Intranasal), or po (by mouth).
4. Record the publication date of each VIS as well as the date it is given to the patient.
5. For combination vaccines, fill in a row for each separate antigen in the combination.

Technical content reviewed by the Centers for Disease Control and Prevention, February 2008. www.immunize.org/catg.d/p2022.pdf • Item #P2022 (2/08)

Distributed by the Immunization Action Coalition • (651) 647-9009 • www.immunize.org • www.vaccineinformation.org

Name_____ **Date**_____ **Score**_____

● COMPETENCY ASSESSMENT

Procedure 27-3: Measuring the Infant: Weight, Length, and Head and Chest Circumference

Task: Obtain an accurate measurement of an infant's weight, length, and head and chest circumference for medical records and to screen for growth abnormalities.

Conditions:
- Infant scale
- Paper protector
- Flexible measuring tape without elasticity
- Growth chart
- Pen
- Ruler
- Biohazard waste container

Standards: Perform the Task within 30 minutes with a minimum score of _____ points, as determined by your instructor.

Time began: _____   **Time ended:** _____   **Total time:** _____

No.	Step	Points	Check #1	Check #2	Check #3
1	Wash hands.				
2	*Introduce yourself to the parents. Identity patient.*				
3	*Speaking at the parents' level of understanding, explain the procedure to the parents. Allay the parents' fears regarding the procedure.*				
4	*Being courteous and respectful,* enlist the assistance of the parents to undress the infant (including the diaper).				
5	Place all of the weights to left of the scale to balance.				
6	*Paying attention to detail,* place a clean utility or paper towel on scale and check balance of scale for accuracy, being sure to compensate for the weight of the towel.				
7	Gently place small infant on her back on the scale. Larger infants can sit on the scale. Place your hand slightly above the infant's body to ensure safety.				
8	Place the bottom weight to its highest measurement that will not cause the balance to drop to the bottom edge.				
9	Slowly move upper weight until the balance bar rests in the center of the indicator. A balanced scale will provide an accurate weight. Read the infant's weight while he or she is lying still.				

No.	Step	Points	Check #1	Check #2	Check #3
10	Return both weights to their resting positions to the extreme left.				
11	Gently remove infant and apply diaper. (Parent can help with diapering and holding infant.)				
12	Discard used protective paper towel per OSHA guidelines.				
13	Sanitize scale.				
14	Wash hands.				
15	Accurately record all information in patient's chart or electronic medical record or in growth chart and patient's booklet, if available. Document according to clinic policy (pounds and ounces or kilograms). Connect dot from previous examination with a ruler to complete the graph.				
Measuring infant length:					
1	Wash hands and follow Standard Precautions.				
2	***Speaking at the parents' level of understanding, explain the procedure to the parents. Allay the parents' fears regarding the procedure.***				
3	***Being courteous and respectful,*** enlist the assistance of the parents to remove the infant's shoes.				
4	Gently place infant on his or her back on the examination table. If the pediatric table has a headboard, ask the parent to hold the infant in place with the head against this board (end) of table at zero mark of ruler while you place the infant's heels against the footboard. Gently straighten infant's back and legs to line up the ruler. If there is no footboard (to place infant's feet against), use your right hand as a guide. If necessary, gently place your left hand over the child's legs at the knees to secure the child in place and straighten the legs so the recumbent length can be read from the head to the heel.				
5	Read length on the measuring device in inches or centimeters.				
6	***Being courteous and respectful,*** enlist the assistance of the parents to dress the infant.				
7	Wash hands.				
8	Accurately record all information in patient's chart or electronic medical record or in growth chart and patient's booklet, if available. Document according to office policy (inches and centimeters). Connect dot from previous examination with a ruler to complete the graph.				

No.	Step	Points	Check #1	Check #2	Check #3
Measuring head circumference:					
1	Wash hands and follow Standard Precautions.				
2	***Speaking at the parents' level of understanding, explain the procedure to the parents. Allay the parents' fears regarding the procedure.***				
3	***Being courteous and respectful, talk to the infant and parents to gain cooperation.*** Infant may be held by parent or placed on the examination table for the measurement. Older children age 2 or 3 years may stand or sit if they will remain still.				
4	Place the measuring tape snugly around the head from the occipital protuberance to the supraorbital prominence. This is the largest part of the head.				
5	Read the measurement, which will be in either inches (to the nearest ½ inch) or centimeters (to the nearest 0.01 cm).				
6	Wash hands.				
7	Accurately record all information in patient's chart or electronic medical record or in growth chart and patient's booklet, if available. Connect dot from previous examination with a ruler to complete the graph.				
Measuring infant's chest circumference:					
1	Wash hands and follow Standard Precautions.				
2	***Speaking at the parents' level of understanding, explain the procedure to the parents. Allay the parents' fears regarding the procedure.***				
3	Use one thumb to hold tape measure with zero mark against the infant's chest at the midsternal area. With the other hand, bring the tape around/under the back to meet the zero mark of the tape in front. Take the measurement of the chest just above the nipples with the tape fitting around the child's chest under the axillary regions. If you need assistance in holding the child still, ask the parent or other assistant. The measurement should be taken when the child is breathing normally and during the resting phase between respirations.				
4	Read the measurement to the nearest 0.01 cm or one-eighth inch.				
5	Wash hands.				

No.	Step	Points	Check #1	Check #2	Check #3
6	Accurately record all information in patient's chart or electronic medical record or in growth chart and patient's booklet if available. Document according to office policy (inches or centimeters).				
Student's Total Points					
Points Possible					
Final Score					
(Student's Total Points/Possible Points)					

Instructor's/Evaluator's Comments and Suggestions:

_____

_____

_____

_____

_____

_____

_____

CHECK #1	
Evaluator's Signature:	Date:

CHECK #2	
Evaluator's Signature:	Date:

CHECK #3	
Evaluator's Signature:	Date:

ABHES Competencies: MA.A.1.9.i Use standard precautions; MA.A.1.9.j Prepare and administer oral and parenteral medications as directed by physician; MA.A.1.9.l Prepare patient for examinations and treatments; MA.A.1.9.p Advise patients of office policies and procedures

CAAHEP Competencies: I.P.10 Assist physician with patient care; I.A.1 Apply critical thinking skills in performing patient assessment and care; I.A.2 Use language/verbal skills that enable patients' understanding; III.P.2 Practice Standard Precautions; III.P.4 Perform handwashing; III.A.2 Explain the rationale for performance of a procedure to a patient; IV.P.8 Document patient care; IV.A.7 Demonstrate recognition of the patient's level understanding in communication; IX.P.7 Document accurately in the patient record

Work Documentation Form(s)

**Birth to 36 months: Boys
Head circumference-for-age and
Weight-for-length percentiles**

NAME _____

RECORD # _____

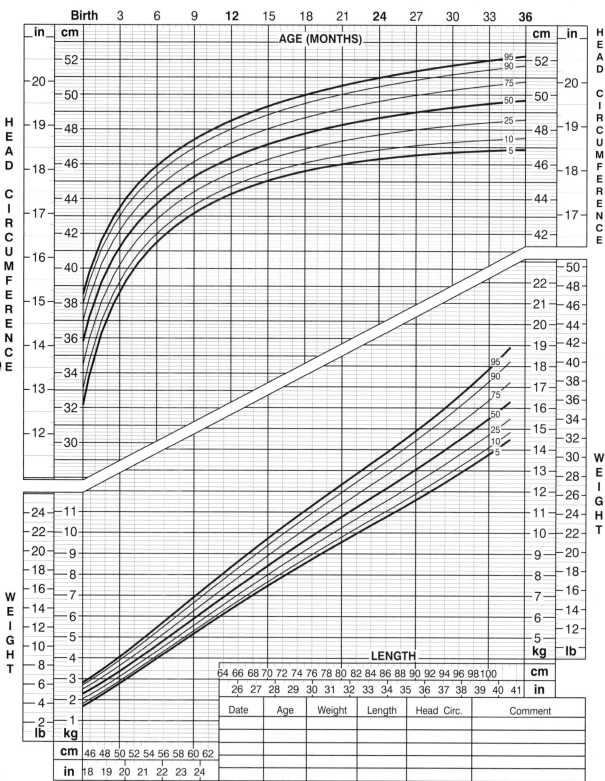

Published May 30, 2000 (modified 10/16/00).
SOURCE: Developed by the National Center for Health Statistics in collaboration with
the National Center for Chronic Disease Prevention and Health Promotion (2000).
http://www.cdc.gov/growthcharts

SAFER·HEALTHIER·PEOPLE™

Courtesy of the Centers for Disease Control and Prevention

Name _____ **Date** _____ **Score** _____

● **COMPETENCY ASSESSMENT**

Procedure 27-4: Taking an Infant's Rectal Temperature with a Digital Thermometer

Task: Obtain a rectal temperature using a digital thermometer.

Conditions:
- Digital thermometer and probe cover
- Lubricating jelly
- 4 × 4 gauze sponges
- Gloves
- Biohazard waste container

Standards: Perform the Task within 15 minutes with a minimum score of _____ points, as determined by your instructor.

Time began: _____   **Time ended:** _____   **Total time:** _____

No.	Step	Points	Check #1	Check #2	Check #3
1	Wash hands and follow Standard Precautions.				
2	*Introduce yourself to the parents. Identity patient.*				
3	*Speaking at the parents' level of understanding, explain the procedure to the parents. Allay the parents' fears regarding the procedure.*				
4	*Paying attention to detail,* assemble equipment.				
5	*Being courteous and respectful,* enlist the assistance of the parents to undress the infant (including the diaper).				
6	Position infant in a prone or supine position having the parent or another medical assistant safeguard the infant.				
7	Place a probe cover on the thermometer.				
8	Lubricate with lubricating jelly.				
9	Apply nonsterile disposable gloves.				
10	Spread buttocks, insert thermometer gently into the rectum past the sphincter; for an infant this is 0.5 inch.				
11	Hold buttocks together while holding the thermometer. If necessary, restrain infant movement by placing your arm across the infant's back. Parent can immobilize infant's legs.				
12	Hold in place until the beep is heard. Do not let go of the thermometer.				

No.	Step	Points	Check #1	Check #2	Check #3
13	Remove thermometer from the rectum.				
14	Provide wipes to remove any additional lubricating jelly.				
15	Have parents attend to infant.				
16	Note temperature reading.				
17	Remove probe cover by ejecting it into a biohazard container.				
18	Wipe probe with antiseptic wipe. Replace thermometer in holder.				
19	Remove gloves and discard in biohazard waste container.				
20	Wash hands.				
21	***Being courteous and respectful***, enlist the parents in dressing the infant.				
22	Accurately record all information in patient's chart or electronic medical record with the designation of (R) indicating a rectal temperature.				
Student's Total Points					
Points Possible					
Final Score **(Student's Total Points/Possible Points)**					

Instructor's/Evaluator's Comments and Suggestions:

_____

_____

_____

_____

_____

_____

_____

CHECK #1	
Evaluator's Signature:	Date:

CHECK #2	
Evaluator's Signature:	Date:

CHECK #3	
Evaluator's Signature:	Date:

Work Documentation Form(s)

*Progress Note Template can be downloaded from the Premium Website

ABHES Competencies: MA.A.1.9.c Take vital signs; MA.A.1.9.i Use standard precautions

CAAHEP Competencies: I.P.1 Obtain vital signs; I.A.1 Apply critical thinking skills in performing patient assessment and care; I.A.2 Use language/verbal skills that enable patient's understanding; 1.A.3 Demonstrate respect for diversity in approaching patients and families; III.P.2 Practice Standard Precautions; III.P.4 Perform handwashing; IV.P.8 Document patient care

Name_____ **Date**_____ **Score**_____

● **COMPETENCY ASSESSMENT**

Procedure 27-5:   Taking an Apical Pulse on an Infant

Task: Obtain an apical pulse rate.

Conditions:
- Stethoscope
- Watch with a second hand
- Alcohol wipes

Standards: Perform the Task within 15 minutes with a minimum score of _____ points, as determined by your instructor.

Time began: _____   **Time ended:** _____   **Total time:** _____

No.	Step	Points	Check #1	Check #2	Check #3
1	Wash hands and follow Standard Precautions.				
2	*Paying attention to detail,* assemble equipment.				
3	*Introduce yourself to the parents. Identity patient.*				
4	*Speaking at the parents' level of understanding, explain the procedure to the parents. Allay the parent's fears regarding the procedure.*				
5	*Being courteous and respectful,* enlist the assistance of the parents to undress the infant (including the diaper).				
6	Provide a drape for the infant's warmth if necessary.				
7	Gently position the infant in a supine position or sitting in the parent's lap.				
8	Locate the fifth intercostal space, midclavicular line, to the left of the sternum.				
9	Place warmed stethoscope on the site and listen for the lub-dub sound of the heart.				
10	Count the pulse for 1 minute; each lub-dub equals one heartbeat or pulse.				
11	Wash hands.				
12	Assist parents as needed to redress the infant.				
13	Clean earpieces and diaphragm of stethoscope with alcohol wipes.				

No.	Step	Points	Check #1	Check #2	Check #3
14	Accurately record all information in patient's chart or electronic medical record. Designate (AP) to indicate apical pulse. Note any arrhythmias.				
	Student's Total Points				
	Points Possible				
	Final Score (Student's Total Points/Possible Points)				

Instructor's/Evaluator's Comments and Suggestions:

_____

_____

_____

_____

_____

_____

_____

CHECK #1 Evaluator's Signature:	Date:

CHECK #2 Evaluator's Signature:	Date:

CHECK #3 Evaluator's Signature:	Date:

Work Documentation Form(s)

*Progress Note Template can be downloaded from the Premium Website

ABHES Competencies: MA.A.1.9.c Take vital signs; MA.A.1.9.i Use standard precautions; MA.A.1.9.l Prepare patient for examinations and treatments

CAAHEP Competencies: I.P.1 Obtain vital signs; III.P.2 Practice standard precautions; III.P.4 Perform handwashing; IX.P.7 Document accurately in the patient record

Name_____ **Date**_____ **Score**_____

● **COMPETENCY ASSESSMENT**

Procedure 27-6: Measuring Infant's Respiratory Rate

Task: Obtain an infant's respiratory rate. It is usually taken after the pulse rate to obtain an accurate respiratory rate.

Conditions: • Watch with a second hand

Standards: Perform the Task within 15 minutes with a minimum score of _____ points, as determined by your instructor.

Time began: _____ **Time ended:** _____ **Total time:** _____

No.	Step	Points	Check #1	Check #2	Check #3
1	Wash hands and follow Standard Precautions.				
2	*Identify the patient and explain the procedure to the parent, speaking at the parent's level of understanding.*				
3	Position infant in a supine position.				
4	Place hand on the chest to feel the rise and fall of the chest wall for 1 minute.				
5	Note depth and rhythm while counting.				
6	Wash hands.				
7	Accurately record all information in patient's chart or electronic medical record. Note any irregularities in depth or rhythm.				
Student's Total Points					
Points Possible					
Final Score (Student's Total Points/Possible Points)					

Instructor's/Evaluator's Comments and Suggestions:

_____

_____

_____

_____

_____

_____

_____

CHECK #1	
Evaluator's Signature:	Date:

CHECK #2	
Evaluator's Signature:	Date:

CHECK #3	
Evaluator's Signature:	Date:

Work Documentation Form(s)

*Progress Note Template can be downloaded from the Premium Website

ABHES Competencies: MA.A.1.9.c Take vital signs; MA.A.1.9.i Use standard precautions; MA.A.1.9.l Prepare patient for examinations and treatments

CAAHEP Competencies: I.P.1 Obtain vital signs; III.P.2 Practice standard precautions; III.P.4 Perform handwashing; IX.P.7 Document accurately in the patient record

Name _____ **Date** _____ **Score** _____

COMPETENCY ASSESSMENT

Procedure 27-7: Obtaining a Urine Specimen from an Infant or Young Child

Task: Obtain a urine specimen from an infant or young child.

Conditions:
- Urine collection bag
- Urine cup
- Laboratory request form
- Biohazard transport bag
- Nonsterile disposable gloves
- Cleansing cloth
- Towel
- Biohazard waste container

Standards: Perform the Task within 2 minutes with a minimum score of _____ points, as determined by your instructor.

Time began: _____   **Time ended:** _____   **Total time:** _____

No.	Step	Points	Check #1	Check #2	Check #3
1	Wash hands and follow Standard Precautions.				
2	*Identify the patient and explain the procedure to the parent, speaking at the parents' level of understanding.*				
3	*Paying attention to detail,* assemble equipment.				
4	*Being courteous and respectful,* enlist the assistance of the parents to disrobe patient and remove the diaper.				
5	Wash and dry perineal area.				
6	Apply collection bag, secure with adhesive tabs. • Girls: spread perineum, place bag over labia. • Boys: place bag over penis and scrotum.				
7	Replace diaper carefully.				
8	Frequently check bag for urine.				
9	Once specimen has been collected, remove bag carefully.				
10	Prepare specimen as required. Send to laboratory in an appropriate container with the appropriate requisition or process the specimen in the clinic laboratory.				
11	Remove gloves and discard in biohazard waste container.				
12	Wash hands.				

No.	Step	Points	Check #1	Check #2	Check #3
13	Accurately record all information in patient's chart or electronic medical record.				
Student's Total Points					
Points Possible					
Final Score (Student's Total Points/Possible Points)					

Instructor's/Evaluator's Comments and Suggestions:

CHECK #1 Evaluator's Signature:	Date:

CHECK #2 Evaluator's Signature:	Date:

CHECK #3 Evaluator's Signature:	Date:

ABHES Competencies: MA.A.1.9.c Take vital signs; MA.A.1.9.i Use standard precautions; MA.A.1.9.l Prepare patient for examinations and treatments

CAAHEP Competencies: I.P.1 Obtain vital signs; III.P.2 Practice standard precautions; III.P.4 Perform handwashing; IX.P.7 Document accurately in the patient record

Work Documentation Form(s)

*Laboratory Requisition form can be downloaded from the Premium Website

Urinalysis Report Form

Patient Name: _____

Age: _____ M _____ F _____

Physician's Name: _____

Collection Date: _____ Test Date: _____ Tester's Initials: _____

Physical Examination

Color: ☐ colorless ☐ yellow ☐ amber ☐ other

Appearance: ☐ clear ☐ hazy ☐ cloudy ☐ turbid

Chemical Examination (circle one)

specific gravity	1.000	1.005	1.010	1.015	1.020	1.025	1.030
pH		5	6	7	8	9	
leukocytes		neg	trace	+	++		
nitrite		neg	pos	(any pink color is considered positive)			
protein (mg/dL)		neg	trace	+/30	++/100	+++/500	
glucose (mg/dL)		normal	50	100	250	500	1000
ketones		neg	+small	++mod	+++large		
urobilinogen (mg/dL)		normal	1	4	8	12	
bilirubin		neg	+	++	+++		
blood (ery/µl)		neg	trace	50	250		
hemoglobin (ery/µl)			10	50	250		

Comments: _____

_____

_____

_____

_____

© Cengage Learning 2014

Name_____ **Date**_____ **Score**_____

● **COMPETENCY ASSESSMENT**

Procedure 28-1:   Instructing Patient in Testicular Self-Examination

Task: Provide a patient with information concerning testicular screening for the presence of a painless mass in the scrotum.

Conditions: • Testicular self-examination card
                • Anatomy illustration

Standards: Perform the Task within 8 minutes with a minimum score of _____ points, as determined by your instructor.

Time began: _____   **Time ended:** _____   **Total time:** _____

No.	Step	Points	Check #1	Check #2	Check #3
1	*Identify yourself and explain the procedure, speaking at the patient's level of understanding. Identify patient.*				
2	*Being courteous and respectful,* instruct the patient to examine his testicles monthly in a warm shower.				
3	Hold the penis out of the way and check one testicle at a time.				
4	Examine each testicle separately with both hands.				
5	Place the index and middle fingers underneath the testicle and the thumbs on top. Roll the testicle gently between the fingers.				
6	Look and feel for any hard lumps, any smooth rounded bumps, or change in the size, shape, or consistency of the testes.				
7	Locate the epididymis. It feels like a small bump on the upper or middle outer side of the testes. Provide a chart to the patient that illustrates the testes and epididymis.				
8	Look for swelling or changes in the scrotal area.				
9	Encourage the patient to report anything unusual to the provider.				
10	Accurately record all information in patient's chart or electronic medical record.				
Student's Total Points					
Points Possible					
Final Score (Student's Total Points/Possible Points)					

Instructor's/Evaluator's Comments and Suggestions:

_____

_____

_____

_____

_____

_____

_____

CHECK #1	
Evaluator's Signature:	Date:

CHECK #2	
Evaluator's Signature:	Date:

CHECK #3	
Evaluator's Signature:	Date:

Work Documentation Form(s)

*Progress Note template can be downloaded from the Premium Website

ABHES Competency: MA.A.1.9.r Teach patients methods of health promotion and disease prevention

CAAHEP Competencies: I.A.2 Use language/verbal skills that enable a patient's understanding; IV.P.5 Instruct patients according to their needs to promote health maintenance and disease prevention; IV.A.7 Demonstrate recognition of patient's level of understanding in communication

Name_____ **Date**_____ **Score**_____

COMPETENCY ASSESSMENT

Procedure 30-1: Assisting the Provider during a Lumbar Puncture for Cerebrospinal Fluid Aspiration

Task: Assemble supplies and position the patient for removal of cerebrospinal fluid from the lumbar area to be sent to the laboratory for analysis.

Conditions:
- Gown
- Sheet or blanket
- Waterproof drape
- Xylocaine 1% to 2%
- Syringe and needle for anesthetic
- Disposable water
- Surgical prep kit (antiseptic soap and sponges)
- Sterile gloves
- Disposable sterile lumbar puncture tray (skin antiseptic [povidone-iodine] with applicator, adhesive bandage, spinal puncture needle, three or four test tubes with corks or tops, drape, manometer, laboratory requisition, examination light, gauze sponge)

Standards: Perform the Task within 30 minutes with a minimum score of _____ points, as determined by your instructor.

Time began: _____ **Time ended:** _____ **Total time:** _____

No.	Step	Points	Check #1	Check #2	Check #3
1	Wash hands.				
2	*Paying attention to detail*, gather appropriate equipment and supplies.				
3	*Introduce yourself and identify patient. Reinforce provider's explanation of the procedure and answer questions, speaking at the patient's level of understanding.*				
4	Verify the patient's signature on the informed consent. If the patient has questions, notify the provider that the patient requires further information.				
5	*If needed, assist the patient* to the restroom to empty bladder and bowel.				
6	Wash hands.				
7	Using a mayo stand as a base, open the sterile lumbar puncture tray in a manner that maintains sterility of contents and establishes a sterile field for the provider.				

No.	Step	Points	Check #1	Check #2	Check #3
8	*Allay the patient's fears and help him to feel safe and comfortable* while positioning him in a lateral recumbent position with his back at the edge of the examination table. Provide a small pillow for comfort under his head.				
9	Drape the patient for warmth and privacy, *protecting the patient's personal boundaries.*				
10	*Attending to any special needs of the patient,* instruct and then assist him to draw the knees up to the abdomen and to grasp the knees to hold them in place. The chin should be angled toward the chest and the back should be arched toward the edge of the examination table.				
11	Instruct the patient that during the procedure, he must remember to breathe slowly and evenly and refrain from talking.				
12	Tuck a waterproof drape under the patient's side in the area to be prepped.				
13	Open the surgical prep tray and pour sterile water into the provided area. Be careful to avoid splashing.				
14	Don sterile gloves.				
15	Prep the puncture site with antiseptic soap solution beginning at puncture location and prepping in a circular manner to a diameter of at least 6 inches. Discard the prep swab and repeat × 3 or per provider's orders. Rinse if required per provider's orders or manufacturer's instructions. Dry with sterile toweling.				
16	Remove sterile gloves and dispose of appropriately.				
17	Assist the provider as needed to swab the puncture site with the providine-iodine solution.				
18	Assist the provider to draw up the anesthetic solution by inverting the vial and holding it stable to be accessed.				
19	Encourage and assist the patient to maintain the knee-chest position until the spinal needle is inserted and a free flow of cerebrospinal fluid is obtained.				
20	When the manometer is attached and measurements are being taken, remind the patient to breathe slowly and evenly and refrain from talking so that an accurate pressure measurement can be obtained.				

No.	Step	Points	Check #1	Check #2	Check #3
21	At the provider's direction, have the patient straighten his legs.				
22	Assist the provider as needed with the vials of CSF.				
23	A sterile dressing will be applied to the puncture site once the procedure is completed. Assist the provider as needed.				
24	Assist the patient to a supine position and instruct him that he must remain in this position for 2–4 hours or per the provider's orders.				
25	Monitor vital signs per office policy or provider's orders. Provide comfort measures and medicate per provider's orders.				
26	At the conclusion of the procedure, don sterile gloves and cap CSF specimens tightly.				
27	Remove gloves and dispose of appropriately.				
28	Wash hands.				
29	Appropriately label the CSF vials with the date, patient's name, and order of collection. Place in biohazard bag for transport.				
30	*Paying attention to detail*, complete the laboratory requisition and following policy, send samples to the selected laboratory.				
31	Don non-sterile disposable gloves.				
32	Dispose of equipment per OSHA guidelines, including disposing of all sharps in approved sharps container.				
33	Follow clinic policy or provider's orders to provide written instructions for after care.				
34	Accurately record procedure per provider's instruction in patient's medical record or EMR. Be sure to include patient education, any medications given, the patient's tolerance of the procedure, any pressure measurements obtained, and the disposition of the CSF samples.				
Student's Total Points					
Points Possible					
Final Score (Student's Total Points/Possible Points)					

Instructor's/Evaluator's Comments and Suggestions:

_____

_____

_____

_____

_____

_____

_____

CHECK #1	
Evaluator's Signature:	Date:

CHECK #2	
Evaluator's Signature:	Date:

CHECK #3	
Evaluator's Signature:	Date:

Work Documentation Form(s)

*Lab Requisition Form and Progress Note Template can be downloaded from the Premium Website

ABHES Competencies: MA.A.1.4.a Document accurately; MA.A.1.9.b Apply principles of aseptic techniques and infection control; MA.A.1.9.d Recognize and understand various treatment protocols; MA.A.1.9.e Recognize emergencies and treatments and minor office surgical procedures; MA.A.1.9.l Prepare patient for examinations and treatments; MA.A.1.9.m Assist physician with routine and specialty examinations and treatments

CAAHEP Competencies: I.P.10 Assist physician with patient care; I.A.2 Use language/verbal skills that enable the patients' understanding; III.P.7 Obtain specimens for microbiological testing; III.A.1 Display sensitivity to patient rights and feelings in collecting specimens; III.A.2 Explain the rationale for performance of a procedure to the patient; III.A.3 Show awareness of patients' concerns regarding their perceptions related to the procedure being performed; IV.P.6 Prepare a patient for procedures and/or treatments; IV.P.8 Document patient care; IV.A.7 Demonstrate recognition of the patient's level of understanding in communication; IX.P.2 Perform within scope of practice; IX.P.7 Document accurately in the patient record

Name_____ **Date**_____ **Score**_____

COMPETENCY ASSESSMENT

Procedure 30-2: Assisting the Provider with a Neurologic Screening Examination

Task: Determine a patient's neurologic status.

Conditions: • Percussion hammer
               • Safety pin or sensory wheel
               • Material for odor identification
               • Cotton ball
               • Tuning fork
               • Flashlight
               • Tongue blade
               • Solid objects such as keys, coins, or paper clips

Standards: Perform the Task within 20 minutes with a minimum score of _____ points, as determined by your instructor.

Time began: _____ **Time ended:** _____ **Total time:** _____

No.	Step	Points	Check #1	Check #2	Check #3
1	Wash hands.				
2	*Paying attention to detail*, gather appropriate equipment and supplies.				
3	*Introduce yourself and identify patient. Speaking at the level of the patient's understanding, explain the procedure and expectations to the patient.*				
4	While taking the patient's medical history, observe the following: • Orientation to person, place, and time • Memory • Mood • Cognition • Appropriate behaviors				
5	Assist the provider as requested when testing reflexes with a percussion hammer.				
6	Assist the provider by assuring the smooth flow of assessment during the neuro exam by providing equipment as requested.				
7	Accurately record findings of neurological exam per provider's instruction in the patient's record or EMR.				
Student's Total Points					
Points Possible					
Final Score (Student's Total Points/Possible Points)					

Instructor's/Evaluator's Comments and Suggestions:

_____

_____

_____

_____

_____

_____

CHECK #1	
Evaluator's Signature:	Date:

CHECK #2	
Evaluator's Signature:	Date:

CHECK #3	
Evaluator's Signature:	Date:

Work Documentation Form(s)

*Progress Note Template can be downloaded from the Premium Website

ABHES Competencies: MA.A.1.4.a Document accurately; MA.A.1.9.d Recognize and understand various treatment protocols; MA.A.1.9.l Prepare patient for examinations and treatments; MA.A.1.9.m Assist physician with routine and specialty examinations and treatments

CAAHEP Competencies: I.P.10 Assist physician with patient care; I.A.1 Apply critical thinking skills in performing patient assessment and care; I.A.2 Use language/verbal skills that enable the patients' understanding; IV.P.8 Document patient care; IV.A.7 Demonstrate recognition of the patient's level of understanding in communication; IX.P.7 Document accurately in the patient record

Name_____ **Date**_____ **Score**_____

COMPETENCY ASSESSMENT

Procedure 30-3: Performing Visual Acuity Testing Using a Snellen Chart

Task: Perform a visual screening test to determine a patient's distance visual acuity.

Conditions:
- Snellen eye chart placed at eye level (appropriate for age and reading ability of the patient)
- Pointer
- Occluder
- Alcohol wipes

Standards: Perform the Task within 15 minutes with a minimum score of _____ points, as determined by your instructor.

Competency Assessment Information

Meredith Moore, aged 27, is seen in the office for a routine annual examination. She wears corrective lenses, but has not seen her eye care professional within the last 18 months. Your provider wants to include visual acuity testing in her exam. Document results using the Progress Note Template (Work Documentation).

Time began: _____   **Time ended:** _____   **Total time:** _____

No.	Step	Points	Check #1	Check #2	Check #3
1	Wash hands. Assemble equipment and supplies, *paying attention to detail*.				
2	Prepare a well-lit room, free from distractions and with a distance mark 20 feet from the eye chart. Be certain there is no glare on the chart.				
3	*Explain the procedure to the patient, speaking at the patient's level of understanding.* Patients should be tested with their glasses or contact lenses, unless otherwise indicated by the provider.				
4	Instruct the patient to stand behind the mark and cover the right eye with the occluder. Instruct the patient to keep the left eye open under the occluder and not to apply pressure to the eyeball.				
5	Stand next to the chart, point to row 3, and instruct the patient to read each letter with the left eye, verbally identifying each letter read. If unable to read line 3, go to line 2 or 1.				
6	Accurately record the results at the smallest line the patient can read with two or fewer errors. Vision is recorded as right eye, left eye, both eyes.				
7	Record the patient's reaction during the test.				
8	Repeat the procedure with the right eye.				

No.	Step	Points	Check #1	Check #2	Check #3
9	Disinfect the occluder with alcohol wipes. Wash hands. Accurately record the results in patient's chart or electronic medical record.				
Student's Total Points					
Points Possible					
Final Score (Student's Total Points/Possible Points)					

Instructor's/Evaluator's Comments and Suggestions:

_____

_____

_____

_____

_____

_____

_____

CHECK #1	
Evaluator's Signature:	Date:

CHECK #2	
Evaluator's Signature:	Date:

CHECK #3	
Evaluator's Signature:	Date:

Work Documentation Form(s)

*Progress Note Template can be downloaded from the Premium Website

ABHES Competency: MA.A.1.9.f Screen and follow up patient test results

CAAHEP Competencies: I.P.6 Perform patient screening using established protocols; I.P.10 Assist physician with patient care; I.A.2 Use language/verbal skills that enable patients' understanding; IV.P.8 Document patient care

Name _____ **Date** _____ **Score** _____

● **COMPETENCY ASSESSMENT**

Procedure 30-4:   Measuring Near Visual Acuity

Task: Measure the near vision of the patient.

Conditions:
- Appropriate near visual acuity chart (Jaegar)
- Occluder
- Measuring tape
- Alcohol wipes

Standards: Perform the Task within 15 minutes with a minimum score of _____ points, as determined by your instructor.

Competency Assessment Information

Meredith Moore, aged 27, is seen in the office for a routine annual examination. She wears corrective lenses, but has not seen her eye care professional within the last 18 months. Your provider wants to include visual acuity testing in her exam. Document results using Progress Note Template (Work Documentation).

Time began: _____   **Time ended:** _____   **Total time:** _____

No.	Step	Points	Check #1	Check #2	Check #3
1	Wash hands.				
2	*Paying attention to detail,* assemble equipment and supplies.				
3	Prepare a well-lit room, free from distractions.				
4	*Identify patient. Explain procedure to patient, speaking at the patient's level of understanding.*				
5	Patients who wear corrective lenses should be tested wearing glasses or contact lenses, unless otherwise indicated by the provider.				
6	Position the near visual acuity card 14 inches from the patient by measuring with a tape measure.				
7	Cover the left eye for right eye measurement. Instruct the patient to keep the left eye open under the occluder and not to apply pressure to the eyeball.				
8	*Demonstrating respect for individual diversity,* provide language appropriate paragraphs printed on a card.				
9	Once patient has reached a line where more than two mistakes are made, note the visual acuity for that line for that eye (allow the patient to repeat the line to verify acuity).				
10	Repeat the process to measure the left eye.				

No.	Step	Points	Check #1	Check #2	Check #3
11	Repeat the process with both eyes open.				
12	Record the patient's reaction during the test.				
13	Disinfect the occluder with alcohol wipes.				
14	Wash hands.				
15	Accurately record the results. Vision is recorded as right eye, left eye, or both eyes. Normal vision using this method is recorded as 14/14.				
Student's Total Points					
Points Possible					
Final Score (Student's Total Points/Possible Points)					

Instructor's/Evaluator's Comments and Suggestions:

_____

_____

_____

_____

_____

_____

_____

CHECK #1

Evaluator's Signature: _____ Date:

CHECK #2

Evaluator's Signature: _____ Date:

CHECK #3

Evaluator's Signature: _____ Date:

Work Documentation Form(s)

*Progress Note Template can be downloaded from the Premium Website

ABHES Competency: MA.A.1.9.f Screen and follow up patient test results

CAAHEP Competencies: I.P.6 Perform patient screening using established protocols; I.P.10 Assist physician with patient care; I.A.2 Use language/verbal skills that enable patients' understanding; IV.P.8 Document patient care

Name_____ **Date**_____ **Score**_____

⬤ COMPETENCY ASSESSMENT

Procedure 30-5: Testing Color Vision Using the Ishihara Plates

Task: Assess a patient's ability to distinguish between the colors red and green.

Conditions: • Ishihara Plates (1–12)
• Measuring tape

Standards: Perform the Task within 15 minutes with a minimum score of _____ points, as determined by your instructor.

Competency Assessment Information

Tim Horner, 10 years old, is in the office for his annual examination. Tim has never been tested for color blindness. Your provider wishes to include this in his exam. Document results using the Progress Note Template (Work Documentation).

Time began: _____ **Time ended:** _____ **Total time:** _____

No.	Step	Points	Check #1	Check #2	Check #3
1	Wash hands.				
2	*Paying attention to detail,* assemble equipment and supplies.				
3	Assure that the plates have been stored covered and protected from sunlight to ensure that no fading of the colors on the plates has occurred. This would invalidate the test.				
4	Prepare a room lit by daylight, free from distractions.				
5	*Explain the procedure to the patient, speaking at the patient's level of understanding.*				
6	Hold each plate 30 inches from the patient and tilted so that the plane of the plate is at a right angle to the line of the patient's vision.				
7	Record the number given by the patient on each plate.				
8	Assess the patient's readings.				
9	*Concisely update the provider with the test results.* Accurately document results in patient's chart or electronic medical record.				
Student's Total Points					
Points Possible					
Final Score (Student's Total Points/Possible Points)					

Instructor's/Evaluator's Comments and Suggestions:

_____

_____

_____

_____

_____

_____

_____

CHECK #1	
Evaluator's Signature:	Date:

CHECK #2	
Evaluator's Signature:	Date:

CHECK #3	
Evaluator's Signature:	Date:

Work Documentation Form(s)

*Progress Note Template can be downloaded from the Premium Website

ABHES Competency: MA.A.1.9.f Screen and follow up patient test results

CAAHEP Competencies: I.P.6 Perform patient screening using established protocols; I.P.10 Assist physician with patient care; I.A.2 Use language/verbal skills that enable patients' understanding; IV.P.8 Document patient care

Name_____ **Date**_____ **Score**_____

● COMPETENCY ASSESSMENT

Procedure 30-6:   Performing Eye Instillation

Task: Treat eye infections, soothe irritation, anesthetize, and dilate pupils.

Conditions:
- Sterile eye dropper for single use
- Sterile ophthalmic medication, either drops or ointment, as ordered by the provider
- Sterile gloves
- Tissues

Standards: Perform the Task within 10 minutes with a minimum score of _____ points, as determined by your instructor.

Competency Assessment Information

Tina Robinson presented in the office today with a history of wearing her contact lenses for 40 hours without removing them. After an eye examination, the provider diagnoses a corneal abrasion and orders antibiotic drops to the left eye. Document the procedure using the Progress Note Template (Work Documentation).

Time began: _____   **Time ended:** _____   **Total time:** _____

No.	Step	Points	Check #1	Check #2	Check #3
1	Wash hands.				
2	*Paying attention to detail,* assemble supplies using sterile technique.				
3	Verify the provider's order and prepare a medication card.				
4	Follow the "Six Rights" of medication administration.				
5	Work in a well-lighted, quiet, clean area.				
6	*Paying attention to detail,* review the medication card. Select the correct medication from the medication area.				
7	Compare the medication label with the medication card (first check).				
8	If unfamiliar with the medication, consult the PDR or other reputable reference.				
9	Check the expiration date.				
10	Compare the medication label with the medication card (second check).				
11	Carefully transport the medication to the patient exam room. Bring the medication card.				
12	Check the medication and medication card at the patient's bedside (third check).				
13	*Introduce yourself and identify patient.*				

No.	Step	Points	Check #1	Check #2	Check #3
14	***Explain procedure to the patient, speaking at the patient's level of understanding.*** State the name of the medication and the purpose of the injection. ***Allay the patient's fears regarding the procedure being performed and help the patient feel safe and comfortable.***				
15	Ask the patient about medication allergies.				
16	Position the patient in a sitting or lying position.				
17	Don gloves. Open the bottle and remove the cap without allowing anything to touch the dropper tip of the medication bottle.				
18	Have the patient look up at the ceiling and expose the lower conjunctival sac of the affected eye by gently pulling downward on the lower lid.				
19	Place the dropper lid as close to the eye as possible (without touching the eye or the lid). Brace the remaining fingers on the nose.				
20	Gently squeeze the bottle and administer one drop or appropriate amount of ointment (or as directed by the provider's order) into the pouch formed by the lower lid.				
21	Instruct the patient to close eye gently and keep closed for at least 60 to 90 seconds to allow the medication to bathe the eye.				
22	With the patient's eye closed, gently place your finger on the lower lid at the nasal corner to occlude the tear duct. This will inhibit the drops and any additional tearing that the eye drops might cause from flowing into the tear draining system.				
23	Blot excess medication and tears from the patient's face with tissues.				
24	Dispose of supplies in appropriate biohazard container.				
25	Wash hands.				
26	If the patient is to continue with medications at home, instruct regarding continued administration of eye preparation.				
27	Accurately record the administration of medication to include name of medication, dose, route, date, time and initials. Also document patient teaching.				
Student's Total Points					
Points Possible					
Final Score (Student's Total Points/Possible Points)					

Instructor's/Evaluator's Comments and Suggestions:

_____

_____

_____

_____

_____

_____

_____

CHECK #1	
Evaluator's Signature:	Date:

CHECK #2	
Evaluator's Signature:	Date:

CHECK #3	
Evaluator's Signature:	Date:

Work Documentation Form(s)

*Progress Note Template can be downloaded from the Premium Website

ABHES Competencies: MA.A.1.6.b Properly utilize PDR, drug handbook, and other drug references to identify a drug's classification, usual dosage, usual side effects, and contraindications; MA.A.1.9.g Maintain medication and immunization records

CAAHEP Competencies: I.P.9 Administer parenteral medications; I.A.2 Use language/verbal skills that enable patient's understanding; III.P.4 Perform hand washing; IV.P.6 Prepare a patient for procedures and/or treatments; IV.P.8 Document patient care

Name_____ **Date**_____ **Score**_____

COMPETENCY ASSESSMENT

Procedure 30-7: Performing Eye Patch Dressing Application

Task: Apply a sterile eye patch.

Conditions:
- Tape
- Sterile eye patch
- Sterile gloves

Standards: Perform the Task within 10 minutes with a minimum score of _____ points, as determined by your instructor.

Competency Assessment Information

Michelle O'Steen is seen in the office today with a history of a foreign body in her right eye. The provider has instructed you, the medical assistant, to apply a sterile eye patch after eye irrigation. Document the procedure using the Progress Note Template (Work Documentation).

Time began: _____ **Time ended:** _____ **Total time:** _____

No.	Step	Points	Check #1	Check #2	Check #3
1	Wash hands. *Paying attention to detail,* gather appropriate equipment and supplies.				
2	*Introduce yourself and identify patient.*				
3	*Explain the procedure, speaking at the patient's level of understanding.* Assure that the patient has a ride home.				
4	Position the patient in a sitting or supine position.				
5	Instruct the patient to close both eyes during the application of the patch. Open package containing the sterile eye patch, observing sterile technique. Don sterile gloves.				
6	Place the patch over the affected eye.				
7	Secure the patch with three to four strips of transparent tape diagonally from mid-forehead to below the ear.				
8	Remove gloves and dispose of in appropriate biohazard waste container.				
9	Instruct patient regarding length of time to wear patch and return visit to provider.				
10	Accurately record the application of a sterile eye patch and patient education in the patient's chart or electronic medical record.				
Student's Total Points					
Points Possible					
Final Score (Student's Total Points/Possible Points)					

Instructor's/Evaluator's Comments and Suggestions:

_____

_____

_____

_____

_____

_____

_____

CHECK #1	
Evaluator's Signature:	Date:

CHECK #2	
Evaluator's Signature:	Date:

CHECK #3	
Evaluator's Signature:	Date:

Work Documentation Form(s)

*Progress Note Template can be downloaded from the Premium Website

ABHES Competencies: MA.A.1.4.a Document accurately; MA.A.1.9.b Apply principles of aseptic techniques and infection control; MA.A.1.9.d Recognize and understand various treatment protocols; MA.A.1.9.m Assist physician with routine and specialty examinations and treatments

CAAHEP Competencies: I.P.10 Assist physician with patient care; I.A.2 Use language/verbal skills that enable the patients' understanding; IV.P.6 Prepare a patient for procedures and/or treatments; IV.P.8 Document patient care; IV.P.9 Document patient education

Name _____   **Date** _____   **Score** _____

● **COMPETENCY ASSESSMENT**

Procedure 30-8:   Performing Eye Irrigation

Task: Irrigate the patient's eye to remove foreign debris, cleanse discharge, remove chemicals, or apply antiseptic.

Conditions:
- Sterile irrigation solution as ordered by the provider
- Sterile bulb syringe (rubber)
- Kidney-shaped basin to catch irrigation solution
- Sterile basin
- Sterile gauze 2 × 2s
- Sterile gloves
- Biohazard waste container
- Towel
- Pillow

Standards: Perform the Task within 15 minutes with a minimum score of _____ points, as determined by your instructor.

Competency Assessment Information

Michelle O'Steen is seen in the office today with a history of a foreign body in her right eye. The provider has instructed you, the medical assistant, to irrigate the right eye. The ordered solution is 0.9% sodium chloride. Document the procedure using the Progress Note Template (Work Documentation).

Time began: _____   **Time ended:** _____   **Total time:** _____

No.	Step	Points	Check #1	Check #2	Check #3
1	Wash hands. *Paying attention to detail,* gather appropriate equipment and supplies.				
2	*Introduce yourself and identify patient.*				
3	*Explain the procedure to the patient, speaking at the patient's level of understanding.*				
4	Position the patient in the supine position.				
5	Check the solution and the provider's order (first check).				
6	Warm the solution to body temperature (98.6°F). Check the expiration date on the solution.				
7	Check the label with the provider's order (second check).				
8	Have the patient turn her head to the side of the affected eye.				
9	Place a towel over that shoulder to absorb any fluid that splashes.				
10	Place the kidney basin along the affected side of the face to catch the irrigation solution.				

No.	Step	Points	Check #1	Check #2	Check #3
11	Open the sterile basin using sterile technique.				
12	Open the sterile bulb syringe and flip into the sterile basin.				
13	Open and flip 3 packages of sterile 2 × 2 gauze sponges onto the sterile field.				
14	Check the label of the irrigation solution against the provider's order (third check).				
15	Carefully pour the sterile solution into the sterile basin.				
16	Don sterile gloves.				
17	Moisten two to three gauze sponges in the sterile saline. If indicated, clean the eyelid and eyelashes of the affected eye from the nasal side to the outer aspect of the eyelid. Discard the sponge after each wipe.				
18	Expose the lower conjunctiva by separating the eyelids with the index finger and the thumb of your non-dominant hand.				
19	Instruct the patient to stare at a fixed spot during the procedure.				
20	Fill the bulb syringe with the sterile irrigation.				
21	Irrigate the affected eye with sterile solution by resting the sterile bulb syringe on the bridge of the patient's nose, being careful not to touch the eye or conjunctival sac with the syringe tip. Gently squeeze the bulb syringe to allow the flow of irrigation from the inner corner to the outer corner of the eye.				
22	Repeat several times until the debris is dislodged.				
23	After irrigation, dry the eyelid and eyelashes with a sterile gauze sponge. Before disposing of the setup, consult the provider. If needed, there may be a stain added to the irrigation to detect corneal abrasions.				
24	Assist the provider as needed.				
25	Discard the supplies as indicated in biohazard waste containers.				
26	Remove and discard gloves appropriately.				
27	Wash hands.				
28	Accurately record the irrigation process in the patient's chart or electronic medical record.				
Student's Total Points					
Points Possible					
Final Score (Student's Total Points/Possible Points)					

Instructor's/Evaluator's Comments and Suggestions:

_____

_____

_____

_____

_____

_____

_____

CHECK #1	
Evaluator's Signature:	Date:

CHECK #2	
Evaluator's Signature:	Date:

CHECK #3	
Evaluator's Signature:	Date:

Work Documentation Form(s)

*Progress Note Template can be downloaded from the Premium Website

ABHES Competencies: MA.A.1.4.a Document accurately; MA.A.1.9.b Apply principles of aseptic techniques and infection control; MA.A.1.9.d Recognize and understand various treatment protocols; MA.A.1.9.m Assist physician with routine and specialty examinations and treatments

CAAHEP Competencies: I.P.10 Assist physician with patient care; I.A.2 Use language/verbal skills that enable the patients' understanding; IV.P.6 Prepare a patient for procedures and/or treatments; IV.P.8 Document patient care; IV.P.9 Document patient education

Name _____ **Date** _____ **Score** _____

● COMPETENCY ASSESSMENT

Procedure 30-9:   Performing Ear Irrigation

Task: Remove impacted cerumen, discharge, or foreign materials from the ear canal as directed by the provider.

Conditions:
• Sterile irrigation solution as ordered by the provider, warmed to 98.6° to 103°F
• Bulb syringe
• Kidney-shaped or emesis (catch) basin
• Sterile basin
• Impervious pad to protect the patient's clothing
• Cotton balls

Standards: Perform the Task within 25 minutes with a minimum score of _____ points, as determined by your instructor.

Competency Assessment Information

Dennis Dinges is a 74-year-old man seen in the office with the complaint of decreased hearing in his left ear. Upon examination by the provider, copious amounts of cerumen are visualized. The provider orders 0.9% solution of sodium chloride at body temperature for irrigation to remove the cerumen. Document the procedure using the Progress Note Template (Work Documentation).

Time began: _____   **Time ended:** _____   **Total time:** _____

No.	Step	Points	Check #1	Check #2	Check #3
1	Wash hands. ***Paying attention to detail,*** gather appropriate equipment and supplies.				
2	***Introduce yourself and identify patient.***				
3	***Explain the procedure and expectations to the patient, speaking at the patient's level of understanding.*** Include the information that the patient might feel a bit of discomfort and that dizziness is not unusual as the fluid comes in contact with the tympanic membrane.				
4	Assist the patient into a comfortable sitting position.				
5	Check the label on the sterile solution and the provider's order (first check).				
6	Check the expiration date.				
7	Place the impervious drape on the patient's shoulder to protect her clothing.				
8	Pour the warmed, sterile irrigation into the sterile basin. Check the label and the provider's order (second check).				
9	Instruct the patient to tilt her head toward the affected side.				
10	Check the label and the provider's order (third check).				

No.	Step	Points	Check #1	Check #2	Check #3
11	Don gloves.				
12	Tilt the patient's head slightly forward and to the affected side.				
13	Place the kidney basin (or emesis basin) under the affected ear and ask the patient to assist by holding it steady.				
14	Fill the bulb syringe with the warmed solution.				
15	With the non-dominant hand, gently pull the auricle upward and back to straighten the ear canal (for adults).				
16	Instruct the patient to immediately inform you of any severe discomfort or pain. If reported, stop immediately and report the findings to the provider.				
17	Expel air from the syringe, leaving the warmed solution filling the bulb and the neck of the syringe. Carefully and gently, insert the syringe tip into the affected ear. Do not insert the tip too deeply. Do not occlude the external auditory canal.				
18	Very gently, squeeze the bulb syringe to deliver a slow, steady stream of warmed fluid in an upward direction into the ear canal. Allow the fluid and debris to drain out into the kidney basin.				
19	Repeat Steps 17 to 18 as ordered by the provider.				
20	Blot the outer ear dry.				
21	Notify the provider to re-examine the ear to assure that the procedure is completed.				
22	If procedure is complete, remove the kidney basin. Discard the contents as indicated per OSHA guidelines.				
23	Instruct the patient to lie on the affected side with a towel under her head to complete drainage of the ear. • Report any pain or dizziness to the provider. • Do not insert any foreign object into the ear canal.				
24	Appropriately dispose of any remaining supplies.				
25	Remove gloves. Wash hands.				
26	Accurately record the type and amount of irrigation utilized. Describe any cerumen noted in irrigation in the patient's paper chart or electronic medical record. Record any complaints of pain or dizziness and provider notification.				
Student's Total Points					
Points Possible					
Final Score (Student's Total Points/Possible Points)					

Instructor's/Evaluator's Comments and Suggestions:

_____

_____

_____

_____

_____

_____

_____

CHECK #1	
Evaluator's Signature:	Date:

CHECK #2	
Evaluator's Signature:	Date:

CHECK #3	
Evaluator's Signature:	Date:

Work Documentation Form(s)

*Progress Note Template can be downloaded from the Premium Website

ABHES Competencies: MA.A.1.4.a Document accurately; MA.A.1.9.b Apply principles of aseptic techniques and infection control; MA.A.1.9.d Recognize and understand various treatment protocols; MA.A.1.9.m Assist physician with routine and specialty examinations and treatments

CAAHEP Competencies: I.P.10 Assist physician with patient care; I.A.2 Use language/verbal skills that enable the patients' understanding; IV.P.6 Prepare a patient for procedures and/or treatments; IV.P.8 Document patient care; IV.P.9 Document patient education

Name_____ **Date**_____ **Score**_____

● COMPETENCY ASSESSMENT

Procedure 30-10: Assisting with Audiometry

Task: Assist in testing patient for hearing loss.

Conditions:
- Audiometer with headphones
- Quiet room

Standards: Perform the Task within 20 minutes with a minimum score of _____ points, as determined by your instructor.

Competency Assessment Information

Seven-year-old Katie McKey is seen in the office for a routine checkup. Her mother reports that recently, her second grade teacher has had to repeat instructions for Katie. The provider wishes to include audiometry in this office visit. Document the procedure using the Progress Note Template (Work Documentation).

Time began: _____ **Time ended:** _____ **Total time:** _____

No.	Step	Points	Check #1	Check #2	Check #3
1	Wash hands. *Paying attention to detail,* gather appropriate equipment and supplies.				
2	*Introduce yourself and identify patient.*				
3	*Explain the procedure and expectations to the patient, speaking at the patient's level of understanding.* Reinforce the instruction to patient to raise her hand when a new frequency is heard.				
4	Assure that the room is quiet without extraneous noises.				
5	Assist the patient into a comfortable sitting position.				
6	Assist the patient to apply the earphones and adjust for fit and comfort.				
7	If the medical assistant has been trained to perform the procedure, the provider may authorize the medical assistant to perform the audiometry. Begin the audiometry with the audiometer set at the lowest frequency. The patient will indicate when the first sound is heard and the medical assistant will plot this information on the appropriate graph (the audiogram).				
8	The frequency is gradually increased and information plotted until the exam is completed.				
9	The other ear is checked in the same manner.				
10	*Accurately and concisely provide the information to the provider* for interpretation.				

No.	Step	Points	Check #1	Check #2	Check #3
11	Clean the equipment as indicated by manufacturer's instructions.				
12	Wash hands.				
13	Accurately record the procedure in the patient's paper chart or electronic medical record.				
Student's Total Points					
Points Possible					
Final Score (Student's Total Points/Possible Points)					

Instructor's/Evaluator's Comments and Suggestions:

_____

_____

_____

_____

_____

_____

_____

CHECK #1	
Evaluator's Signature:	Date:

CHECK #2	
Evaluator's Signature:	Date:

CHECK #3	
Evaluator's Signature:	Date:

Work Documentation Form(s)

*Progress Note Template can be downloaded from the Premium Website

ABHES Competencies: MA.A.1.4.a Document accurately; MA.A.1.9.d Recognize and understand various treatment protocols; MA.A.1.9.m Assist physician with routine and specialty examinations and treatments

CAAHEP Competencies: I.P.10 Assist physician with patient care; I.A.2 Use language/verbal skills that enable the patients' understanding; IV.P.6 Prepare a patient for procedures and/or treatments; IV.P.8 Document patient care; IV.P.9 Document patient education; IX.P.2 Perform within scope of practice

Name_____ **Date**_____ **Score**_____

● **COMPETENCY ASSESSMENT**

Procedure 30-11: Performing Ear Instillation

Task: Soften impacted cerumen, fight infection with antibiotics, or relieve pain by instilling medication into ear.

Conditions:
- Otic medication as prescribed by the provider
- Sterile ear dropper
- Cotton balls
- Gloves

Standards: Perform the Task within 15 minutes with a minimum score of _____ points, as determined by your instructor.

Competency Assessment Information

After Sean Mitchell has been examined by the provider, it is determined that Sean has swimmer's ear. Dr. Thompson has ordered an instillation of Burow's solution in the office and education for Sean's mother to continue these instillations at home. Document the procedure using the Progress Note Template (Work Documentation).

Time began: _____ **Time ended:** _____ **Total time:** _____

No.	Step	Points	Check #1	Check #2	Check #3
1	Wash hands. *Paying attention to detail,* gather appropriate equipment and supplies.				
2	*Introduce yourself and identify patient.*				
3	*Explain procedure to the patient, speaking at the patient's level of understanding.*				
4	Ask patient either to lie on unaffected side or to sit with head tilted toward unaffected ear.				
5	*Paying attention to detail,* check otic medication three times against the provider's order and check expiration date of the medication.				
6	Put on gloves.				
7	Draw up the prescribed amount of medication.				
8	Gently pull the top of the ear upward and back (adult) or pull earlobe downward and backward (child).				
9	Instill prescribed dose of medication (number of drops) by squeezing rubber bulb on dropper into the affected ear.				
10	Have the patient maintain the position for about 5 minutes to retain medication.				
11	When instructed by the provider, insert moistened cotton ball into external ear canal for 15 minutes.				
12	Dispose of supplies.				

No.	Step	Points	Check #1	Check #2	Check #3
13	Remove gloves and wash hands.				
14	Accurately document procedure in patient's chart or electronic medical record.				
Student's Total Points					
Points Possible					
Final Score (Student's Total Points/Possible Points)					

Instructor's/Evaluator's Comments and Suggestions:

_____

_____

_____

_____

_____

_____

_____

CHECK #1 Evaluator's Signature:	Date:

CHECK #2 Evaluator's Signature:	Date:

CHECK #3 Evaluator's Signature:	Date:

Work Documentation Form(s)

*Progress Note Template can be downloaded from the Premium Website

ABHES Competencies: MA.A.1.4.a Document accurately; MA.A.1.6.a Demonstrate accurate occupational math and metric conversions for proper medication administration; MA.A.1.9.d Recognize and understand various treatment protocols; MA.A.1.9.g Maintain medication and immunization records; MA.A.1.9.j Prepare and administer oral and parenteral medications as directed by physician

CAAHEP Competencies: I.P.9 Administer parenteral (excluding IV) medications; I.P.10 Assist physician with patient care; I.A.2 Use language/verbal skills that enable the patients' understanding; II.P.1 Prepare proper dosages of medication for administration; II.A.1 Verify ordered doses/dosages prior to administration; III.P.4 Perform hand washing; III.A.2 Explain the rationale for performance of a procedure to the patient; IV.P.6 Prepare a patient for procedures and/or treatments; IV.P.8. Document patient care; IX.P.7 Document accurately in the patient record

Name_____ **Date**_____ **Score**_____

● **COMPETENCY ASSESSMENT**

Procedure 30-12:   Assisting with Nasal Examination

Task: Assist the provider with the nasal examination when looking for polyps and engorged superficial blood vessels, and assist in the possible removal of a foreign body.

Conditions: • Nasal speculum
                • Light source
                • Disposable, nonsterile gloves
                • Bayonet forceps
                • Kidney basin

Standards: Perform the Task within 15 minutes with a minimum score of _____ points, as determined by your instructor.

Competency Assessment Information

Three-year-old LaWanda Green was playing with marbles. Her mother noticed that LaWanda's left nare was distorted and upon examination, saw that LaWanda had inserted a marble in her nose. They are in your provider's office in order to have the marble removed. Document the procedure using the Progress Note Template (Work Documentation).

Time began: _____   **Time ended:** _____   **Total time:** _____

No.	Step	Points	Check #1	Check #2	Check #3
1	Wash hands. ***Paying attention to detail,*** gather appropriate equipment and supplies.				
2	***Introduce yourself and identify patient.***				
3	***Explain the procedure and expectations to the patient, speaking at the patient's level of understanding.***				
4	Assist the patient to sit in a comfortable position.				
5	***Allay the patient's fears regarding the procedure being performed and help him feel safe and comfortable.***				
6	Put on gloves.				
7	Assist the provider by handing the equipment and supplies as needed/requested.				
8	Appropriately discard disposable supplies according to OSHA guidelines.				
9	Sanitize non-disposable instruments following office procedures.				
10	Remove gloves and dispose of appropriately. Wash hands.				
11	Accurately document procedure in patient's chart or electronic medical record, noting foreign object if applicable.				
Student's Total Points					
Points Possible					
Final Score (Student's Total Points/Possible Points)					

Instructor's/Evaluator's Comments and Suggestions:

_____

_____

_____

_____

_____

_____

_____

CHECK #1	
Evaluator's Signature:	Date:

CHECK #2	
Evaluator's Signature:	Date:

CHECK #3	
Evaluator's Signature:	Date:

Work Documentation Form(s)

*Progress Note Template can be downloaded from the Premium Website

ABHES Competencies: MA.A.1.4.a Document accurately; MA.A.1.9.d Recognize and understand various treatment protocols; MA.A.1.9.l Prepare patient for examinations and treatments; MA.A.1.9.m Assist physician with routine and specialty examinations and treatments

CAAHEP Competencies: I.P.10 Assist physician with patient care; I.A.1 Apply critical thinking skills in performing patient assessment and care; I.A.2 Use language/verbal skills that enable the patients' understanding; III.A.2 Explain the rationale for performance of a procedure to the patient; IV.P.6 Prepare a patient for procedures and/or treatments; IV.P.8 Document patient care; IX.P.7 Document accurately in the patient record

Name_____ **Date**_____ **Score**_____

● **COMPETENCY ASSESSMENT**

Procedure 30-13: Cautery Treatment of Epistaxis

Task: Assist the provider with treatment and control of nose bleeding.

Conditions:
- Patient gown and drapes
- Syringe and needles
- Kidney basin
- Tissues
- Vienna nasal speculum
- Light source (hands free)
- Electrocautery
- Gloves, and other PPE if bleeding is severe
- Bayonet forceps
- Epinephrine
- Silver nitrate sticks
- Cotton balls or 2 × 2 gauze sponges
- Nasal packaging or nasal tampons
- Absorbable packaging
- Medicine cups
- Local anesthetic (such as Xylocaine [lidocaine] with epinephrine or cocaine 4%)
- Antibiotic/antiseptic ointment (such as triamcinolone)

Standards: Perform the Task within 20 minutes with a minimum score of _____ points, as determined by your instructor.

Competency Assessment Information

Ethel Hodgens is in the office today c/o prolonged nose bleed. She lives in a home with forced air, gas heat. It has had a severe drying effect on her nasal mucosa. Your provider instructs you to set up a tray and assist him in attempting to control the bleeding. Document the procedure using the Progress Note Template (Work Documentation).

Time began: _____   **Time ended:** _____   **Total time:** _____

No.	Step	Points	Check #1	Check #2	Check #3
1	Wash hands. ***Paying attention to detail,*** gather appropriate equipment and supplies.				
2	Provide kidney basin and tissues to allow the patient to manage bleeding until provider can intervene.				
3	Instruct the patient to pinch all the soft structures of the nose between the thumb and index finger and press against the bones of the face. Have the patient lean forward with his head tilted forward until the provider can intervene.				
4	***Introduce yourself and identify the patient. Explain the procedure and expectations, speaking at the patient's level of understanding. Allay the patient's fears regarding the procedure being performed and help them feel safe and comfortable.***				

No.	Step	Points	Check #1	Check #2	Check #3
5	Assist the patient into a comfortable sitting position.				
6	Monitor patient to assure maintenance of airway and breathing.				
7	Don non-sterile, disposable gloves.				
8	Assist the provider by handing the equipment and supplies as needed/requested.				
9	If instructed by the provider, use a syringe and needle to withdraw the prescribed amount of anesthetic and inject it carefully into a medicine cup being careful to avoid splashing. Soak cotton balls or gauze sponges in the anesthetic agent.				
10	As instructed by provider, hand instruments and medication soaked packaging as needed.				
11	Remain with patient as anesthesia takes effect.				
12	Assist the provider as needed to apply vasoconstrictive medication on cotton balls or 2 × 2s to the site of the bleeding.				
13	Apply pressure to the external aspect of the nose if instructed by the provider.				
14	If the bleeding is controlled, skip to Step 16. If the bleeding is not controlled, prepare electrocautery or silver nitrate sticks per provider preference.				
15	If bleeding is controlled, skip to Step 16. If the bleeding continues, prepare nasal packaging or nasal tampons per provider preference.				
16	***Speaking at the patient's level of understanding and including the patient's support system***, instruct patient per provider's orders regarding post-epistaxis care. • Nasal packaging should remain in place for 24 to 48 hours • A follow-up appointment must be made with an otolaryngologist for further treatment • Avoid aspirin or anti-inflammatory medications				
17	Gather and dispose of equipment per OSHA guidelines. Sanitize non-disposable instruments following office procedures.				
18	Remove gloves and dispose of appropriately. Wash hands.				
19	Accurately document the procedure in the patient's chart or electronic medical record. Include medications, dose, route, time and date, and initials. Document patient education.				
Student's Total Points					
Points Possible					
Final Score (Student's Total Points/Possible Points)					

Instructor's/Evaluator's Comments and Suggestions:

_____
_____
_____
_____
_____
_____
_____

CHECK #1	
Evaluator's Signature:	Date:

CHECK #2	
Evaluator's Signature:	Date:

CHECK #3	
Evaluator's Signature:	Date:

Work Documentation Form(s)

*Progress Note Template can be downloaded from the Premium Website

ABHES Competencies: MA.A.1.4.a Document accurately; MA.A.1.9.d Recognize and understand various treatment protocols; MA.A.1.9.e Recognize emergencies and treatments and minor office surgical procedures; MA.A.1.9.i Use standard precautions; MA.A.1.9.l Prepare patient for examinations and treatments; MA.A.1.9.m Assist physician with routine and specialty examinations and treatments; MA.A.1.9.n Assist physician with minor office surgical procedures

CAAHEP Competencies: I.P.9 Administer parenteral (excluding IV) medications; I.P.10 Assist physician with patient care; I.A.2 Use language/verbal skills that enable the patients' understanding; II.P.1 Prepare proper dose/dosages of medication; III.P.3 Select appropriate barrier/personal protective equipment (PPE) for potentially infectious situations; III.A.2 Explain the rationale for performance of a procedure to the patient; IV.P.6 Prepare a patient for procedures and/or treatments; IV.P.8 Document patient care; IV.P.9 Document patient education; IX.P.4 Practice within the standard of care for a medical assistant; IX.P.7 Document accurately in the patient record; XI.P.10 Perform first aid procedures

Name_____ **Date**_____ **Score**_____

● COMPETENCY ASSESSMENT

Procedure 30-14: Performing Nasal Instillation

Task: Provide medication to the nasal membranes as ordered by the provider.

Conditions: • Nasal medication, drops or spray, as ordered by provider
                 • Medicine dropper (sterile)
                 • Tissues
                 • Nonsterile disposable gloves

Standards: Perform the Task within 15 minutes with a minimum score of _____ points, as determined by
                 your instructor.

Competency Assessment Information

Ryan Adams has allergic rhinitis. Your provider has instructed you to assist Ryan with the first dose of his medication. Document the procedure using the Progress Note Template (Work Documentation).

Time began: _____   **Time ended:** _____   **Total time:** _____

No.	Step	Points	Check #1	Check #2	Check #3
1	Wash hands. ***Paying attention to detail,*** gather appropriate equipment and supplies.				
2	***Introduce yourself and identify patient.***				
3	***Explain procedure and expectations to the patient, speaking at the patient's level of understanding.***				
4	Assist the patient to sit comfortably with the head tilted back slightly.				
5	***Paying attention to detail,*** compare the nasal medication to the provider's order (first check).				
6	Check the expiration date.				
7	If the medication is not a single-user, self-contained dropper, calculate the medication.				
8	Compare the medication and the provider's order (second check).				
9	Don nonsterile disposable gloves if indicated.				
10	Compare the medication and the provider's order (third check).				
11	Utilize the sterile dropper or the self-contained dropper with the medication ready into the center of the nostril. Take care not to touch the inside of the nasal passage.				
12	Instruct the patient to inhale during the instillation of the nasal drops.				
13	Instill the prescribed dose.				

No.	Step	Points	Check #1	Check #2	Check #3
14	Repeat the procedure for the other nostril if ordered. Provide tissues to the patient for management of any drainage.				
15	*Speaking at the level of the patient's understanding,* instruct the patient not to blow nose after treatment in order to keep the medication in contact with the mucous membranes of the nasal passages.				
16	If utilizing a dropper, dispose of properly per OSHA guidelines. If non-disposable, follow office procedure for sanitization and sterilization. If utilizing a self-contained medication, recap using sterile technique.				
17	Remove gloves and dispose of appropriately.				
18	Wash hands.				
19	Accurately record the administration of medication to include name of medication, dose, route, date, time and initials.				
Student's Total Points					
Points Possible					
Final Score (Student's Total Points/Possible Points)					

Instructor's/Evaluator's Comments and Suggestions:

_____
_____
_____
_____
_____
_____
_____

CHECK #1	
Evaluator's Signature:	Date:

CHECK #2	
Evaluator's Signature:	Date:

CHECK #3	
Evaluator's Signature:	Date:

Work Documentation Form(s)

*Progress Note Template can be downloaded from the Premium Website

ABHES Competencies: MA.A.1.4.a Document accurately; MA.A.1.9.d Recognize and understand various treatment protocols; MA.A.1.9.g Maintain medication and immunization records; MA.A.1.9.j Prepare and administer oral and parenteral medications as directed by physician; MA.A.1.9.l Prepare patient for examinations and treatments

CAAHEP Competencies: I.P.9 Administer parenteral (excluding IV) medications; I.P.10 Assist physician with patient care; I.A.2 Use language/verbal skills that enable the patients' understanding; II.P.1 Prepare proper dose/dosages of medication; II.A.1 Verify ordered doses/dosages prior to administration; III.P.4 Perform hand washing; III.A.2 Explain the rationale for performance of a procedure to the patient; IV.P.6 Prepare a patient for procedures and/or treatments; IV.P.8 Document patient care; IX.P.7 Document accurately in the patient record

Name_____ **Date**_____ **Score**_____

COMPETENCY ASSESSMENT

Procedure 30-15:   Administer Oxygen by Nasal Cannula for Minor Respiratory Distress

Task: Provide a low dose of concentrated oxygen to a patient during periods of respiratory distress (e.g., chronic obstructive pulmonary disease).

Conditions: • Portable D cylinder oxygen tank with stand
                 • Disposable nasal cannula with 6 ft tubing
                 • Flowmeter with Christmas tree adapter
                 • Pressure regulator with gauge

Standards: Perform the task within 15 minutes with a minimum score of _____ points, as determined by your instructor.

Competency Assessment Information

Mr. Edwards has COPD. It has been determined using a pulse oximeter that his O_2 sat upon exertion is 86%. Dr. Wagner has ordered O_2 via nasal cannula at 2 liters/min. You are following the provider's orders and applying oxygen prior to the patient leaving the office. Document the procedure using the Progress Note Template (Work Documentation).

Time began: _____   **Time ended:** _____   **Total time:** _____

No.	Step	Points	Check #1	Check #2	Check #3
1	Wash hands.				
2	*Paying attention to detail,* gather appropriate equipment and supplies.				
3	*Introduce yourself and identify patient. Explain procedure and expectations to the patient, speaking at the patient's level of understanding. Allay the patient's fears regarding the procedure and help him feel safe and comfortable.*				
4	Open the cylinder with one full turn in a counterclockwise direction.				
5	Check the pressure gauge to assure that oxygen is present in the tank.				
6	Attach the nasal cannula and tubing to the Christmas tree adapter on the flowmeter.				
7	Adjust the flow rate according to the provider's order (first check).				
8	Check the nasal cannula to assure that oxygen is flowing. Check the flow rate and provider's order (second check).				

No.	Step	Points	Check #1	Check #2	Check #3
9	Carefully place the nasal cannula into the nares of the patient with the tips curving inward to follow the curve of the nasal passage and the tab resting below the nose. Check with patient for comfort. Compare the flow rate and the provider's order (third check).				
10	Adjust the tubing around the patient's ears and adjust slide for comfort under the chin.				
11	Instruct the patient to breathe slowly through his nose in order to achieve the maximum benefit from oxygen therapy.				
12	Oxygen is flammable. Instruct the patient and family members that smoking is not allowed near the patient.				
13	Wash hands.				
14	Accurately document the procedure in patient's chart or electronic medical record to include name of medication, dose, route, date, time and initials.				
Student's Total Points					
Points Possible					
Final Score (Student's Total Points/Possible Points)					

Instructor's/Evaluator's Comments and Suggestions:

_____

_____

_____

_____

_____

_____

_____

CHECK #1	
Evaluator's Signature:	Date:

CHECK #2	
Evaluator's Signature:	Date:

CHECK #3	
Evaluator's Signature:	Date:

Work Documentation Form(s)

*Progress Note Template can be downloaded from the Premium Website

ABHES Competencies: MA.A.1.4.a Document accurately; MA.A.1.9.d Recognize and understand various treatment protocols; MA.A.1.9.g Maintain medication and immunization records; MA.A.1.9.l Prepare patient for examinations and treatments; MA.A.1.9.j Prepare and administer oral and parenteral medications as directed by physician

CAAHEP Competencies: I.P.9 Administer parenteral (excluding IV) medications; I.P.10 Assist physician with patient care; I.A.2 Use language/verbal skills that enable the patients' understanding; II.P.1 Prepare proper dose/dosages of medication; II.A.1 Verify ordered doses/dosages prior to administration; III.P.4 Perform hand washing; III.A.2 Explain the rationale for performance of a procedure to the patient; IV.P.6 Prepare a patient for procedures and/or treatments; IV.P.8 Document patient care; IV.P.9 Document patient education; IX.P.7 Document accurately in the patient record

Name_____ **Date**_____ **Score**_____

● **COMPETENCY ASSESSMENT**

Procedure 30-16: Instructing Patient in the Use of a Metered Dose Inhaler With and Without a Spacer

Task: Instruct patient on the use of a handheld device known as a metered dose inhaler.

Conditions: • Handheld inhaler with mouthpiece
• Spacer
• Medication as ordered by provider

Standards: Perform the Task within 20 minutes with a minimum score of _____ points, as determined by your instructor.

Competency Assessment Information

Tyler Shiflett has exercise-induced asthma. Dr. Miller has ordered Albuterol 2 puffs prior to football practice. You are in charge of teaching Tyler how to use his meter dose inhaler. Document the procedure using the Progress Note Template (Work Documentation).

Time began: _____ **Time ended:** _____ **Total time:** _____

No.	Step	Points	Check #1	Check #2	Check #3
1	Wash hands. ***Paying attention to detail***, gather appropriate equipment and supplies.				
2	Check the medication and the provider's order (first check).				
3	***Introduce yourself and identify patient. Speaking at the level of the patient's understanding, explain the procedure and expectations to the patient.***				
4	Check the medication and the provider's order (second check).				
5	Instruct the patient regarding: • The purpose of using the medication via the metered dose inhaler as it relates to the diagnosis • The dose and frequency of the medication • Breathing out completely prior to administering the dose • Shaking the inhaler to mobilize the medication • Inserting the mouthpiece between the teeth and closing the lips to create a seal • Breathing in slowly while simultaneously pressing the top of the inhaler once • Removing the inahler from the mouth • Holding breath for at least 10 seconds • Breathing out completely • Waiting 30 seconds if an additional dose is required • Shaking the inhaler again and repeating steps • Rinsing the mouth, especially if the inhaled medication contains a steroid				

No.	Step	Points	Check #1	Check #2	Check #3
6	Check the medication and the provider's order (third check).				
7	If a spacer is to be used, skip to Step 12.				
8	Review and simulate the use of the metered dose inhaler (MDI) and then have the patient return the demonstration.				
9	After administration of the dose, note any patient condition changes or comments. Record in the patient record.				
10	Replace the cap on the MDI when finished.				
11	Instruct the patient on the care of the MDI to include: • Storing at room temperature • After use, removing the metal canister from the plastic mouth piece and spacer (if utilized) and cleaning with mild soap and water and leaving to dry overnight • Never using water on the metal canister • Reassembling the MDI • Reloading the MDI by spraying a puff into the air prior to the next dose				
12	If a spacer is to be used, instruct the patient on assembly: • Remove the cap on the MDI • Insert the MDI into the appropriate end of the spacer				
13	Follow Steps 5 to 10 above.				
14	Accurately document in patient's chart or electronic medical record the administration of medication to include name of medication, dose, route, date, time and initials. Document patient education.				
Student's Total Points					
Points Possible					
Final Score (Student's Total Points/Possible Points)					

Instructor's/Evaluator's Comments and Suggestions:

_____

_____

_____

_____

_____

_____

_____

CHECK #1	
Evaluator's Signature:	Date:

CHECK #2	
Evaluator's Signature:	Date:

CHECK #3	
Evaluator's Signature:	Date:

Work Documentation Form(s)

*Progress Note Template can be downloaded from the Premium Website

ABHES Competencies: MA.A.1.4.a Document accurately; MA.A.1.9.d Recognize and understand various treatment protocols; MA.A.1.9.g Maintain medication and immunization records; MA.A.1.9.j Prepare and administer oral and parenteral medications as directed by physician; MA.A.1.9.l Prepare patient for examinations and treatments; MA.A.1.9.m Assist physician with routine and specialty examinations and treatments

CAAHEP Competencies: I.P.9 Administer parenteral (excluding IV) medications; I.P.10 Assist physician with patient care; I.A.2 Use language/verbal skills that enable the patients' understanding; II.P.1 Prepare proper dose/dosages of medication; II.A.1 Verify ordered doses/dosages prior to administration; III.P.4 Perform hand washing; III.A.2 Explain the rationale for performance of a procedure to the patient; IV.P.5 Instruct patients according to their needs to promote health maintenance and disease prevention; IV.A.7 Demonstrate recognition of the patient's level of understanding in communication; IV.P.6 Prepare a patient for procedures and/or treatments; IV.P.8. Document patient care; IV.P.9 Document patient education; IX.P.7 Document accurately in the patient record

Name_____ **Date**_____ **Score**_____

⬤ **COMPETENCY ASSESSMENT**

Procedure 30-17: Spirometry

Task: Prepare a patient for a spirometry to obtain optimal test results. Assist with diagnosis of asthma and chronic obstructive pulmonary disease (COPD).

Conditions:
- Spirometer
- Disposable mouthpiece

Standards: Perform the Task within 20 minutes with a minimum score of _____ points, as determined by your instructor.

Competency Assessment Information

After using Albuterol, 2 puffs from a meter dose inhaler, Dr. Miller wants you to perform spirometry for Tyler Shiflett to assess the effectiveness of the medication. Document the procedure using the Progress Note Template (Work Documentation).

Time began: _____ **Time ended:** _____ **Total time:** _____

No.	Step	Points	Check #1	Check #2	Check #3
1	Wash hands. ***Paying attention to detail,*** gather appropriate equipment and supplies.				
2	***Introduce yourself and identify the patient.***				
3	***Explain the procedure and expectations to the patient, speaking at the patient's level of understanding. Allay the patient's fears regarding the procedure and help the patient feel safe and comfortable.***				
4	Include the following in the patient education: • The patient should not have eaten a large meal before the test. • The use of tobacco products must have been avoided 4–6 hours prior to the spirometry. • The patient will have received instructions from the provider regarding the use of bronchodilators or other inhalers prior to the testing. • When exhaling into the mouthpiece, the lips must form a tight seal. • Maximum effort is required for accurate test results.				
5	Allow the patient to practice several times to become familiar with the machine and the feel of the testing.				
6	Enter patient demographic data as required by the spirometry program. This will include the patient's height and weight.				

No.	Step	Points	Check #1	Check #2	Check #3
7	Place the nose clip on the patient's nose to assure that all exhalation occurs via the oral airway.				
8	Place the disposable mouthpiece on the spirometer.				
9	Instruct the patient that several readings may be needed to assure accurate test results for interpretation by the provider.				
10	Remind the patient to exhale forcibly and rapidly until unable to exhale any more air.				
11	Coach the patient during the inhalation and exhalation in order to achieve maximum results. Instruct the patient that he must continue to exhale until instructed to stop.				
12	Remind the patient to remain upright during the exhalation.				
13	***Be supportive and encouraging throughout the test. Attend to any special needs of the patients.***				
14	At the conclusion of the procedure, discard the disposable mouthpiece into biohazard container. Disinfect and sanitize the equipment per policy.				
15	Wash hands.				
16	***Concisely update the provider*** with the results of the spirometry for interpretation.				
17	Accurately record the procedure, the patient's tolerance of the procedure, and patient education. Affix the record of the spirometry in the patient's chart or scan into the medical record.				
Student's Total Points					
Points Possible					
Final Score (Student's Total Points/Possible Points)					

Instructor's/Evaluator's Comments and Suggestions:

_____

_____

_____

_____

_____

_____

_____

CHECK #1	
Evaluator's Signature:	Date:

CHECK #2	
Evaluator's Signature:	Date:

CHECK #3	
Evaluator's Signature:	Date:

Work Documentation Form(s)

*Progress Note Template can be downloaded from the Premium Website

ABHES Competencies: MA.A.1.4.a Document accurately; MA.A.1.9.d Recognize and understand various treatment protocols; MA.A.1.9.f Screen and follow up patient test results; MA.A.1.9.l Prepare patient for examinations and treatments; MA.A.1.9.m Assist physician with routine and specialty examinations and treatments; MA.A.1.9.o (2) Perform respiratory testing

CAAHEP Competencies: I.P.4 Perform pulmonary function testing; I.P.6 Perform patient screening using established protocols; I.P.10 Assist physician with patient care; I.A.1 Apply critical thinking skills in performing patient assessment and care; I.A.2 Use language/verbal skills that enable the patients' understanding; III.P.4 Perform hand washing; III.A.2 Explain the rationale for performance of a procedure to the patient; IV.P.5 Instruct patients according to their needs to promote health maintenance and disease prevention; IV.A.7 Demonstrate recognition of the patient's level of understanding in communication; IV.P.6 Prepare a patient for procedures and/or treatments; IV.P.8 Document patient care; IV.P.9 Document patient education; IX.P.7 Document accurately in the patient record

Name_____ **Date**_____ **Score**_____

● **COMPETENCY ASSESSMENT**

Procedure 30-18: Pulse Oximetry

Task: Measure arterial oxyhemoglobin saturation within seconds by using an external sensor.

Conditions:
- Pulse oximeter
- Sensor
- Soap and water or alcohol wipe
- Nail polish remover, if needed

Standards: Perform the Task within 3 minutes with a minimum score of _____ points, as determined by your instructor.

Competency Assessment Information

Ms. Tomalina Hastings is at the clinic for management of her COPD. In order for Dr. Miller to assess her status, he orders an O$_2$ saturation using a pulse oximeter. Document the procedure using the Progress Note Template (Work Documentation).

Time began: _____ **Time ended:** _____ **Total time:** _____

No.	Step	Points	Check #1	Check #2	Check #3
1	Wash hands. ***Paying attention to detail,*** gather appropriate equipment and supplies.				
2	***Introduce yourself and identify patient.***				
3	***Explain the procedure and expectations to the patient, speaking at the patient's level of understanding.***				
4	Select a site for the sensor (finger commonly used). Adequate circulation is required for an accurate reading, so move to other sites if fingers are cold or peripheral vascular disease limits circulation to the hands.				
5	Make sure the site is clean. If fingers are to be utilized, have the patient wash hands with soap and water. If fingernail polish is present, remove. If a site other than the hands is to be utilized, clean with an alcohol prep pad.				
6	Secure the sensor to the cable. Assure a tight connection between the cable and the pulse oximeter.				
7	Apply the sensor to the selected site. If applied to a finger, insert the finger into the sensor clip. For an earlobe, insert as much of the earlobe as possible into the specialized sensor. If a forehead is to be utilized, apply the appropriate sensor and secure with adhesive strip provided.				

No.	Step	Points	Check #1	Check #2	Check #3
8	Turn the pulse oximeter on. A tone can be heard and a pulse fluctuation can be seen on the digital readout. Adjust the volume.				
9	Review the alarm parameters.				
10	Palpate the patient's pulse and compare to the digital representation of the pulse to assure an accurate reading.				
11	Refer to manufacturer's information if trouble-shooting is required.				
12	*Accurately and concisely update the provider* with results.				
13	Accurately document procedure in patient's chart or electronic medical record, noting type of sensor used, site of application, and results.				
14	Plug in oximeter for recharging when not in use so that the battery does not get low.				
Student's Total Points					
Points Possible					
Final Score (Student's Total Points/Possible Points)					

Instructor's/Evaluator's Comments and Suggestions:

_____

_____

_____

_____

_____

_____

_____

CHECK #1	
Evaluator's Signature:	Date:

CHECK #2	
Evaluator's Signature:	Date:

CHECK #3	
Evaluator's Signature:	Date:

Work Documentation Form(s)

*Progress Note Template can be downloaded from the Premium Website

ABHES Competencies: MA.A.1.4.a Document accurately; MA.A.1.9.d Recognize and understand various treatment protocols; MA.A.1.9.f Screen and follow up patient test results; MA.A.1.9.l Prepare patient for examinations and treatments; MA.A.1.9.m Assist physician with routine and specialty examinations and treatments

CAAHEP Competencies: I.P.6 Perform patient screening using established protocols; I.P.10 Assist physician with patient care; I.A.1 Apply critical thinking skills in performing patient assessment and care; I.A.2 Use language/verbal skills that enable the patients' understanding; III.A.2 Explain the rationale for performance of a procedure to the patient; IV.A.7 Demonstrate recognition of the patient's level of understanding in communication; IV.P.6 Prepare a patient for procedures and/or treatments; IV.P.8 Document patient care; IX.P.7 Document accurately in the patient record

Name _____ **Date** _____ **Score** _____

● **COMPETENCY ASSESSMENT**

Procedure 30-19: Assisting with Plaster Cast Application

Task: Assist provider in cast application.

Conditions:
- Plaster or fiberglass casting material
- Container of warm water, lined with plastic or cloth to catch loose plaster
- Stockinette (diameter based on limb to be immobilized)
- Webril (sheet wadding) padding material
- Bandage scissors
- Rubber gloves
- Sponge rubber for padding

Standards: Perform the Task within 25 minutes with a minimum score of _____ points, as determined by your instructor.

Competency Assessment Information

14-year-old Thomas Myers fell while skateboarding and sustained a Colles fracture of his right wrist. Dr. McDonald plans to sedate Thomas and reduce the fracture and apply a short arm cast to his right arm. Dr. McDonald asks you to set up the cast room for the procedure. Document the procedure using the Progress Note Template (Work Documentation).

Time began: _____   **Time ended:** _____   **Total time:** _____

No.	Step	Points	Check #1	Check #2	Check #3
1	Wash hands.				
2	*Paying attention to detail*, gather appropriate equipment and supplies.				
3	*Introduce yourself and identify patient. Explain the procedure and expectations to the patient, speaking at the patient's level of understanding. Allay the patient's fears and help him feel safe and comfortable.*				
4	Remove clothing that could interfere with cast application and provide a gown, sheet, and warm blanket to the patient.				
5	*Attending to any special needs of the patient*, assist him into position per provider's orders for comfort and ease of cast application.				
6	Medicate per provider's orders.				
7	Drape the area of cast application, including applying a waterproof pad under the extremity to be casted.				
8	Don non-sterile disposable casting gloves.				
9	Cleanse the area to be casted per provider's orders. Dry the area completely.				

No.	Step	Points	Check #1	Check #2	Check #3
10	Accurately document any areas of skin lesions, soft-tissue injuries and neurovascular status as indicated per provider in the patient's chart or electronic medical record.				
11	Select the appropriate diameter of stockinette for the extremity to be casted. If too tight, it can cause neurovascular impairment. If too large, it can wrinkle and contribute to skin breakdown.				
12	Measure stockinette to length long enough to cover the area to be casted. Add 2 to 3 inches to each end of the measurement to allow for stockinette to fold back over the casting material and provide a smooth finish and padded edge.				
13	Assist the provider with the correct width of Webril or other padded roll material.				
14	Assist the provider with the alignment and immobilization of the extremity while applying the stockinette and padding, This will provide comfort for the patient.				
15	When instructed by the provider, immerse the chosen casting material in water per manufacturer's instructions.				
16	Upon removal from the water bath, gently squeeze the cast material roll to remove excess water. Do not wring.				
17	Assist with the application of casting material per provider's request/instruction.				
18	***Reassure patient as needed.***				
19	After completion of cast material application, support the extremity in a manner that will not distort the molding of the cast material.				
20	Clean the care. Remove any plaster from the patient's exposed skin.				
21	Evaluate the neurovascular status of the affected area. Document in the patient's chart of electronic medical record. ***Notify the provider immediately*** of any abnormal findings.				
22	Per office policy or provider order, furnish and review written cast care and after care instructions with the patient, ***including the patient's support system.***				
23	Discard the water bath in the sink or hopper using extreme care not to allow any casting material to enter the drain.				
24	Discard the liner containing the plaster or other residue in the trash receptacle.				
25	Remove gloves and dispose of appropriately. Wash hands.				
26	Schedule follow up appointment for cast check.				

No.	Step	Points	Check #1	Check #2	Check #3
27	Accurately record the casting procedure, the neurovascular status of the affected limb, all patient education, and the date for follow up in the patient's chart or electronic medical record.				
Student's Total Points					
Points Possible					
Final Score (Student's Total Points/Possible Points)					

Instructor's/Evaluator's Comments and Suggestions:

_____

_____

_____

_____

_____

_____

_____

CHECK #1	
Evaluator's Signature:	Date:

CHECK #2	
Evaluator's Signature:	Date:

CHECK #3	
Evaluator's Signature:	Date:

Work Documentation Form(s)

*Progress Note Template can be downloaded from the Premium Website

ABHES Competencies: MA.A.1.4.a Document accurately; MA.A.1.9.d Recognize and understand various treatment protocols; MA.A.1.9.l Prepare patient for examinations and treatments; MA.A.1.9.m Assist physician with routine and specialty examinations and treatments; MA.A.1.9.o (5) Perform first aid and CPR

CAAHEP Competencies: I.P.10 Assist physician with patient care; I.A.1 Apply critical thinking skills in performing patient assessment and care; I.A.2 Use language/verbal skills that enable the patients' understanding; III.A.2 Explain the rationale for performance of a procedure to the patient; IV.A.7 Demonstrate recognition of the patient's level of understanding in communication; IV.P.6 Prepare a patient for procedures and/or treatments; IV.P.8 Document patient care; IV.P.9 Document patient education; IX.P.7 Document accurately in the patient record

Name_____ **Date**_____ **Score**_____

● COMPETENCY ASSESSMENT

Procedure 30-20: Assisting with Cast Removal

Task: Assist the provider with removal of a cast.

Conditions: • Cast cutter
              • Cast spreader
              • Bandage scissors
              • Bag for disposing of cast materials
              • Drape

Standards: Perform the Task within 20 minutes with a minimum score of _____ points, as determined by your instructor.

Competency Assessment Information

Six weeks have passed since Thomas Myers fractured his right forearm in a skateboarding accident. It is now time for his cast to be removed. Dr. McDonald instructs you to assist in the removal of the cast. Document the procedure using the Progress Note Template (Work Documentation).

Time began: _____ **Time ended:** _____ **Total time:** _____

No.	Step	Points	Check #1	Check #2	Check #3
1	Wash hands.				
2	*Paying attention to detail,* gather appropriate equipment and supplies.				
3	*Introduce yourself and identify patient. Explain the procedure and expectations to the patient, speaking at the patient's level of understanding. Allay the patient's fears and help him feel safe and comfortable.* Explain that the cast cutter will not damage soft tissue as it vibrates, it does not spin.				
4	Explain that there may be a sensation of warmth and some pressure during the cutting of the cast.				
5	Assist the provider by handing instruments and supplies as requested.				
6	Once the cast has been removed, cleanse the area under the cast of excess skin and dry completely.				
7	Wash hands.				
8	Follow clinic policy or provider's orders to provide written instructions for after care.				
9	*Follow up with collateral allied health professionals to optimize the patient's plan of care by* arranging physical therapy follow up.				

No.	Step	Points	Check #1	Check #2	Check #3
10	Accurately record removal of the cast. Be sure to document skin, neurovascular, and bony assessment per provider's orders. Document patient teaching.				
Student's Total Points					
Points Possible					
Final Score (Student's Total Points/Possible Points)					

Instructor's/Evaluator's Comments and Suggestions:

_____

_____

_____

_____

_____

_____

_____

CHECK #1	
Evaluator's Signature:	Date:

CHECK #2	
Evaluator's Signature:	Date:

CHECK #3	
Evaluator's Signature:	Date:

Work Documentation Form(s)

*Progress Note Template can be downloaded from the Premium Website

ABHES Competencies: MA.A.1.4.a Document accurately; MA.A.1.9.d Recognize and understand various treatment protocols; MA.A.1.9.l Prepare patient for examinations and treatments; MA.A.1.9.m Assist physician with routine and specialty examinations and treatments

CAAHEP Competencies: I.P.10 Assist physician with patient care; I.A.1 Apply critical thinking skills in performing patient assessment and care; I.A.2 Use language/verbal skills that enable the patients' understanding; III.A.2 Explain the rationale for performance of a procedure to the patient; IV.A.7 Demonstrate recognition of the patient's level of understanding in communication; IV.P.6 Prepare a patient for procedures and/or treatments; IV.P.8 Document patient care; IV.P.9 Document patient education; IX.P.7 Document accurately in the patient record

Name _____ **Date** _____ **Score** _____

● **COMPETENCY ASSESSMENT**

Procedure 30-21:   Fecal Occult Blood Test

Task: Test feces for occult blood.

Conditions: *Fecal occult blood test:*
                   • Three occult slide test kits containing three slides, applicators, and envelope

                   Developing the fecal occult slide:
                   • Prepared fecal slides from patient
                   • Occult blood developer
                   • Reference card that accompanies kit
                   • Nonsterile disposable gloves
                   • Biohazard waste container
                   • Clock or watch with a second hand

Standards: Perform the Task within 15 minutes with a minimum score of _____ points, as determined by
                   your instructor.

Competency Assessment Information

Dr. Burke's patient, Mr. Eugene Dixon, is being seen in the office today for complaints of fatigue and dark stools. Dr. Burke orders a Fecal Occult Blood (Hemacult) test. After the stool specimen is supplied, you are to perform the testing. Document the procedure using the Progress Note Template (Work Documentation).

● **Time began:** _____   **Time ended:** _____   **Total time:** _____

No.	Step	Points	Check #1	Check #2	Check #3
1	***Paying attention to detail,*** check the expiration dates on the slides.				
2	***Introduce yourself and identify patient.***				
3	Complete the information on the front flap of all three slide packages.				
4	***Explain the procedure, speaking at the patient's level of understanding*** as follows: • Keep slides at room temperature. • Obtain a stool specimen in a clean, dry container. • Write date of collection on the front flap and then open the packet. • Use one end of the wooden applicator to apply a thin smear of the stool sample from the toilet to Box "A" on the slide. • Repeat the procedure using the other end of the applicator, obtaining a sample from a different area of the stool specimen and applying a thin smear to Box "B." • Dispose of the applicator appropriately. • Close the cover after air drying overnight. • Repeat the process with the next two bowel movements, on subsequent days.				

No.	Step	Points	Check #1	Check #2	Check #3
5	Provide the patient with an envelope to return the slides to the provider's office. Review with the patient instructions on diet and medication. Instruct the patient not to mail the slides to the provider's office.				
6	Accurately record all information regarding instructions and provisions of test kits in patient's chart or electronic medical record.				
Developing the Fecal Occult Slide:					
1	Wash hands and check the expiration date on the label of the developer, *paying attention to detail*.				
2	Don nonsterile disposable gloves.				
3	Establish a work area in a well-lit environment by covering a flat, dry surface with surface protections such as paper towels.				
4	Refer to package directions if unsure of the procedure.				
5	Open the window flap on the back of the slide packet.				
6	Apply two drops of the developer to each Box "A" and "B," directly over each smear.				
7	Using a watch with a second hand, interpret the results within 30 to 60 seconds or per manufacturer's instructions.				
8	A positive reaction consists of a blue halo appearing around the perimeter of the specimen. Any blue color is positive.				
9	Perform the quality-control procedure by processing the positive and negative monitor strip on each slide to confirm the test system is functional.				
10	Dispose of all supplies according to OSHA guidelines.				
11	Remove gloves and dispose in appropriate biohazard waste container.				
12	Wash hands.				
13	Accurately record all information in patient's chart or electronic medical record.				
Student's Total Points					
Points Possible					
Final Score (Student's Total Points/Possible Points)					

Instructor's/Evaluator's Comments and Suggestions:

_____

_____

_____

_____

_____

_____

CHECK #1	
Evaluator's Signature:	Date:

CHECK #2	
Evaluator's Signature:	Date:

CHECK #3	
Evaluator's Signature:	Date:

Work Documentation Form(s)

*Progress Note Template can be downloaded from the Premium Website

ABHES Competencies: MA.A.1.9.f Screen and follow up patient test results; MA.A.1.10.a Practice quality control; MA.A.1.10.b Perform selected CLIA-waived tests that assist with diagnosis and treatment; MA.A.1.10.d Collect, label, and process specimens; MA.A.1.10.f Instruct patients in the collection of a fecal specimen

CAAHEP Competencies: I.P.6 Perform patient screening using established protocols; I.P.11 Perform quality control measures; I.P.16 Screen test results; I.A.1 Apply critical thinking skills in performing patient assessment and care; IA.2 Use language/verbal skills that enable patients' understanding; IV.P.6 Prepare patients for procedures and/or treatments; IV.P.8 Document patient care; IV.P.9 Document patient education

Name _____ **Date** _____ **Score** _____

COMPETENCY ASSESSMENT

Procedure 30-22:   Urinary Catheterization of a Male Patient

Task: Obtain a sterile urine specimen for analysis or to relieve urinary retention.

Conditions: Catheterization kit (commercially available) containing:
* Sterile gloves
* Fenestrated drape (sterile)
* Betadine solution or swabs
* Lubricant
* Sterile cotton balls
* Sterile urine container with label
* Sterile 2 × 2 gauze sponges
* Forceps (sterile)
* Sterile absorbent plastic pad

Additional items needed:
* Sterile catheter (size and type as ordered by provider)
* Biohazard waste container
* Laboratory requisition form
* Waxed paper bag

Standards: Perform the Task within 15 minutes with a minimum score of _____ points, as determined by your instructor.

Competency Assessment Information

Your patient, Mr. Michael Sheppard, is seen in the office for difficulty urinating. He had an outpatient procedure earlier today with general anesthesia and after returning home, he has been unable to void. Dr. Morris has ordered a straight catheterization for Mr. Sheppard. Document the procedure using the Progress Note Template (Work Documentation).

Time began: _____   **Time ended:** _____   **Total time:** _____

No.	Step	Points	Check #1	Check #2	Check #3
1	Wash hands and follow Standard Precautions.				
2	*Introduce yourself and identify patient. Explain the procedure, speaking at the patient's level of understanding. Allay the patient's fears and help him to feel safe and comfortable.*				
3	Wash hands. *Paying attention to detail,* assemble equipment.				
4	Place unopened catheter kit on Mayo stand near the patient.				
5	Provide good lighting.				
6	*Being courteous and respectful,* have the patient disrobe below the waist and provide a drape, *respecting patient's personal boundaries.* Cover from umbilical area to pubic hairline.				

No.	Step	Points	Check #1	Check #2	Check #3
7	***Attending to any special needs of the patient,*** assist the patient into position lying on his back with knees slightly bent and legs separated on the examination table.				
8	Drape patient with sheet exposing only the external genitalia.				
9	Wash hands.				
10	Open outer wrapping of the sterile kit. This becomes the sterile field.				
11	Utilizing sterile principles, place sterile absorbent plastic pad under patient's buttocks. Touching only the corners, empty contents of tray onto sterile field. Drape perineal area with fenestrated drape. Add sterile catheter to field.				
12	This will place the sterile catheter tray between the patient's legs. Open catheter using sterile technique and place on the sterile field.				
13	Ask patient to keep knees apart.				
14	Apply sterile gloves.				
15	Open fenestrated drape and, being careful not to contaminate drape or gloves, position drape opening over penis.				
16	Pour Betadine over three cotton balls in appropriate compartment of the kit or open Betadine swabs.				
17	Open urine specimen container.				
18	Apply sterile lubricant to a sterile gauze sponge and place tip of catheter in lubricant.				
19	Instruct patient to breathe slowly and deeply during procedure.				
20	With nondominant hand, hold the penis just below the glans. In uncircumcised males, the glans must be pulled back to expose the meatus. This is done entirely with the nondominant hand.				
21	With the dominant hand, take the Betadine swabs or sterile forceps and a cotton ball that has been saturated with Betadine, cleanse the meatus in a circular motion from the center to the outside of the glans. Use all three cotton balls or swabs.				
22	Using the dominant, sterile gloved hand, pick up the catheter. While holding the head of the penis upright and straight with the nondominant hand, insert the catheter slowly approximately 6 inches until the urine begins to flow.				
23	Interrupt urine flow by clamping or pinching off.				

No.	Step	Points	Check #1	Check #2	Check #3
24	Position end of catheter into urine specimen container.				
25	Collect specimen by releasing clamp and collecting approximately 60 mL of urine.				
26	Allow remaining urine to flow into basin until flow ceases. Pinch catheter closed.				
27	Remove catheter gently and slowly.				
28	Clean Betadine from penis with remaining cotton balls.				
29	Tighten lid on the urine specimen container.				
30	Remove procedure items and dispose of appropriately in biohazard waste container.				
31	Position patient for comfort.				
32	*Attending to any special needs*, assist the patient to sit on the edge of the table or relaxing in a horizontal recumbent position.				
33	Offer tissues for cleanup of lubricant.				
34	When patient is ready for sitting up, assess patient's color and pulse. Take blood pressure if indicated.				
35	Remove gloves and wash hands.				
36	Don nonsterile disposable gloves.				
37	Dispose of items utilized per OSHA guidelines.				
38	If collecting urine specimen for analysis, label specimen container and attach to completed laboratory requisition form. Place in biohazard transportation bag.				
39	Remove gloves and dispose of appropriately. Wash hands.				
40	Assist patient from examination table.				
41	Don nonsterile disposable gloves.				
42	Clean room and table. Remove gloves and discard appropriately.				
43	Wash hands.				
44	Accurately record all information in patient's chart or electronic medical record, noting the amount of urine collected. Document that specimen was sent to outside laboratory (if appropriate).				
Student's Total Points					
Points Possible					
Final Score (Student's Total Points/Possible Points)					

Instructor's/Evaluator's Comments and Suggestions:

CHECK #1	
Evaluator's Signature:	Date:

CHECK #2	
Evaluator's Signature:	Date:

CHECK #3	
Evaluator's Signature:	Date:

Work Documentation Form(s)

*Lab Requisition form and Progress Note Template can be downloaded from the Premium Website

ABHES Competencies: MA.A.1.4.a Document accurately; MA.A.1.9.l Prepare patient for examinations and treatments; MA.A.1.9.m Assist physician with routine and specialty examinations and treatments

CAAHEP Competencies: I.A.2 Use language/verbal skills that enable a patient's understanding; IV.P.5 Instruct patients according to their needs to promote health maintenance and disease prevention; IV.A.7 Demonstrate recognition of patient's level of understanding in communication

Name_____ **Date**_____ **Score**_____

● COMPETENCY ASSESSMENT

Procedure 30-23: Urinary Catheterization of a Female Patient

Task: Obtain a sterile urine specimen for analysis or to relieve urinary retention.

Conditions: Catheterization kit (commercially available) containing:
- Sterile gloves
- Betadine solution or swabs
- Lubricant
- Sterile fenestrated drape
- Sterile cotton balls
- Sterile urine container with label
- Sterile 2 × 2 gauze sponges
- Forceps (sterile)
- Sterile absorbent plastic pad

Additional items needed:
- Sterile catheter (size and type as ordered by provider)
- Biohazard waste container
- Laboratory requisition form
- Waxed paper bag

Standards: Perform the Task within 20 minutes with a minimum score of _____ points, as determined by your instructor.

● Competency Assessment Information

Teresa Wood is exhibiting signs and symptoms of a urinary tract infection including frequency, burning, and hesitancy when voiding. Dr. Miller orders a straight catheterization for culture and sensitivity. Document the procedure using the Progress Note Template (Work Documentation).

Time began: _____ **Time ended:** _____ **Total time:** _____

No.	Step	Points	Check #1	Check #2	Check #3
1	Wash hands and follow Standard Precuations.				
2	*Introduce yourself and identify patient. Explain the procedure, speaking at the patient's level of understanding.*				
3	Wash hands. *Paying attention to detail,* assemble equipment.				
4	Place unopened catheter kit on Mayo stand near the patient.				
5	Provide good lighting.				
6	*Being courteous and respectful,* have the patient disrobe below the waist and provide a drape, *protecting the patient's personal boundaries.*				
7	*Attending to any special needs of the patient,* assist the patient into the dorsal lithotomy position on the examination table.				

No.	Step	Points	Check #1	Check #2	Check #3
8	Drape patient with sheet exposing only the external genitalia.				
9	Wash hands.				
10	Open outer wrapping of the sterile kit. This becomes a sterile field.				
11	Utilizing sterile principles, place sterile absorbent plastic pad under patient's buttocks. Touching only the corners, empty contents of tray onto sterile field. Drape perineal area with fenestrated drape. Add sterile catheter to field.				
12	This will place the sterile catheter trap between the patient's legs. Open catheter using sterile technique and place on the sterile field.				
13	Ask patient to keep knees apart.				
14	Apply sterile gloves.				
15	Pour Betadine over three cotton balls in appropriate compartment of the kit or open Betadine swabs.				
16	Open urine specimen container.				
17	Apply sterile lubricant to a gauze sponge and place tip of catheter in lubricant.				
18	Instruct patient to breathe slowly and deeply during procedure.				
19	Spread labia with nondominant hand. Dominant hand remains sterile. With dominant hand and sterile forceps, wipe genitalia with each of three antiseptic soaked cotton balls or Betadine swabs with a front to back motion. First wipe the right labia using a front to back motion. Discard cotton ball or swab into biohazard waste container. Second, wipe the left labia with cotton ball or swab and discard. Lastly, wipe down the center with the cotton ball or swab. Discarding after each wipe. Discard forceps if used. Continue to hold labia apart until catheter is inserted.				
20	Using sterile gloved hand, pick up the catheter and hold it 3 to 4 inches from lubricated end. The other end of the catheter should remain in the sterile tray.				
21	Gently insert lubricated tip of the catheter into the urinary meatus approximately 6 inches or until urine begins to flow.				
22	Interrupt urine flow by clamping or pinching off.				
23	Position end of catheter into urine specimen container.				

No.	Step	Points	Check #1	Check #2	Check #3
24	If urinalysis is required, wait until catheterization is complete and pour urine into sterile container.				
25	Collect specimen by releasing clamp and collect approximately 60 mL of urine.				
26	Allow remaining urine to flow into basin until flow ceases. Pinch catheter closed.				
27	Remove catheter gently and slowly.				
28	Clean Betadine from perineum with remaining cotton balls.				
29	Tighten lid on the urine specimen container.				
30	Remove procedure items and dispose of appropriately in biohazard waste containers.				
31	Remove sterile gloves and discard appropriately in biohazard waste container.				
32	Position patient for comfort.				
33	*Attending to any special needs of the patient,* assist the patient to sit on the edge of the table or relax in a horizontal recumbent position. Offer tissues for cleanup of lubricant.				
34	When patient is ready for sitting up, assess patient's color and pulse. Take blood pressure if indicated.				
35	Don nonsterile disposable gloves.				
36	Discard items utilized per OSHA guidelines.				
37	If collecting urine specimen for analysis, label specimen container and attach to completed laboratory requisition form. Place in biohazard transportation bag.				
38	Remove gloves and dispose of appropriately. Wash hands.				
39	Assist patient from examination table.				
40	Don nonsterile disposable gloves.				
41	Clean room and table. Remove gloves and discard appropriately.				
42	Wash hands.				
43	Accurately record all information in patient's chart or electronic medical record, noting the amount of urine collected. Document that specimen was sent to outside laboratory (if appropriate).				
Student's Total Points					
Points Possible					
Final Score (Student's Total Points/Possible Points)					

Instructor's/Evaluator's Comments and Suggestions:

CHECK #1	
Evaluator's Signature:	Date:

CHECK #2	
Evaluator's Signature:	Date:

CHECK #3	
Evaluator's Signature:	Date:

Work Documentation Form(s)

*Lab Requisition form and Progress Note Template can be downloaded from the Premium Website

ABHES Competencies: MA.A.1.4.a Document accurately; MA.A.1.9.l Prepare patient for examinations and treatments; MA.A.1.9.m Assist physician with routine and specialty examinations and treatments

CAAHEP Competencies: I.A.2 Use language/verbal skills that enable a patient's understanding; IV.P.5 Instruct patients according to their needs to promote health maintenance and disease prevention; IV.A.7 Demonstrate recognition of patient's level of understanding in communication

Name _____ **Date** _____ **Score** _____

COMPETENCY ASSESSMENT

Procedure 31-1: Applying Sterile Gloves

Task: To correctly apply sterile gloves.

Conditions:
- Prepackaged pair of sterile gloves in the appropriate size
- Flat, clean, dry surface

Standards: Perform the Task within 5 minutes with a minimum score of ___ points, as determined by your instructor.

Time began: _____ **Time ended:** _____ **Total time:** _____

No.	Step	Points	Check #1	Check #2	Check #3
1	Remove rings and watch. Wash hands using surgical asepsis.				
2	Inspect glove package for tears or stains.				
3	Place the glove package on a clean, dry, flat surface above waist level.				
4	*Paying attention to detail,* peel open the package taking care not to touch the sterile inner surface of the package. Do not allow the gloves to slide beyond the sterile inner border.				
5	The gloves should be opened with the cuffs toward you, the palms up, and the thumbs pointing outward. If the gloves are not positioned properly, turn the package around, being careful not to reach over the sterile area or touch the inner surface or the gloves.				
6	With the index finger and thumb of the nondominant hand, grasp the *inner* cuffed edge of the opposite glove. The glove should be picked straight up from the package surface without dragging or dangling the fingers over any nonsterile area.				
7	With the palm up on the dominant hand, carefully slide the hand into the glove. Do not allow the outside of the glove to come in contact with anything and stand away from the sterile package. Always hold the hands above the waist and away from the body with palms up.				
8	With the gloved hand, pick up the glove for the remaining hand by slipping four fingers under the outside of the cuff. Lift the second glove up, keeping it held above the waist and away from the body. Do not allow the glove to drag across the package or touch nonsterile surfaces.				

No.	Step	Points	Check #1	Check #2	Check #3
9	With the palm up, slip the second hand into the glove. Do not allow the outside of the gloves to touch nonsterile skin and be especially mindful of the thumb.				
10	Adjust the gloves on the hands as needed, but avoid touching the wrist area. Keep gloved hands above the waist and away from the body. Do not touch nonsterile surfaces with the gloved hands.				
Student's Total Points					
Points Possible					
Final Score (Student's Total Points/Possible Points)					

Instructor's/Evaluator's Comments and Suggestions:

_____

_____

_____

_____

_____

_____

CHECK #1 Evaluator's Signature:	Date:

CHECK #2 Evaluator's Signature:	Date:

CHECK #3 Evaluator's Signature:	Date:

ABHES Competency: MA.A.1.9.b Apply principles of aseptic techniques and infection control

CAAHEP Competency: III.P.3 Select appropriate barrier/personal protective equipment (PPE) for potentially infectious situations

Name_____ **Date**_____ **Score**_____

● **COMPETENCY ASSESSMENT**

Procedure 31-2:   Chemical "Cold" Sterilization of Endoscopes

Task: To sterilize heat-sensitive items such as fiber-optic endoscopes and delicate cutting instruments using appropriate chemical solutions.

Conditions:
- Chemical solution such as Cidex® Steris® System (Liquid Chemical Sterilant)
- Airtight container
- Timer
- Sterile water
- Gloves (heavy duty)
- Sterile towel
- Plastic-lined sterile drapes
- Sterile transfer forceps
- Sterile basin

Standards: Perform the Task within 30 minutes with a minimum score of ___ points, as determined by your instructor.

Time began: _____   **Time ended:** _____   **Total time:** _____

No.	Step	Points	Check #1	Check #2	Check #3
1	Sanitize items that require chemical sterilization. Rinse and dry.				
2	*Paying attention to detail,* read manufacturer's instructions on original container of chemical sterilization solution.				
3	Put on gloves.				
4	*Paying attention to detail,* prepare solution as indicated by manufacturer; place the date of opening or preparation on the container and initial it.				
5	Pour solution carefully to avoid splashing into a container large enough to accommodate the instrument and allow complete immersion in the sterilizing solution. Be sure the container has an airtight lid.				
6	Place sanitized and dried instruments into the solution, completely submerging item(s). Avoid splashing when placing items into airtight container.				
7	Close lid of container; label with name of solution, date, and time required for sterilization to complete per manufacturer's instructions, and initial.				
8	Do not open lid of container or add additional items during the processing time.				

No.	Step	Points	Check #1	Check #2	Check #3
9	Following the recommended processing time, lift item(s) from the container using sterile gloved hands or sterile transfer forceps. Carefully hold item above sterile basin and pour copious amounts of sterile water over it and through it (endoscopes) until adequately rinsed of chemical solution.				
10	Hold item(s) upright for a few seconds to allow excess sterile water to drip off.				
11	Place the sterile time on a sterile towel (which has been placed on a sterile field) and dry with another sterile towel. The towel used for drying is removed from the sterile field. The use of sterile drapes that have a plastic polylined barrier layer between two layers of paper is recommended for the sterile field.				
Student's Total Points					
Points Possible					
Final Score (Student's Total Points/Possible Points)					

Instructor's/Evaluator's Comments and Suggestions:

_____

_____

_____

_____

_____

_____

CHECK #1	
Evaluator's Signature:	Date:

CHECK #2	
Evaluator's Signature:	Date:

CHECK #3	
Evaluator's Signature:	Date:

ABHES Competencies: MA.A.1.9.b Apply principles of aseptic techniques and infection control; MA.A.1.9.o (1) Perform sterilization techniques

CAAHEP Competencies: III.P.3 Select appropriate barrier/personal protective equipment (PPE) for potentially infectious situations; III.P.6 Perform sterilization procedures

Name _____ **Date** _____ **Score** _____

⬤ **COMPETENCY ASSESSMENT**

Procedure 31-3: Preparing Instruments for Sterilization in an Autoclave

Task: To properly wrap sanitized instruments for sterilization in an autoclave.

Conditions:
- Sanitized instruments
- Wrapping material (muslin or disposable wrapping paper)
- Sterilization indicator
- 2 × 2 gauze or cotton balls (if instruments have hinges)
- Autoclave wrapping tape
- Permanent marker or felt-tipped pen

Standards: Perform the Task within 10 minutes with a minimum score of ___ points, as determined by your instructor.

Time began: _____ **Time ended:** _____ **Total time:** _____

No.	Step	Points	Check #1	Check #2	Check #3
1	*Paying attention to detail,* prepare a clean, dry, flat surface of adequate size to lay the wrapping material upon.				
2	Select two wraps of adequate size in which to wrap the instruments.				
3	Place one square of wrapping material at an angle in front of you on the dry surface with one corner pointing directly toward you.				
4	Place the sanitized instrument or articles to be placed in the autoclave just below the center of the wrap. Open instruments with hinges as wide as possible and place a 2 × 2 gauze or cotton ball in the opening.				
5	Place one sterilization indicator with the instrument(s).				
6	Bring the corner of the wrap closest to you up and over the article(s) toward the center. Bring the tip of the same corner back toward you until it reaches the folded edge, creating a fan-fold effect. Smooth the edges of the fold. The article should remain completely covered.				
7	Fold one side edge toward the center line; fan-fold back to side and crease.				
8	Repeat step 7 for the other side edge.				
9	Fold the package up from the bottom.				
10	Fold the top edge down and over the entire package.				

No.	Step	Points	Check #1	Check #2	Check #3
11	To "wrap twice," place this package into the center of the second wrap. Repeat Steps 7 through 10.				
12	Tape with autoclave tape across the point left exposed.				
13	Label the tape with the name of the instrument or type of pack (i.e., laceration tray), date of sterilization, and your initials.				
14	Place wrapped instruments in the autoclave.				
Student's Total Points					
Points Possible					
Final Score (Student's Total Points/Possible Points)					

Instructor's/Evaluator's Comments and Suggestions:

_____

_____

_____

_____

_____

_____

CHECK #1	
Evaluator's Signature:	Date:

CHECK #2	
Evaluator's Signature:	Date:

CHECK #3	
Evaluator's Signature:	Date:

ABHES Competency: MA.A.1.9.h Wrap items for autoclaving

CAAHEP Competency: III.P.6 Perform sterilization procedures

Name_____ **Date**_____ **Score**_____

● **COMPETENCY ASSESSMENT**

Procedure 31-4: Sterilization of Instruments (Autoclave)

Task: To rid items for use in invasive procedures of all forms of microbial life (microorganisms).

Conditions:
- Steam sterilizer (autoclave)
- Timer
- Autoclave manufacturer's instructions
- Wrapped sanitized instrument package(s) with sterilization indicators placed inside package (or unwrapped item if removed with sterile forceps)
- Sterile transfer forceps

Standards: Perform the Task within 30 minutes with a minimum score of ___ points, as determined by your instructor.

Time began: _____   **Time ended:** _____   **Total time:** _____

No.	Step	Points	Check #1	Check #2	Check #3
1	*Paying attention to detail,* check water level in the autoclave reservoir and add distilled water to the fill line if necessary.				
2	Depending on your autoclave, turn the knob to "fill" line and allow water into the chamber until it reaches the "fill" line. Turn the knob to the next position. This stops water from continuing to enter the chamber.				
3	Load packages into autoclave tray; allow room for steam to circulate. • Load jars of dressing or cups on their sides, with tops ajar or loosely in place. • Load unwrapped instruments flat with handles opened, exposing all surfaces.				
4	Close autoclave door and seal.				
5	Turn on autoclave. When temperature dial indicates 270°F (118°C) and 15 pounds of pressure has been achieved inside the autoclave, begin necessary exposure time by setting timer. • Wrapped instrument packages or trays: 30 minutes • Unwrapped items: 15 minutes • Unwrapped items covered with cloth: 20 minutes				
6	After completion of the autoclave cycle, vent exhaust steam pressure from the autoclave by following the manufacturer's instructions.				

No.	Step	Points	Check #1	Check #2	Check #3
7	Open the door approximately 1 inch after the pressure gauge indicates zero (0) pressure and the temperature gauge indicates a decrease to at least 212°F.				
8	Allow the contents to completely dry, approximately 30 to 45 minutes; do NOT touch contents until completely dry.				
9	Remove wrapped contents with dry, clean hands and store in clean, dry, closed cupboard or drawer.				
10	Remove unwrapped contents with sterile transfer forceps; resanitize and resterilize the transfer forceps following use.				
11	Perform quality control on a regular basis, based on usage. • Monitor sterilization indicators with each use of sterilized instruments. • On a weekly basis, perform quality control by documenting sterilization indicator outcome in a log; date and initial quality-control log entries.				
12	Clean and service the autoclave regularly according to the manufacturer's guidelines. When sterilization is not being achieved, take equipment out of service and contact a qualified service agency for repair.				
13	Maintain a log of cleaning, service, and quality-control measures performed.				
Student's Total Points					
Points Possible					
Final Score (Student's Total Points/Possible Points)					

Instructor's/Evaluator's Comments and Suggestions:

_____

_____

_____

_____

_____

_____

CHECK #1	
Evaluator's Signature:	Date:

CHECK #2	
Evaluator's Signature:	Date:

CHECK #3	
Evaluator's Signature:	Date:

ABHES Competencies: MA.A.1.9.o (4) Perform sterilization techniques; MA.A.1.10.a Practice quality control

CAAHEP Competency: III.P.6 Perform sterilization procedures

Name _____ **Date** _____ **Score** _____

● **COMPETENCY ASSESSMENT**

Procedure 31-5:   Setting Up and Covering a Sterile Field

Task: To properly set up and cover a sterile field.

Conditions: • Disposable sterile polylined field drapes (two) or reusable sterile towels (two) (muslin or linen with water-repellent finish)
• Mayo instrument tray/stand positioned above the waist with the stem to the right
• Sterile transfer forceps (if needed)
• Nonsterile disposable gloves

Standards: Perform the Task within 15 minutes with a minimum score of ___ points, as determined by your instructor.

Time began: _____   **Time ended:** _____   **Total time:** _____

No.	Step	Points	Check #1	Check #2	Check #3
1	Wash hands. Put on nonsterile disposable gloves.				
2	Sanitize and disinfect a Mayo instrument tray. Adjust tray to above waist level and have the stem to the right.				
3	Remove gloves and dispose of properly. Wash hands again.				
4	Select an appropriate disposable sterile field drape and place the drape package on a clean, dry, flat surface.				
5	Open the package exposing the fan-folded drape. Ensure that the cut corners of the drape are toward you; turn the package if necessary.				
6	With thumb and forefinger of one hand, carefully grasp the top cut corner without touching the rest of the drape or towel and pick the drape or towel up high enough to ensure that as it unfolds it does not drag across a nonsterile area.				
7	Holding the drape or towel above waist level and away from the body, grasp the opposing corner so that both the corners along the long edge of the drape are being held.				
8	Keeping the drape or towel above waist level and away from the body, reach over the Mayo tray with the drape or towel. Take care that the lower edge of the drape or towel does not drag across the tray.				

No.	Step	Points	Check #1	Check #2	Check #3
9	Gently pull the drape or towel toward you as it is laid onto the tray. If adjustment is needed to center the drape or towel, do not touch the center of the drape or towel, or reach over the sterile field. Walk around or reach underneath the tray to move it or make adjustments.				
10	After setting the instruments and supplies on the tray, it must be covered.				
11	To cover the sterile field with a second sterile drape or towel, follow Steps 5 through 8; then instead of pulling the drape or towel toward you (as described in Step 9), which would necessitate reaching over the sterile field, apply the covering drape or towel by holding it up in front of the field. Adjust the lower edge so it is even with the lower edge of the field drape or towel. With a forward motion, carefully lay the cover over the sterile field.				
Student's Total Points					
Points Possible					
Final Score (Student's Total Points/Possible Points)					

Instructor's/Evaluator's Comments and Suggestions:

_____

_____

_____

_____

_____

_____

CHECK #1	
Evaluator's Signature:	Date:

CHECK #2	
Evaluator's Signature:	Date:

CHECK #3	
Evaluator's Signature:	Date:

ABHES Competencies: MA.A.9.1.b Apply principles of aseptic techniques and infection control; MA.A.1.9.n Assist physician with minor office surgical procedures

CAAHEP Competency: I.P.10 Assist the physician with patient care

Name _____ **Date** _____ **Score** _____

● **COMPETENCY ASSESSMENT**

Procedure 31-6: Opening Sterile Packages of Instruments and Supplies and Applying Them to a Sterile Field

Task: To open sterile packages of surgical instruments and supplies and place them onto a sterile field using sterile technique.

Conditions:
- Mayo instrument tray draped with sterile field
- Sterile gloves
- Wrapped-twice sterile surgical instruments
- Prepackaged sterile surgical supplies

Standards: Perform the Task within 20 minutes with a minimum score of ___ points, as determined by your instructor.

Time began: _____ **Time ended:** _____ **Total time:** _____

No.	Step	Points	Check #1	Check #2	Check #3
1	*Paying attention to detail,* assemble supplies.				
2	Wash hands and set up sterile field (see Procedure 31-5).				
3	Position package of surgical instruments on palm of nondominant hand with outer envelope flap on top.				
4	Grasping the taped end of the top flap, open the first flap away from you. Do not touch the inside of the flap.				
5	Grasping just the folded-back tips of the side flaps, pull the right-sided flap to the right. Then pull the left-sided flap to the left, taking care not to reach over the package.				
6	Pull the last flap toward you by grasping the folded-back tip, taking care not to touch the inner contents of the package.				
7	Gather all of the loose edges together to obtain a snug cover over the nondominant hand. Close your covered hand over the inner package and carefully apply the inner package to the sterile field.				
8	Open peel-apart packages using sterile technique by grasping both edge of the flaps and pulling them apart in a rolling down motion, keeping both hands together. The sterile item should be exposed gradually between the two peel-apart edges. The sterile inner contents may then be offered to the sterile-gloved provider or applied to the sterile field using a flipping motion, or dropped, taking care not to contaminate either the package contents or the field.				

No.	Step	Points	Check #1	Check #2	Check #3
9	Apply sterile gloves. Arrange instruments and supplies in an organized and logical manner according to the provider's preference.				
10	Apply the sterile field cover if the tray is not going to be immediately utilized.				
Student's Total Points					
Points Possible					
Final Score (Student's Total Points/Possible Points)					

Instructor's/Evaluator's Comments and Suggestions:

_____

_____

_____

_____

_____

_____

CHECK #1	
Evaluator's Signature:	Date:

CHECK #2	
Evaluator's Signature:	Date:

CHECK #3	
Evaluator's Signature:	Date:

ABHES Competencies: MA.A.1.9.b Apply principles of aseptic techniques and infection control; MA.A.1.9.k Prepare and maintain examination and treatment area

CAAHEP Competency: I.P.10 Assist the physician with patient care

Name _____ **Date** _____ **Score** _____

● **COMPETENCY ASSESSMENT**

Procedure 31-7: Pouring a Sterile Solution into a Cup on a Sterile Field

Task: To pour a sterile solution into a cup on a sterile tray in a sterile manner.

Conditions: • Covered sterile surgical tray with a sterile cup in the upper right corner
  • Container of sterile solution (as ordered)

Standards: Perform the Task within 5 minutes with a minimum score of ___ points, as determined by your instructor.

Time began: _____ **Time ended:** _____ **Total time:** _____

No.	Step	Points	Check #1	Check #2	Check #3
1	Wash hands.				
2	*Paying attention to detail,* transport the surgical tray into the surgical area before pouring the solution; or, the surgical tray can be set up for immediate use in the surgical area.				
3	Read the label of the solution container three times and check the expiration date.				
4	Remove the cap from the solution container, taking care not to touch the inner surface of the cap. Place the cap upside down on a nonsterile surface to avoid touching the inner surface of the cap with a nonsterile surface. When the cap is held in the hand, hold it right side up.				
5	*Paying attention to detail,* read the label again to ensure accuracy. Place palm over the label to protect from stains. Pour a small amount of the solution into a bowl, cup, or sink that is outside of the sterile field.				
6	Carefully pull back the upper right corner of the tray cover to expose the cup. Take care to only touch the corner tip of the cover and not to reach over the exposed field.				
7	Approaching from the corner of the tray and using the cleansed side of the lip of the container, pour the needed amount of solution into the sterile cup. Precaution should be taken to avoid splashing, spilling, reaching over the field, or touching any of the sterile surfaces.				
8	Replace the corner of the drape cover using sterile technique or cover with a sterile drape or towel.				

No.	Step	Points	Check #1	Check #2	Check #3
9	Replace the cap of the solution container using sterile technique.				
10	Read the label again, *paying attention to detail*.				
Student's Total Points					
Points Possible					
Final Score (Student's Total Points/Possible Points)					

Instructor's/Evaluator's Comments and Suggestions:

_____

_____

_____

_____

_____

_____

CHECK #1 Evaluator's Signature:	Date:

CHECK #2 Evaluator's Signature:	Date:

CHECK #3 Evaluator's Signature:	Date:

ABHES Competencies: MA.A.1.9.b Apply principles of aseptic techniques and infection control; MA.A.1.9.k Prepare and maintain examination and treatment area

CAAHEP Competency: I.P.10 Assist the physician with patient care

Name _____ **Date** _____ **Score** _____

● **COMPETENCY ASSESSMENT**

Procedure 31-8:   Assisting with Office/Ambulatory Surgery

Task: To maintain sterility during surgical procedures that require surgical excision.

Conditions: **Mayo stand**
- Needles and syringe for anesthesia
- Prep bowl/cup
- Gauze sponges
- Scalpel and blade
- Operating scissors
- Fenestrated drape
- Hemostats (curved and straight)
- Thumb dressing forceps
- Thumb tissue forceps
- Needle holder
- Suture pack
- Transfer forceps

Side table (unsterile field)
- Sterile gloves (in package)
- Labeled biopsy containers with formalin
- Appropriate laboratory requisition
- Anesthesia vial
- Alcohol wipes
- Dressing, tape, bandages
- Biohazard container
- Betadine® solution

Standards: Perform the Task within 30 minutes with a minimum score of ___ points, as determined by your instructor.

Time began: _____   **Time ended:** _____   **Total time:** _____

No.	Step	Points	Check #1	Check #2	Check #3
1	Check room and equipment for readiness and cleanliness.				
2	Wash hands.				
3	*Paying attention to detail,* set up side table of nonsterile items.				
4	Perform surgical asepsis hand cleansing.				
5	Set up sterile field on a sanitized and disinfected Mayo stand or on a clean, dry, flat surface.				
6	*Paying attention to detail,* add sterile items.				
7	Apply sterile gloves or use sterile transfer forceps. Arrange instruments according to provider's instructions. Remove sterile gloves and dispose of appropriately or remove forceps from area.				

No.	Step	Points	Check #1	Check #2	Check #3
8	Wash hands.				
9	Cover the sterile field with a sterile towel if not being used immediately.				
10	*Introduce yourself. Identify the patient and explain the procedure at the patient's level of understanding.*				
11	Prepare the patient based on the procedure to be performed and per provider's preference.				
12	Use appropriate skin prep.				
13	*Paying attention to detail,* remove the sterile cover from the sterile setup as the provider applies sterile gloves. Lift the towel by grasping the tips of the corners farthest away from you and lifting toward you. Do not allow arms to pass over the sterile field.				
14	*Working within your scope of practice,* assist the provider as necessary, being certain to follow the principles of surgical asepsis. • Appropriately hold the vial of anesthetic agent while the provider withdraws the required dose. • The provider injects the local anesthetic, applies the Betadine® or other antiseptic to the surgical site, applies the sterile drapes, and begins the surgery. Apply sterile gloves to assist as requested. • Adjust the instrument tray and equipment around the provider. • Ensure a good light source. • *Allay the patient's fears regarding the procedure being performed and help the patient to feel safe and comfortable.*				
15	Hand instruments to the provider and receive used instruments from the provider and place in a basin or container out of the patient's line of sight.				
16	If necessary, hold biopsy container to receive specimen being excised. Do not contaminate the inside of the container. Assist with or apply sterile dressing to the operative site.				
17	*Being courteous and respectful,* assist the patient as necessary. *Attend to any special needs of the patient.*				
18	The specimen container must be tightly covered; labeled with the patient's name, date, type, and source of specimen; and sent to the laboratory accompanied by the appropriate laboratory requisition.				

No.	Step	Points	Check #1	Check #2	Check #3
19	Wearing appropriate personal protective equipment (PPE), clean surgical or examination room. • Dispose of used gauze sponges in biohazard container and knife blades and other disposable sharps in puncture-proof sharps container. • Rinse used surgical instruments; soak, sanitize, and sterilize for reuse. • Remove gloves and other PPE and dispose of per OSHA guidelines.				
20	Wash hands.				
21	Accurately document in patient's chart or electronic medical record that the specimen was sent to the laboratory.				
Student's Total Points					
Points Possible					
Final Score (Student's Total Points/Possible Points)					

Instructor's/Evaluator's Comments and Suggestions:

_____

_____

_____

_____

_____

_____

CHECK #1	
Evaluator's Signature:	Date:

CHECK #2	
Evaluator's Signature:	Date:

CHECK #3	
Evaluator's Signature:	Date:

Work Documentation Form(s)

*Lab Requisition form and Progress Note Template can be downloaded from the Premium Website

ABHES Competencies: MA.A.1.9.b Apply principles of aseptic techniques and infection control; MA.A.1.9.d Recognize and understand various treatment protocols; MA.A.1.9.k Prepare and maintain examination and treatment area; MA.A.1.9.l Prepare patient for examinations and treatments; MA.A.1.9.n Assist physician with minor office surgical procedures

CAAHEP Competencies: I.P.10 Assist the physician with patient care; I.A.2 Use language/verbal skills that enable patients' understanding; III.A.2 Explain the rationale for performance of a procedure to the patient; III.A.3 Show awareness of patient' concerns regarding their perceptions related to the procedure being performed; III.P.3 Select appropriate barrier/personal protective equipment (PPE) for potentially infectious situations; IV.P.6 Prepare a patient for procedures and/or treatments; IV.P.8 Document patient care; IX.P.2 Perform within scope of practice; IX.P.7 Document accurately in the patient record

Name_____ **Date**_____ **Score**_____

● COMPETENCY ASSESSMENT

Procedure 31-9: Dressing Change

Task: To remove a wound dressing and apply a dry sterile dressing.

Conditions: **Sterile field:**
- Several sterile gauze sponges and other dressing material as needed or prepackaged sterile dressing kit
- Sterile bowl with Betadine® solution or sterile Betadine® swab sticks
- Sterile dressing forceps
- Sponge forceps

Side table (unsterile field):
- Nonsterile gloves
- Sterile gloves
- Hydrogen peroxide
- Container of sterile water
- Cotton-tipped applicators
- Adhesive strips
- Antibacterial ointment/cream as ordered
- Tape
- Sponge forceps
- Bandage scissors
- Waterproof waste bag
- Biohazard waste container

Standards: Perform the Task within 20 minutes with a minimum score of ___ points, as determined by your instructor.

Time began: _____ **Time ended:** _____ **Total time:** _____

No.	Step	Points	Check #1	Check #2	Check #3
1	Check provider's order.				
2	Wash hands.				
3	*Paying attention to detail,* prepare the sterile field. Add gauze sponges, bowl with solution, and forceps.				
4	Position a waterproof bag away from the sterile area.				
5	Pour Betadine® solution into sterile bowl or use Betadine® swab sticks.				
6	*Introduce yourself. Identify the patient and explain the procedure, speaking at the patient's level of understanding.*				
7	*Allay the patient's fears regarding the procedure being performed and help the patient to feel safe and comfortable.*				
8	Don nonsterile gloves or use forceps.				

No.	Step	Points	Check #1	Check #2	Check #3
9	Loosen tape on dressing by pulling tape toward wound, or cut off bandage if necessary.				
10	Carefully remove bandage; place in biohazard waste container. Do not pass over sterile field.				
11	Remove dressing, taking care not to cause stress on the wound. • If the dressing is stuck to the wound, pour small amounts of sterile water or saline over the dressing; allow to soak for a short time. Remove dressing when loose enough to remove without resistance. Note type and amount of drainage.				
12	Place used dressing in waterproof bag without touching the inside or outside of the bag.				
13	Assess wound and note any drainage or signs of infection. Remove and discard gloves in waterproof bag.				
14	Wash hands.				
15	Don sterile gloves.				
16	Clean the wound with antiseptic solution as ordered. Gauze may be held with forceps, or use swabs.				
17	Dispose of used gauze in waterproof bag.				
18	Using sterile cotton-tipped applicators, apply ointment/cream as ordered. Using sterile forceps or sterile gloves, apply sterile gauze sponge(s) to wound.				
19	Remove gloves and dispose of appropriately. Wash hands.				
20	Secure dressing with roller bandage and adhesive tape or elastic bandage.				
21	Wash hands.				
22	Accurately document procedure in patient's chart or electronic medical record, describing wound appearance (i.e., discharge, signs of infection, healing, etc.).				
Student's Total Points					
Points Possible					
Final Score (Student's Total Points/Possible Points)					

Instructor's/Evaluator's Comments and Suggestions:

_____

_____

_____

_____

_____

_____

CHECK #1	
Evaluator's Signature:	Date:

CHECK #2	
Evaluator's Signature:	Date:

CHECK #3	
Evaluator's Signature:	Date:

Work Documentation Form(s)

*Progress Note Template can be downloaded from the Premium Website

ABHES Competencies: MA.A.1.9.b Apply principles of aseptic techniques and infection control; MA.A.1.9.d Recognize and understand various treatment protocols; MA.A.1.9.l Prepare patient for examinations and treatments; MA.A.1.9.m Assist physician with routine and specialty examinations and treatments

CAAHEP Competencies: I.P.10 Assist physician with patient care; I.A.2 Use language/verbal skills that enable patients' understanding; III.A.3 Show awareness of patient' concerns regarding their perceptions related to the procedure being performed; IV.P.6 Prepare a patient for procedures and/or treatments; IV.P.8 Document patient care; IX.P.7 Document accurately in the patient record

Name_____ **Date**_____ **Score**_____

COMPETENCY ASSESSMENT

Procedure 31-10:   Wound Irrigation

Task: To irrigate a wound to remove the accumulation of exudate that impairs and delays healing.

Conditions: **On Mayo Tray:**
- Sterile gloves in package
- Sterile irrigation kit (irrigating syringe, basin, and container for solution)
- Sterile dressing material in package

Side Area/Unsterile Field:
- Waterproof pad
- Sterile solution for irrigation (per provider's orders)
- Nonsterile gloves
- Waterproof waste bag

Standards: Perform the Task within 20 minutes with a minimum score of ___ points, as determined by your instructor.

Time began: _____   Time ended: _____   Total time: _____

No.	Step	Points	Check #1	Check #2	Check #3
1	Check the provider's order. Select the correct solution and appropriate solution strength. It should be at least body temperature.				
2	*Introduce yourself. Identify the patient and explain the procedure, speaking at the patient's level of understanding. Allay the patient's fears regarding the procedure being performed and help him to feel safe and comfortable.*				
3	Wash hands.				
4	Place the waterproof pad under the body part that will be irrigated.				
5	Position the patient in such a way that directs the flow of the solution into the wound. The basin catches the flow from the wound.				
6	Don nonsterile gloves, remove the dressing, and dispose into the waterproof waste bag.				
7	Note the wound's appearance, color, amount of discharge, and odor to the discharge.				
8	Remove and discard gloves into biohazard container.				
9	Wash hands.				
10	Maintain sterile technique, open the sterile irrigation tray and the dressings. Use the inner kit wrapping as a sterile field.				

No.	Step	Points	Check #1	Check #2	Check #3
11	Pour the irrigation solution into the sterile solution bowl or container. (Should be at least room temperature.)				
12	Don sterile gloves.				
13	Place the sterile basin against the edge of the wound.				
14	Fill the irrigating syringe (or bulb syringe) with the solution and carefully wash out the wound with the flow of solution.				
15	Continue to fill the syringe and continue to wash out the wound until the solution becomes clear and there is no drainage noted.				
16	Dry the wound edge with sterile gauze.				
17	Reassess the wound.				
18	Apply a sterile dressing.				
19	Remove gloves. Dispose in biohazard container.				
20	Wash hands.				
21	Accurately document procedure in patient's chart or electronic medical record.				
Student's Total Points					
Points Possible					
Final Score (Student's Total Points/Possible Points)					

Instructor's/Evaluator's Comments and Suggestions:

_____

_____

_____

_____

_____

_____

CHECK #1	
Evaluator's Signature:	Date:

CHECK #2	
Evaluator's Signature:	Date:

CHECK #3	
Evaluator's Signature:	Date:

Work Documentation Form(s)

*Progress Note Template can be downloaded from the Premium Website

ABHES Competencies: MA.A.1.9.b Apply principles of aseptic techniques and infection control; MA.A.1.9.d Recognize and understand various treatment protocols; MA.A.1.9.l Prepare patient for examinations and treatments; MA.A.1.9.m Assist physician with routine and specialty examinations and treatments

CAAHEP Competencies: I.P.10 Assist the physician with patient care; I.A.2 Use language/verbal skills that enable patients' understanding; III.A.2 Explain the rationale for performance of a procedure to the patient; IV.P.6 Prepare a patient for procedures and/or treatments; IV.P.8 Document patient care; IX.P.7 Document accurately in the patient record

Name _____ **Date** _____ **Score** _____

● **COMPETENCY ASSESSMENT**

Procedure 31-11: Preparation of Patient's Skin before Surgery

Task: To remove as many microorganisms as possible from the patient's skin immediately before surgery.

Conditions:
- Absorbent pads
- Drape
- Disposable prep kit (includes antiseptic solution, several sponges, razor, a container for water, or self-contained skin prep unit)
- Sterile water
- Sterile bowl
- Sterile gloves for the medical assistant and the provider

If kit is unavailable, equipment needed is:
- Sterile bowls (two)
- Antiseptic solution
- Sterile gauze sponges
- Sterile razor
- Basin for soiled sponges
- Sterile transfer forceps

Standards: Perform the Task within 20 minutes with a minimum score of ___ points, as determined by your instructor.

● **Time began:** _____ **Time ended:** _____ **Total time:** _____

No.	Step	Points	Check #1	Check #2	Check #3
1	Wash hands.				
2	Assemble equipment.				
3	*Introduce yourself. Identify patient.*				
4	*Speaking at the patient's level of understanding, explain the procedure.*				
5	*Remaining courteous, patient, and respectful to the patient, provide privacy,* and drape patient if appropriate. Prior to prepping and draping for the procedure, verify the location of the procedure by asking the patient to state or indicate the surgical site. Some facilities require that the appropriate site be marked with an indelible ink pen to be certain that the correct site is identified.				
6	Provide a good light source.				
7	Position patient for comfort and exposure of site.				
8	Wash hands.				

No.	Step	Points	Check #1	Check #2	Check #3
9	Insert waterproof absorbent toweling under the patient in the area to be prepped.				
10	Open kit or individual items required for prep.				
11	Don sterile gloves or use sterile transfer forceps.				
12	Apply Betadine® or other antiseptic to the sponges or gauze being careful to avoid splashing. ***Paying attention to detail,*** beginning at the site that the incision is to be made, cleanse in an outward circular motion from the site of the incision. Do not return to the center with the same sponge.				
13	Discard used sponges as necessary.				
14	Hold skin taut to avoid nicks, shave hair away from the operative site, following the hair growth pattern.				
15	When hair has been removed, scrub again in a circular fashion as in Step 12 for at least 3 minutes or per provider's orders.				
16	Rinse shaved area with sterile water and dry with a sterile 4 × 4 gauze sponge.				
17	Remove and appropriately discard absorbent pad, 4 × 4 sponges, disposable prep kit, and gloves.				
18	Wash hands.				
19	Don sterile gloves, place a sterile towel under the operative site taking care not to contaminate sterile hands.				
20	Instruct patient not to touch the area.				
21	Pour antiseptic solution (Betadine®) into the sterile bowl. Avoid splashing. If instructed by the provider, don sterile gloves and prep the area with antiseptic solution. Using the same approach as in Step 12, paint the operative site with antiseptic three times, discarding the sponge after creating a cleansed area much larger than the intended incisional area.				
22	Allow the area to completely dry prior to proceeding.				
23	The provider will cover the patient with the fenestrated drape and begin the surgical procedure.				
24	Accurately document the skin prep in patient's chart or EMR if instructed by the provider.				
Student's Total Points					
Points Possible					
Final Score (Student's Total Points/Possible Points)					

Instructor's/Evaluator's Comments and Suggestions:

_____

_____

_____

_____

_____

_____

CHECK #1	
Evaluator's Signature:	Date:

CHECK #2	
Evaluator's Signature:	Date:

CHECK #3	
Evaluator's Signature:	Date:

Work Documentation Form(s)

*Progress Note Template can be downloaded from the Premium Website

ABHES Competencies: MA.A.1.9.b Apply principles of aseptic techniques and infection control; MA.A.1.9.d Recognize and understand various treatment protocols; MA.A.1.9.l Prepare patient for examinations and treatments; MA.A.1.9.m Assist physician with routine and specialty examinations and treatments

CAAHEP Competencies: I.P.10 Assist physician with patient care; I.A.2 Use language/verbal skills that enable patients' understanding; III.A.2 Explain the rationale for performance of a procedure to the patient; III.A.3 Show awareness of patient' concerns regarding their perceptions related to the procedure being performed; IV.P.6 Prepare a patient for procedures and/or treatments; IV.P.8 Document patient care; IX.P.7 Document accurately in the patient record

Name_____ **Date**_____ **Score**_____

● COMPETENCY ASSESSMENT

Procedure 31-12: Suturing of Laceration or Incision Repair

Task: To set up and assist with the procedure of suturing a wound.

Conditions: **Surgical Tray:**
- Appropriately sized syringe and gauge of needles for administering anesthesia
- Hemostats (curved)
- Adson tissue forceps
- Iris scissors (curved)
- Suture material as ordered by provider
- Needle holder
- Gauze sponges
- Sterile water or saline

Side Table (Unsterile Field):
- Anesthetic as ordered by the provider
- Dressings, bandages, and tape
- Splint/brace/sling (optional)
- Sterile gloves in package (appropriate sizes for medical assistant and provider)

Standards: Perform the Task within 30 minutes with a minimum score of ___ points, as determined by your instructor.

● Time began: _____   Time ended: _____   Total time: _____

No.	Step	Points	Check #1	Check #2	Check #3
1	Wash hands.				
2	Assemble equipment.				
3	*Introduce yourself. Identify the patient and explain the procedure, speaking at the patient's level of understanding.* Obtain a signed consent for the procedure.				
4	*Being courteous, patient, and respectful to the patient, provide privacy,* and drape patient if appropriate.				
5	*Allay the patient's fears regarding the procedure being performed and help the patient to feel safe and comfortable.*				
6	Assess cause of wound and its severity. *Accurately and concisely update the provider.* • Inquire regarding allergies and last tetanus shot. Document appropriately. • *Using active listening skills,* review health history to avoid possible complications. Share information with provider. • *Paying attention to any special needs of the patient,* assist her to a supine position. • Soak wound in an antiseptic solution as ordered by provider. • Clean and dry wound.				

No.	Step	Points	Check #1	Check #2	Check #3
7	Assist the provider as requested.				
8	*Being courteous, patient, and respectful,* support the patient as needed.				
Postoperative Care:					
9	Don sterile gloves.				
10	Using sterile water or saline and a 4 × 4 sponge, clean the area around the wound and dry with a 4 × 4 sponge or sterile towels.				
11	Dress/bandage/splint wound following provider's preference.				
12	Remove gloves and dispose of in a biohazard waste container.				
13	Wash hands.				
14	Obtain vital signs to assess patient stability post-procedure. Document in the patient's chart or EMR.				
15	Educate patient regarding care of the wound per provider's orders. *Include the patient's support system as indicated.* Provide written instructions that include the signs and symptoms of infection and an after-hours contact number.				
16	*Demonstrating respect for individual diversity,* assist the patient with any questions or concerns.				
17	Arrange for a follow-up appointment and post-operative medication as ordered.				
18	Accurately document procedure in patient's chart or EMR.				
19	Don PPE.				
20	Dispose of supplies as per OSHA guidelines. Clean room, sanitize instruments, and sterilize for reuse.				
21	Wash hands.				
Student's Total Points					
Points Possible					
Final Score (Student's Total Points/Possible Points)					

Instructor's/Evaluator's Comments and Suggestions:

_____

_____

_____

_____

_____

_____

CHECK #1	
Evaluator's Signature:	Date:

CHECK #2	
Evaluator's Signature:	Date:

CHECK #3	
Evaluator's Signature:	Date:

Work Documentation Form(s)

*Progress Note Template can be downloaded from the Premium Website

ABHES Competencies: MA.A.1.9.a Obtain chief complaint, recording patient history; MA.A.1.9.b Apply principles of aseptic techniques and infection control; MA.A.1.9.c Take vital signs; MA.A.1.9.d Recognize and understand various treatment protocols; MA.A.1.9.e Recognize emergencies and treatments and minor office surgical procedures; MA.A.1.9.l Prepare patient for examinations and treatments; MA.A.1.9.m Assist physician with routine and specialty examinations and treatments; MA.A.1.9.p Advise patients of office policies and procedures

CAAHEP Competencies: I.P.1 Obtain vital signs; I.P.10 Assist physician with patient care; I.A.1 Apply critical thinking skills in performing patient assessment and care; I.A.2 Use language/verbal skills that enable patients' understanding; III.A.2 Explain the rationale for performance of a procedure to the patient; III.A.3 Show awareness of patient' concerns regarding their perceptions related to the procedure being performed; IV.P.6 Prepare a patient for procedures and/or treatments; IV.P.8 Document patient care; IV.A.1 Demonstrate empathy in communicating with patients, family, and staff; IX.P.2 Perform within scope of practice; IX.P.4 Practice within the standard of care for a medical assistant; IX.P.7 Document accurately in the patient record

Name_____ **Date**_____ **Score**_____

● **COMPETENCY ASSESSMENT**

Procedure 31-13: Sebaceous Cyst Excision

Task: To remove an inflamed or infected sebaceous cyst. To remove a sebaceous cyst that is not inflamed or infected but is located on an area of the body where the cyst is unsightly or where it may become irritated from rubbing.

Conditions: **Sterile Field:**
  • Appropriate size syringe and gauge of needle for administering anesthesia
  • Iris scissors (curved)
  • Mosquito hemostat (curved)
  • Knife handle and blade
  • Needle holder
  • Suture material as ordered by provider
  • Tissue forceps (two)
  • Mayo scissors (curved)
  • Sterile 4 × 4 gauze sponges
  • Fenestrated drape
  • Antiseptic solution as per provider preference

Side Area (Unsterile Field):
  • Skin prep supplies
  • Nonsterile disposable gloves
  • Personal protective equipment (PPE)
  • Anesthetic as ordered by the provider
  • Dressings, bandages, and tape
  • Splint/brace/sling as indicated
  • Alcohol pads
  • Tube for culture
  • Biohazard specimen transport bag
  • Appropriate lab requisitions

Standards: Perform the Task within 30 minutes with a minimum score of ___ points, as determined by your instructor.

Time began: _____   **Time ended:** _____   **Total time:** _____

No.	Step	Points	Check #1	Check #2	Check #3
1	Wash hands.				
2	*Paying attention to detail*, assemble equipment.				
3	*Introduce yourself. Identify the patient and explain the procedure, speaking at the patient's level of understanding.*				
4	Obtain a signed consent for the procedure.				
5	*Being courteous, patient, and respectful to the patient, provide privacy,* and drape patient if appropriate.				
6	*Allay the patient's fears regarding the procedure being performed and help the patient to feel safe and comfortable.*				

No.	Step	Points	Check #1	Check #2	Check #3
7	Inquire regarding allergies and last tetanus shot. Document appropriately.				
8	*Using active listening skills,* review health history to avoid possible complications. Share information with provider.				
9	*Paying attention to any special needs of the patient,* assist the patient to a supine position.				
10	Don appropriate PPE including goggles if indicated.				
11	Don sterile gloves.				
12	Perform skin prep as ordered by provider.				
13	Remove gloves and dispose of in biohazard waste container.				
14	Assist the provider to withdraw the ordered anesthetic by holding the vial in an inverted position. Assist provider as needed during the procedure.				
Give Postoperative Care:					
15	Don sterile gloves.				
16	Using sterile water or saline and a 4 × 4 sponge, clean the area around the wound and dry with a 4 × 4 sponge or sterile towels.				
17	Dress and bandage wound per provider's orders.				
18	Dispose of items utilized during the procedure according to OSHA guidelines.				
19	Remove gloves and dispose of in biohazard waste container.				
20	Wash hands.				
21	Obtain vital signs to assess patient stability post-procedure. Document in the patient's chart or EMR.				
22	*Explain wound care to the patient (and caregiver), speaking at the patient's level of understanding, and provide written instructions* including symptoms of infection.				
23	*Demonstrating respect for individual diversity,* assist the patient with any questions or concerns.				
24	Arrange for a follow-up appointment and post-operative medication as required.				
25	Document procedure in patient's chart or electronic medical record, noting that the culture specimen was sent to laboratory, if appropriate.				
26	Don PPE, including nonsterile disposable gloves.				
27	Clean room, sanitize instruments, and sterilize for reuse.				
28	Remove PPE and dispose of appropriately.				
29	Wash hands.				
Student's Total Points					
Points Possible					
Final Score (Student's Total Points/Possible Points)					

Instructor's/Evaluator's Comments and Suggestions:

CHECK #1	
Evaluator's Signature:	Date:

CHECK #2	
Evaluator's Signature:	Date:

CHECK #3	
Evaluator's Signature:	Date:

Work Documentation Form(s)

*Lab Requisition form and Progress Note Template can be downloaded from the Premium Website

ABHES Competencies: MA.A.1.9.a Obtain chief complaint, recording patient history; MA.A.1.9.b Apply principles of aseptic techniques and infection control; MA.A.1.9.c Take vital signs; MA.A.1.9.d Recognize and understand various treatment protocols; MA.A.1.9.e Recognize emergencies and treatments and minor office surgical procedures; MA.A.1.9.l Prepare patient for examinations and treatments; MA.A.1.9.m Assist physician with routine and specialty examinations and treatments

CAAHEP Competencies: I.P.1 Obtain vital signs; I.P.10 Assist physician with patient care; I.A.1 Apply critical thinking skills in performing patient assessment and care; I.A.2 Use language/verbal skills that enable patients' understanding; III.A.2 Explain the rationale for performance of a procedure to the patient; III.A.3 Show awareness of patient' concerns regarding their perceptions related to the procedure being performed; IV.P.6 Prepare a patient for procedures and/or treatments; IV.P.8 Document patient care; IV.A.1 Demonstrate empathy in communicating with patients, family, and staff; IX.P.2 Perform within scope of practice; IX.P.4 Practice within the standard of care for a medical assistant; IX.P.7 Document accurately in the patient record

Name_____ **Date**_____ **Score**_____

● COMPETENCY ASSESSMENT

Procedure 31-14:   Incision and Drainage of Localized Infection

Task: To incise and drain an abscess or other localized infection.

Conditions: **Surgical Tray:**
- Appropriate size syringe and gauge of needle for administering anesthesia
- Knife handle and blade
- Mosquito hemostat (curved)
- Fenestrated drape
- Tissue forceps (two)
- Mayo scissors (curved)
- Iris scissors (curved)
- Antiseptic solution as per provider preference
- Suture material as ordered by provider
- Needle holder
- Sterile 4 × 4 gauze sponges
- Sterile culture swabs
- Iodoform® gauze or Penrose drain

Side Area (Unsterile Field):
- Skin prep supplies
- Prepackaged sterile gloves (appropriate sizes for medical assistant and provider)
- Nonsterile disposable gloves
- Personal protective equipment (PPE)
- Anesthetic as ordered by the provider
- Dressings, bandages, and tape
- Splint/brace/sling as indicated
- Biohazard specimen transport bag
- Alcohol pads
- Appropriate lab requisitions

Standards: Perform the Task within 30 minutes with a minimum score of ____ points, as determined by your instructor.

Time began: _____   **Time ended:** _____   **Total time:** _____

No.	Step	Points	Check #1	Check #2	Check #3
1	Wash hands.				
2	*Paying attention to detail*, assemble equipment.				
3	*Introduce yourself. Identify the patient and explain the procedure, speaking at the patient's level of understanding*				
4	Obtain a signed consent for the procedure.				
5	*Being courteous, patient, and respectful to the patient, provide privacy,* and drape patient if appropriate.				
6	*Allay the patient's fears regarding the procedure being performed and help the patient to feel safe and comfortable.*				
7	Inquire regarding allergies and last tetanus shot. Document appropriately.				

No.	Step	Points	Check #1	Check #2	Check #3
8	*Using active listening skills,* review health history to avoid possible complications. Share information with provider.				
9	*Paying attention to any special needs of the patient,* assist the patient to the appropriate position.				
10	Don appropriate PPE, including goggles if indicated.				
11	Don sterile gloves.				
12	Perform skin prep as ordered by provider.				
13	Remove gloves and dispose of in biohazard waste container.				
14	Assist the provider as needed to inject the anesthesia by holding the vial while the appropriate amount is aspirated for injection. The provider incises the abscess and inserts either Iodoform gauze or a latex Penrose drain into the wound to encourage drainage. No sutures are used. A specimen is taken for culture and sensitivity.				
15	*Being courteous, patient, and respectful,* support the patient as needed.				
Postoperative Care:					
16	Don sterile gloves.				
17	Using sterile water or saline and a 4 × 4 sponge, clean the area around the wound and dry with a 4 × 4 sponge or sterile towels.				
18	Dress and bandage as directed. Several thicknesses of dressing material will be needed to absorb exudate, or the accumulated fluid in the cavity.				
19	Dispose of items utilized during the procedure according to OSHA guidelines.				
20	Remove gloves and dispose of in biohazard waste container.				
21	Wash hands.				
22	Obtain vital signs to assess patient stability post-procedure. Document in the patient's chart or EMR.				
23	*Explain wound care to the patient (and caregiver), speaking at the patient's level of understanding,* and provide written instructions such as to apply warm moist compresses to wound. Explain to watch for symptoms of infection. Stress caution when handling contaminated items.				
24	*Demonstrating respect for individual diversity,* assist the patient with any questions or concerns.				
25	Arrange for a follow-up appointment and post-operative medication as required.				
26	Accurately document procedure in patient's chart or electronic medical record.				
27	Don PPE including nonsterile disposable gloves.				
28	Clean room, sanitize instruments, and sterilize for reuse.				

No.	Step	Points	Check #1	Check #2	Check #3
29	Remove PPE and dispose of appropriately.				
30	Wash hands.				
Student's Total Points					
Points Possible					
Final Score (Student's Total Points/Possible Points)					

Instructor's/Evaluator's Comments and Suggestions:

_____

_____

_____

_____

_____

_____

CHECK #1 Evaluator's Signature:	Date:

CHECK #2 Evaluator's Signature:	Date:

CHECK #3 Evaluator's Signature:	Date:

Work Documentation Form(s)

*Lab Requisition form and Progress Note Template can be downloaded from the Premium Website

ABHES Competencies: MA.A.1.9.a Obtain chief complaint, recording patient history; MA.A.1.9.b Apply principles of aseptic techniques and infection control; MA.A.1.9.c Take vital signs; MA.A.1.9.d Recognize and understand various treatment protocols; MA.A.1.9.e Recognize emergencies and treatments and minor office surgical procedures; MA.A.1.9.l Prepare patient for examinations and treatments; MA.A.1.9.m Assist physician with routine and specialty examinations and treatments

CAAHEP Competencies: I.P.1 Obtain vital signs; I.P.10 Assist physician with patient care; I.A.1 Apply critical thinking skills in performing patient assessment and care; I.A.2 Use language/verbal skills that enable patients' understanding; III.A.2 Explain the rationale for performance of a procedure to the patient; III.A.3 Show awareness of patient' concerns regarding their perceptions related to the procedure being performed; IV.P.6 Prepare a patient for procedures and/or treatments; IV.P.8 Document patient care; IV.A.1 Demonstrate empathy in communicating with patients, family, and staff; IX.P.2 Perform within scope of practice; IX.P.4 Practice within the standard of care for a medical assistant; IX.P.7 Document accurately in the patient record

Name _____   **Date** _____   **Score** _____

● **COMPETENCY ASSESSMENT**

Procedure 31-15:   Aspiration of Joint Fluid

Task: To remove excess synovial fluid from a joint after injury.

Conditions: **Surgical Tray:**
- Appropriate size syringe and gauge of needle for administering anesthesia
- Sterile 4 × 4 gauze sponges
- Sterile basin for aspirated fluid
- Fenestrated drape
- Appropriate size syringe and gauge of needle for joint aspiration per provider preference
- Hemostat
- Antiseptic solution as per provider preference

Side Area (Unsterile Field):
- Skin prep supplies
- Prepackaged sterile gloves (appropriate sizes for medical assistant and provider)
- Nonsterile disposable gloves
- Personal protective equipment (PPE)
- Anesthetic as ordered by the provider
- Medication for joint infection per provider's orders
- Splint/brace/sling as indicated
- Alcohol pads
- Specimen container
- Appropriate lab requisitions
- Supplies to obtain culture of joint fluid
- Dressing, bandages, and tape
- Biohazard specimen transport bag

Standards: Perform the Task within 30 minutes with a minimum score of ___ points, as determined by your instructor.

Time began: _____   **Time ended:** _____   **Total time:** _____

No.	Step	Points	Check #1	Check #2	Check #3
1	Wash hands.				
2	*Paying attention to detail,* assemble equipment.				
3	*Introduce yourself. Identify the patient and explain the procedure, speaking at the patient's level of understanding.*				
4	Obtain a signed consent for the procedure.				
5	*Being courteous, patient, and respectful to the patient, provide privacy,* and drape patient if appropriate.				
6	*Allay the patient's fears regarding the procedure being performed and help the patient to feel safe and comfortable.*				
7	Inquire regarding allergies and last tetanus shot. Document appropriately.				
8	*Using active listening skills,* review health history to avoid possible complications. Share information with provider.				

No.	Step	Points	Check #1	Check #2	Check #3
9	*Paying attention to any special needs of the patient,* assist the patient to the supine position.				
10	Don appropriate PPE, including goggles if indicated.				
11	Don sterile gloves.				
12	Perform skin prep as ordered by provider.				
13	Remove gloves and dispose of in biohazard waste container.				
14	Assist the provider by holding the vial as anesthesia is aspirated. The provider injects anesthesia; inserts a long, sturdy needle into the synovial sac; and aspirates fluid with a large syringe. The aspirated fluid is put into a sterile bowl as the syringe fills with fluid. A hemostat is used to remove the syringe from the needle, leaving the needle in the joint. The syringe is reapplied to the needle, and the process continues until excess fluid is removed.				
15	*Being courteous, patient, and respectful,* support the patient as needed.				
Give Postoperative Care:					
16	Don sterile gloves.				
17	Using sterile water or saline and a 4 × 4 sponge, clean the area around the wound and dry with a 4 × 4 sponge or sterile towels.				
18	Dress and bandage wound per provider's instructions. Dress to absorb exudates.				
19	Dispose of items utilized during the procedure according to OSHA guidelines.				
20	Remove gloves and dispose of in biohazard waste container.				
21	Wash hands.				
22	Obtain vital signs to assess patient stability post-procedure. Document in the patient's chart or EMR.				
23	*Explain wound care to the patient (and caregiver), speaking at the patient's level of understanding, and provide written instructions* including symptoms of infection.				
24	*Demonstrating respect for individual diversity,* assist the patient with any questions or concerns.				
25	Arrange for a follow-up appointment and post-operative medication as required.				
26	Apply gloves and eye/mouth protection if sending specimen to laboratory. Place aspirated fluid into a sterile container and cover tightly.				
27	Send labeled specimen container and requisition to the pathology laboratory after placing specimen in biohazard transport bag.				
28	Accurately document the procedure in patient's chart or electronic medical record.				
Student's Total Points					
Points Possible					
Final Score (Student's Total Points/Possible Points)					

Instructor's/Evaluator's Comments and Suggestions:

_____

_____

_____

_____

_____

_____

CHECK #1	
Evaluator's Signature:	Date:

CHECK #2	
Evaluator's Signature:	Date:

CHECK #3	
Evaluator's Signature:	Date:

Work Documentation Form(s)

*Lab Requisition form and Progress Note Template can be downloaded from the Premium Website

ABHES Competencies: MA.A.1.9.a Obtain chief complaint, recording patient history; MA.A.1.9.b Apply principles of aseptic techniques and infection control; MA.A.1.9.c Take vital signs; MA.A.1.9.d Recognize and understand various treatment protocols; MA.A.1.9.e Recognize emergencies and treatments and minor office surgical procedures; MA.A.1.9.l Prepare patient for examinations and treatments; MA.A.1.9.m Assist physician with routine and specialty examinations and treatments

CAAHEP Competencies: I.P.1 Obtain vital signs; I.P.10 Assist physician with patient care; I.A.1 Apply critical thinking skills in performing patient assessment and care; I.A.2 Use language/verbal skills that enable patients' understanding; III.A.2 Explain the rationale for performance of a procedure to the patient; III.A.3 Show awareness of patient' concerns regarding their perceptions related to the procedure being performed; IV.P.6 Prepare a patient for procedures and/or treatments; IV.P.8 Document patient care; IV.A.1 Demonstrate empathy in communicating with patients, family, and staff; IX.P.2 Perform within scope of practice; IX.P.4 Practice within the standard of care for a medical assistant; IX.P.7 Document accurately in the patient record

Name_____ Date_____ Score_____

● **COMPETENCY ASSESSMENT**

Procedure 31-16: Hemorrhoid Thrombectomy

Task: To incise inflamed hemorrhoids and remove thrombus. To remove hemorrhoids with laser, electrosurgery, cryosurgery, or banding.

Conditions: **Surgical Tray:**
- Appropriate size syringe and gauge of needle for administering anesthesia
- Mosquito hemostat (curved)
- Sterile basin
- Sterile 4 × 4 gauze sponges
- Rubber band
- Fenestrated drape
- Appropriate size syringe and gauge of needle for joint aspiration per provider preference
- Antiseptic solution as per provider preference

Side Area (Unsterile Field):
- Skin prep supplies
- Prepackaged sterile gloves (appropriate sizes for medical assistant and provider)
- Nonsterile disposable gloves
- Personal protective equipment (PPE)
- Anesthetic as ordered by the provider
- Biohazard specimen transport bag
- Soft absorbent pad, similar to sanitary napkin
- T-bandage (to hold pad in place)
- Medication for joint injection per provider's orders
- Specimen container
- Appropriate lab requisition

Standards: Perform the Task within 30 minutes with a minimum score of ___ points, as determined by your instructor.

Time began: _____ **Time ended:** _____ **Total time:** _____

No.	Step	Points	Check #1	Check #2	Check #3
1	Wash hands.				
2	*Paying attention to detail,* assemble equipment.				
3	*Introduce yourself. Identify the patient and explain the procedure, speaking at the patient's level of understanding.*				
4	Obtain a signed consent for the procedure.				
5	*Allay the patient's fears regarding the procedure being performed and help the patient to feel safe and comfortable.*				
6	Inquire regarding allergies and last tetanus shot. Document appropriately.				
7	*Using active listening skills,* review health history to avoid possible complications. Share information with provider.				
8	*Attending to any special needs of the patient,* position the patient per provider's preference (Sim's position).				

No.	Step	Points	Check #1	Check #2	Check #3
9	***Being courteous, patient, and respectful to the patient, provide privacy,*** and drape patient if appropriate, ***being sure to protect the patient's personal boundaries.***				
10	Don appropriate PPE, including goggles if indicated.				
11	Don sterile gloves.				
12	Perform skin prep as ordered by provider.				
13	Remove gloves and dispose of in biohazard waste container.				
14	Assist the provider to aspirate the appropriate amount of local anesthesia. After administering the anesthesia, the provider either bands or excises the hemorrhoids with a scalpel. Suturing is usually not necessary.				
15	***Being courteous, patient, and respectful,*** support the patient as needed.				
Give Postoperative Care:					
16	Don nonsterile disposable gloves.				
17	Assist the provider in placing the soft absorbent pad against the wound. It may be held in place with the T-shaped bandage.				
18	Dress and bandage wound per provider's instructions. Dress to absorb exudates.				
19	Dispose of items utilized during the procedure according to OSHA guidelines.				
20	Remove gloves and dispose of in biohazard waste container.				
21	Wash hands.				
22	Obtain vital signs to assess patient stability post-procedure. Document in the patient's chart or EMR.				
23	***Explain wound care to the patient (and caregiver), speaking at the patient's level of understanding,*** per provider. Sitting in a tub of warm water is soothing and aids healing. ***Provide written instructions*** including signs of complications such as excessive bleeding or pain.				
24	***Demonstrating respect for individual diversity,*** assist the patient with any questions or concerns.				
25	Arrange for a follow-up appointment and post-operative medication as ordered.				
26	***Demonstrating respect for individual diversity,*** assist the patient with any questions or concerns.				
27	Don PPE including nonsterile disposable gloves.				
28	Clean room, sanitize instruments, and sterilize for reuse.				
29	Remove PPE and dispose of appropriately.				
30	Wash hands.				
Student's Total Points					
Points Possible					
Final Score (Student's Total Points/Possible Points)					

Instructor's/Evaluator's Comments and Suggestions:

_____
_____
_____
_____
_____
_____

CHECK #1	
Evaluator's Signature:	Date:

CHECK #2	
Evaluator's Signature:	Date:

CHECK #3	
Evaluator's Signature:	Date:

Work Documentation Form(s)

*Lab Requisition form and Progress Note Template can be downloaded from the Premium Website

ABHES Competencies: MA.A.1.9.a Obtain chief complaint, recording patient history; MA.A.1.9.b Apply principles of aseptic techniques and infection control; MA.A.1.9.c Take vital signs; MA.A.1.9.d Recognize and understand various treatment protocols; MA.A.1.9.e Recognize emergencies and treatments and minor office surgical procedures; MA.A.1.9.l Prepare patient for examinations and treatments; MA.A.1.9.m Assist physician with routine and specialty examinations and treatments

CAAHEP Competencies: I.P.1 Obtain vital signs; I.P.10 Assist physician with patient care; I.A.1 Apply critical thinking skills in performing patient assessment and care; I.A.2 Use language/verbal skills that enable patients' understanding; III.A.2 Explain the rationale for performance of a procedure to the patient; III.A.3 Show awareness of patient' concerns regarding their perceptions related to the procedure being performed; IV.P.6 Prepare a patient for procedures and/or treatments; IV.P.8 Document patient care; IV.A.1 Demonstrate empathy in communicating with patients, family, and staff; IX.P.2 Perform within scope of practice; IX.P.4 Practice within the standard of care for a medical assistant; IX.P.7 Document accurately in the patient record

Name_____ **Date**_____ **Score**_____

● **COMPETENCY ASSESSMENT**

Procedure 31-17: Suture/Staple Removal

Task: To remove sutures from a healed surgical wound (as per provider).

Conditions:
- Gauze sponges
- Bandage scissors
- Biohazard waste container
- Tape
- Forceps
- Suture removal kit (suture scissors or staple remover, thumb forceps, and 4 × 4s)
- Sterile latex gloves
- Antibiotic ointment/cream as per provider's orders

Standards: Perform the Task within 15 minutes with a minimum score of ___ points, as determined by your instructor.

Time began: _____ **Time ended:** _____ **Total time:** _____

No.	Step	Points	Check #1	Check #2	Check #3
1	Wash hands.				
2	*Paying attention to detail*, assemble equipment.				
3	*Introduce yourself. Identify patient. Speaking at the level of the patient's understanding, explain the procedure to the patient.*				
4	*Allay the patient's fears regarding the procedure being performed and help the patient to feel safe and comfortable.*				
5	Apply nonsterile gloves and remove bandage. Dispose of bandage and gloves in biohazard waste container.				
6	Wash hands.				
7	Open suture or staple removal kit.				
8	Apply sterile gloves.				
9	*If removing sutures:* • If the sutures are covered with dried fluids, don sterile gloves, soak a sterile 4 × 4 gauze sponge with sterile water or saline and gently place on the suture line to allow removal of dried fluids in order to visualize the sutures. • Using thumb forceps, gently pick up one knot of a suture. Gently pull upward toward suture line. • Using suture removal scissors, cut ONLY one side of the suture as close to skin as possible. • Grasping the knot, pull slowly and continuously until the suture is free of the skin. • Repeat until all sutures are removed. • CAUTION: If suture line opens as sutures are removed, **STOP** and consult provider.				

No.	Step	Points	Check #1	Check #2	Check #3
10	*If removing staples:* • If the staples are covered with dried fluids, don sterile gloves, soak a sterile 4 × 4 gauze sponge with sterile water or saline and gently place on the suture line to allow removal of dried fluids in order to visualize the staples. • Gently insert staple remover under the first staple with the two prongs positioned below the staple and the single prong on top of the staple. • With slow, continuous pressure, close the staple remover handles to remove the staple. • Repeat until all staples are removed. • CAUTION: If incision line opens as staples are removed, **STOP** and consult provider.				
11	Apply antibiotic ointment/cream per provider's orders.				
12	Place sterile dressing over wound per provider's orders.				
13	Remove sterile gloves and dispose of in biohazard waste container.				
14	Wash hands.				
Postoperative Care					
15	Don nonsterile disposable gloves.				
16	Dispose of items utilized during the procedure according to OSHA guidelines.				
17	Remove gloves and dispose of in biohazard waste container.				
18	Wash hands.				
19	Obtain vital signs to assess patient stability post-procedure. Document in the patient's chart or EMR.				
20	**Demonstrating respect for individual diversity,** assist the patient with any questions or concerns.				
21	Arrange for a follow-up appointment and post-operative medication as required.				
22	Accurately document procedure in patient's chart or electronic medical record.				
Student's Total Points					
Points Possible					
Final Score (Student's Total Points/Possible Points)					

Instructor's/Evaluator's Comments and Suggestions:

CHECK #1	
Evaluator's Signature:	Date:

CHECK #2	
Evaluator's Signature:	Date:

CHECK #3	
Evaluator's Signature:	Date:

Work Documentation Form(s)

*Progress Note Template can be downloaded from the Premium Website

ABHES Competencies: MA.A.1.9.b Apply principles of aseptic techniques and infection control; MA.A.1.9.c Take vital signs; MA.A.1.9.d Recognize and understand various treatment protocols; MA.A.1.9.e Recognize emergencies and treatments and minor office surgical procedures

CAAHEP Competencies: I.P.1 Obtain vital signs; I.P.10 Assist physician with patient care; I.A.1 Apply critical thinking skills in performing patient assessment and care; I.A.2 Use language/verbal skills that enable patients' understanding; III.A.2 Explain the rationale for performance of a procedure to the patient; III.A.3 Show awareness of patient' concerns regarding their perceptions related to the procedure being performed; IV.P.6 Prepare a patient for procedures and/or treatments; IV.P.8 Document patient care; IV.A.1 Demonstrate empathy in communicating with patients, family, and staff; IX.P.4 Practice within the standard of care for a medical assistant; IX.P.7 Document accurately in the patient record

Name_____ **Date**_____ **Score**_____

● **COMPETENCY ASSESSMENT**

Procedure 31-18: Application of Sterile Adhesive Skin Closure Strips

Task: To approximate the edges of a wound after the removal of sutures. Sometimes used in lieu of sutures or to give additional support along with sutures.

Conditions: **Sterile Field:**
- Suture removal instruments (if indicated)
- Sterile adhesive skin closure devices
- Iris scissors (straight)
- Adson dressing forceps
- Tincture of benzoin per provider's preference
- Sterile cup
- Sterile cotton-tipped applicators (for tincture of benzoin)

Side Area (Unsterile Field):
- Prepackaged sterile gloves in the appropriate size
- Dressings, bandages, and tape
- Waterproof bag

Standards: Perform the Task within 15 minutes with a minimum score of ___ points, as determined by your instructor.

Time began: _____ **Time ended:** _____ **Total time:** _____

No.	Step	Points	Check #1	Check #2	Check #3
1	Wash hands.				
2	*Paying attention to detail*, assemble equipment.				
3	*Introduce yourself. Identify patient. Explain the procedure, speaking at the patient's level of understanding.*				
4	*Allay the patient's fears regarding the procedure being performed and help the patient to feel safe and comfortable.*				
5	*Considering any special needs of the patient,* position the patient comfortably.				
6	Using existing sterile field, open strips and drop onto sterile field.				
7	Open sterile cup and cotton-tipped applicators (or use prepackaged swabs) and drop onto sterile field.				
8	Carefully pour a small amount of tincture benzoin into cup. (Skip step if using prepackaged swabs.)				
9	Don sterile gloves.				
10	Clean and dry wound.				
11	Apply tincture of benzoin to wound edges using sterile cotton-tipped applicator or swab stick. *DO NOT* allow benzoin to come into contact with the incision. Allow to dry.				

No.	Step	Points	Check #1	Check #2	Check #3
12	Cut strips to size if needed. Carefully peel strips from backing using thumb forceps.				
13	Place the first strip at the center of the wound.				
14	Apply one end of the skin closure strip to one side of the wound, and using slight tension, apply to the other side of the wound. *Do not pucker the skin.*				
15	Secure the strip to the skin by pressing gently.				
16	Apply the strips as needed to reinforce the suture line per provider's instructions.				
Give Postoperative Care:					
17	Dress and bandage if necessary.				
18	Dispose of used items per OSHA guidelines.				
19	Remove gloves and wash hands.				
20	Check the patient's vital signs, if indicated.				
21	***Explain wound care to the patient (and caregiver), speaking at the patient's level of understanding, and provide written instructions*** including symptoms of infection.				
22	***Demonstrating respect for individual diversity,*** assist the patient with any questions or concerns.				
23	Arrange for follow-up appointment and medication as ordered.				
24	Accurately document procedure in patient's chart or electronic medical record.				
Student's Total Points					
Points Possible					
Final Score (Student's Total Points/Possible Points)					

Instructor's/Evaluator's Comments and Suggestions:

_____

_____

_____

_____

_____

_____

CHECK #1	
Evaluator's Signature:	Date:

CHECK #2	
Evaluator's Signature:	Date:

CHECK #3	
Evaluator's Signature:	Date:

Work Documentation Form(s)

*Progress Note Template can be downloaded from the Premium Website

ABHES Competencies: MA.A.1.9.b Apply principles of aseptic techniques and infection control; MA.A.1.9.d Recognize and understand various treatment protocols; MA.A.1.9.e Recognize emergencies and treatments and minor office surgical procedures

CAAHEP Competencies: I.P.1 Obtain vital signs; I.P.10 Assist physician with patient care; I.A.1 Apply critical thinking skills in performing patient assessment and care; I.A.2 Use language/verbal skills that enable patients' understanding; III.A.2 Explain the rationale for performance of a procedure to the patient; III.A.3 Show awareness of patient' concerns regarding their perceptions related to the procedure being performed; IV.P.6 Prepare a patient for procedures and/or treatments; IV.P.8 Document patient care; IV.A.1 Demonstrate empathy in communicating with patients, family, and staff; IX.P.4 Practice within the standard of care for a medical assistant; IX.P.7 Document accurately in the patient record

Name_____ **Date**_____ **Score**_____

● COMPETENCY ASSESSMENT

Procedure 33-1:   Transferring Patient from Wheelchair to Examination Table

Task:　　　　To move a patient safely from a wheelchair to the examination table.

Conditions:　　• Footstool with hand rail and non-skid rubber tips
　　　　　　　　• Gait belt

Standards:　　Perform the Task within 15 minutes with a minimum score of ___ points, as determined by your instructor.

Time began: _____　　Time ended: _____　　Total time: _____

No.	Step	Points	Check #1	Check #2	Check #3
1	Wash hands.				
2	*Introduce yourself and identify patient. Speaking at the patient's level of understanding, explain the process of transfer* so that the patient is able to assist as much as possible.				
3	Place the wheelchair next to the examination table and lock the brakes.				
4	Assure that the wheelchair is parked with the patient's strongest side near the exam table. The patient can balance on this leg during the transfer.				
5	Place the gait belt snugly around the patient's waist and tuck the excess belting under the belt to avoid tripping or entanglement.				
6	Move the wheelchair's footrests up and out of the way. If the footrests are removable, that is preferred.				
7	Instruct the patient to place their feet flat on the floor. *Assist patient* if needed.				
8	Position the stool in front of the examination table as close to the wheelchair as possible.				
9	Instruct the patient to move forward to the edge of the wheelchair.				
10	Remind the patient of instructions and signal.				
11	Stand directly in front of the patient with your feet slightly apart. Remember and use good body mechanics.				
12	Bend at the hips and knees. Grasp the gait belt from underneath. Have the patient place his or her hands on the armrests of the wheelchair. At your signal, have your patient push on the armrests to assist in lifting himself to a standing position.				

No.	Step	Points	Check #1	Check #2	Check #3
13	Steady the patient momentarily and observe for strength, balance, and skin color. If there are any changes, or as indicated by patient statements, carefully lower the patient to a sitting position in the wheelchair and check vital signs.				
14	If the patient appears steady, stable and balanced, proceed by standing slightly behind and on the weakest side of the patient.				
15	Grasp the gait belt with one hand and place the other hand on the patient's bent arm for support.				
16	Still grasping the gait belt, have the patient grasp the handle of the footstool. Instruct the patient to carefully step up on the footstool. Assist the patient to pivot so that his back is toward the examination table.				
17	The buttocks should be slightly above the edge of the bed. Steady the patient.				
18	Instruct the patient to place one hand on the safety handle of the footstool and one hand on the examination table.				
19	***Considering any special needs of the patient***, gently ease the patient onto the examination table.				
20	Position the examination table as necessary.				
21	Move the wheelchair and foot stool out of the way.				
Two-Person Transfer					
1	Follow Steps 1 to 7 above.				
2	Position one staff member in front of the patient and one on the patient's weakest side.				
3	Both persons should grasp the gait belt from underneath.				
4	Remind the patient and your assistant of your instructions and have the patient place his hands on the armrests of the wheelchair. At your signal, have your patient push on the armrests to assist in lifting himself to a standing position.				
5	Upon your signal, coordinate the upward motion gripping the gait belt.				
6	The person nearest the examination table should move the wheelchair out of the way. The other person should assist the patient to pivot.				
7	Have the patient grasp the handle of the footstool. Instruct and assist the patient to place the foot on his strongest side upon the footstool.				

No.	Step	Points	Check #1	Check #2	Check #3
8	On yours signal, both persons lift the patient onto the examination table.				
9	*Considering any special needs of the patient*, position the patient on the examination table as necessary.				
Student's Total Points					
Points Possible					
Final Score (Student's Total Points/Possible Points)					

Instructor's/Evaluator's Comments and Suggestions:

_____

_____

_____

_____

_____

_____

_____

CHECK #1 Evaluator's Signature:	Date:

CHECK #2 Evaluator's Signature:	Date:

CHECK #3 Evaluator's Signature:	Date:

ABHES Competency: MA.A.1.9.1 Prepare patient for examinations and treatments

CAAHEP Competencies: I.A.2 Use language/verbal skills that enable patients' understanding; IV.P.6 Prepare a patient for procedures and/or treatments; IV.A.7 Demonstrate recognition of the patient's level of understanding; XI.P.11 Use proper body mechanics

Name _____ **Date** _____ **Score** _____

● COMPETENCY ASSESSMENT

Procedure 33-2:   Transferring Patient from Examination Table to Wheelchair

Task: To move a patient safely from the examination table to a wheelchair.

Conditions:
- Safety handrail footstool with non-slip rubber tips
- Gait belt

Standards: Perform the Task within 15 minutes with a minimum score of _____ points, as determined by your instructor.

Time began: _____   **Time ended:** _____   **Total time:** _____

No.	Step	Points	Check #1	Check #2	Check #3
1	Wash hands.				
2	*Introduce yourself and identify patient. Speaking at the patient's level of understanding, explain the procedure.*				
3	*Allay the patient's fears regarding the procedure being performed and help the patient to feel safe and comfortable.*				
4	Position the wheelchair next to the examination table and lock the brakes.				
5	Park the wheelchair so that it is closest to the patient's strongest side. This will allow the transfer of weight onto the strongest leg when descending from the examination table.				
6	Position the stool next to the wheelchair.				
7	*Considering any special patient needs,* assist the patient into a sitting position. Place the gait belt snugly around the patient's waist. Tuck the excess end under the belt to avoid tripping or entaglement.				
8	Position your arm under the patient's arm and around her shoulders, and your other arm under her knees. Pivot the patient so that her legs are dangling over the edge of the examination table.				
9	Instruct the patient that upon your signal the patient should push off the examination table and grasp the handrail of the stool for support.				
10	Give the signal and pull the patient slightly toward you so that her feet land squarely on the foot stool.				
11	Still grasping the gait belt, instruct and then assist the patient to step to the floor with the strongest leg and pivot at the same time so that she is facing away from the wheelchair.				

No.	Step	Points	Check #1	Check #2	Check #3
12	Bending from your knees and hips, gently lower the patient into the wheelchair controlling her rate of descent with the gait belt. Assist her to attain comfort in the seated position.				
13	Lower or replace the footrests. Assist the patient to comfortably place her feet on the footrests.				
Student's Total Points					
Points Possible					
Final Score (Student's Total Points/Possible Points)					

Instructor's/Evaluator's Comments and Suggestions:

_____

_____

_____

_____

_____

_____

_____

_____

CHECK #1	
Evaluator's Signature:	Date:

CHECK #2	
Evaluator's Signature:	Date:

CHECK #3	
Evaluator's Signature:	Date:

ABHES Competency: MA.A.1.9.1 Prepare patient for examinations and treatments

CAAHEP Competencies: I.A.2 Use language/verbal skills that enable patients' understanding; IV.P.6 Prepare a patient for procedures and/or treatments; IV.A.7 Demonstrate recognition of the patient's level of understanding; XI.P.11 Use proper body mechanics

Name_____ **Date**_____ **Score**_____

● **COMPETENCY ASSESSMENT**

Procedure 33-3: Assisting the Patient to Stand and Walk

Task: To help a patient ambulate safely.

Conditions: • Gait belt

Standards: Perform the Task within 20 minutes with a minimum score of ____ points, as determined by your instructor.

Time began: _____ **Time ended:** _____ **Total time:** _____

No.	Step	Points	Check #1	Check #2	Check #3
1	Wash hands.				
2	*Introduce yourself and identify the patient. Speaking at the patient's level of understanding, explain the procedure.*				
3	Lock the brakes on the wheelchair, if the patient is using one. *Considering any special needs of the patient*, place the patient's feet on the floor and move the foot plates out of the way.				
4	Instruct and/or assist the patient to slide forward to the edge of the wheelchair.				
5	Place the gait belt snugly around the patient's waist. Tuck the excess end under the belt to avoid tripping or entanglement.				
6	Remembering the principles of good body mechanics, stand directly in front of the patient.				
7	Bend at the hips and knees. Grasp the gait belt from underneath.				
8	Have the patient place his hands on the armrest of the wheelchair. At your signal, have your patient push on the armrests to assist in lifting himself to a standing position.				
9	Steady the patient momentarily and observe for balance, strength, and skin color. If there are any changes or as indicated by patient statements, carefully lower the patient to a sitting position in the wheelchair and check vital signs.				
10	If the patient appears steady, stable, and is balanced, proceed by standing slightly behind and to the side of the patient's weaker side.				
11	Grasp the gait belt with one hand and place the other hand on the patient's bent arm for support. *NOTE:* The gait belt is to be grasped with fingers under the belt, palm facing upwards, and elbow bent.				

No.	Step	Points	Check #1	Check #2	Check #3
12	Indicate when you are ready to begin ambulation. Step forward with the same leg as the patient and remain in step.				
13	Accurately document the procedure in the patient's chart or electronic medical record, including date, time, duration of ambulation, response of patient, and instructions given.				
Two-Person Assist with Ambulation					
1	Perform the preceding Steps 1 through 5.				
2	Position a person on either side of the patient. Utilizing good body mechanics, bending at hips and knees, grasp the gait belt from underneath with one hand, and place the other hand on the patient's back for support.				
3	During ambulation each person should remain on either side and slightly behind the patient. Both people must retain a grip on the gait belt throughout the ambulation.				
4	Accurately document the procedure in the patient's chart or electronic medical record, including date, time, duration of ambulation, and any gait disturbances noted response of patient, vital signs if taken, and patient education.				
Student's Total Points					
Points Possible					
Final Score (Student's Total Points/Possible Points)					

Instructor's/Evaluator's Comments and Suggestions:

_____

_____

_____

_____

_____

_____

_____

CHECK #1	
Evaluator's Signature:	Date:

CHECK #2	
Evaluator's Signature:	Date:

CHECK #3	
Evaluator's Signature:	Date:

Work Documentation Form(s)

*Progress Note Template can be downloaded from the Premium Website

ABHES Competency: MA.A.1.9.1 Prepare patient for examinations and treatments

CAAHEP Competencies: I.A.2 Use language/verbal skills that enable patients' understanding; IV.P.6 Prepare a patient for procedures and/or treatments; IV.A.7 Demonstrate recognition of the patient's level of understanding; XI.P.11 Use proper body mechanics

Name _____ **Date** _____ **Score** _____

● **COMPETENCY ASSESSMENT**

Procedure 33-4:   Care of the Falling Patient

Task: To help the patient fall safely to prevent injury.

Conditions: • Gait belt (should already be on patient)

Standards: Perform the Task within 5 minutes with a minimum score of _____ points, as determined by your instructor.

Time began: _____   **Time ended:** _____   **Total time:** _____

No.	Step	Points	Check #1	Check #2	Check #3
1	Firmly grip the gait belt. Never grab clothing as it can shift and become unstable.				
2	If the patient falls backward, widen your stance to become a more stable base of support to accept the person's weight. Gently guide the patient to the floor, call for assistance, and assess vital signs.				
3	If the patient falls to either side, attempt to assist the patient back to center of gravity by moving your foot in the direction of the fall.				
4	Assess the patient to determine whether to terminate the ambulation session. Call for assistance if needed. Assess vital signs.				
5	If the patient falls forward, provide support by utilizing a firm grip on the gait belt.				
6	Gently lower patient to the floor. Call for assistance. Assess vital signs.				
7	Notify the provider of the need for assessment prior to moving patient.				
8	Accurately document in the patient's chart or electronic medical record indicating date, time, factual description of the event, response of patient, vital signs if taken, and any injuries noted by provider. Complete occurrence report if required.				
Student's Total Points					
Points Possible					
Final Score (Student's Total Points/Possible Points)					

Instructor's/Evaluator's Comments and Suggestions:

_____

_____

_____

_____

_____

_____

_____

_____

CHECK #1	
Evaluator's Signature:	Date:

CHECK #2	
Evaluator's Signature:	Date:

CHECK #3	
Evaluator's Signature:	Date:

Work Documentation Form(s)

*Progress Note Template can be downloaded from the Premium Website

ABHES Competency: MA.A.1.9.1 Prepare patient for examinations and treatments

CAAHEP Competencies: I.A.2 Use language/verbal skills that enable patients' understanding; IV.P.6 Prepare a patient for procedures and/or treatments; IV.A.7 Demonstrate recognition of the patient's level of understanding; XI.P.11 Use proper body mechanics

Name_____ **Date**_____ **Score**_____

● **COMPETENCY ASSESSMENT**

Procedure 33-5: Assisting a Patient to Ambulate with a Walker

Task: To allow a patient to ambulate independently and safely with a walker.

Conditions:
- Walker
- Gait belt

Standards: Perform the Task within 20 minutes with a minimum score of ____ points, as determined by your instructor.

Time began: _____ **Time ended:** _____ **Total time:** _____

No.	Step	Points	Check #1	Check #2	Check #3
1	Wash hands.				
2	*Introduce yourself and identify patient. Explain to the patient what you are going to do, speaking at the patient's level of understanding.*				
3	Notify the provider of the need for assessment prior to moving patient.				
4	Place the gait belt snugly around the patient's waist and tuck the excess belting under the belt to avoid tripping or entanglement.				
5	Check the walker to be sure the rubber suction tips are secure on all the legs. Check the handles for rough and damaged edges that could injure the patient. Assure that the walker is locked in the open position.				
6	Check the height of the walker. The hand rests should be level with the patient's hip joint. When placing hands on the hand rest, the elbows should be bent at an approximately 30-degree angle.				
7	Position the patient inside the walker, and instruct the patient to hold onto the handles while keeping the walker in front.				
8	Position yourself behind and slightly to the side of the patient. (If one side is weaker, choose that side for your placement.)				
9	Check the patient's footwear. It must be sturdy with a flat, non-slip sole.				
10	Have the patient step into the walker and have her hold onto the hand rests. Instruct the patient to keep the walker out in front of her as she begins to ambulate.				

No.	Step	Points	Check #1	Check #2	Check #3
11	Position yourself behind and slightly to the side of the patient. If one side is weaker, choose that side for your placement.				
12	Instruct the patient to lift the walker and place all four legs of the walker in front of herself. The back legs of the walker should be even with the patient's toes.				
13	The patient should then lean forward placing hands on the hand rest. Have the patient utilize her arms to transfer some of the weight to the walker.				
14	Have the patient step into the walker using the stronger leg, then the weaker leg. Ensure that the patient's stronger leg is within the embrace of the walker.				
15	Steady the patient momentarily and observe for strength, balance, and skin color. If there are any changes, or as indicated by patient statements, rest and make a decision about continuing to ambulate.				
16	If the walker has rollers, the patient simply rolls the walker ahead a comfortable distance, then walks into it. The patient can also walk normally with a rolling walker by simply rolling it in front and leaning into the gait, using the walker for support.				
17	Accurately document in the patient's chart or electronic medical record indicating the date, time, duration of ambulation, response of patient, vital signs if taken, and any injuries noted by provider.				
Student's Total Points					
Points Possible					
Final Score (Student's Total Points/Possible Points)					

Instructor's/Evaluator's Comments and Suggestions:

_____
_____
_____
_____
_____
_____
_____

CHECK #1 Evaluator's Signature:	Date:

CHECK #2 Evaluator's Signature:	Date:

CHECK #3 Evaluator's Signature:	Date:

Work Documentation Form(s)

*Progress Note Template can be downloaded from the Premium Website

ABHES Competency: MA.A.1.9.1 Prepare patient for examinations and treatments

CAAHEP Competencies: I.A.2 Use language/verbal skills that enable patients' understanding; IV.P.6 Prepare a patient for procedures and/or treatments; IV.A.7 Demonstrate recognition of the patient's level of understanding; XI.P.11 Use proper body mechanics

Name _____ **Date** _____ **Score** _____

● **COMPETENCY ASSESSMENT**

Procedure 33-6:   Teaching the Patient to Ambulate with Crutches

Task: To teach the patient how to ambulate safely using crutches.

Conditions: • Crutches
                   • Gait belt

Standards: Perform the Task within 20 minutes with a minimum score of ____ points, as determined by your instructor.

Time began: _____   **Time ended:** _____   **Total time:** _____

No.	Step	Points	Check #1	Check #2	Check #3
1	Wash hands.				
2	*Introduce yourself and identify patient. Explain to the patient what you are going to do, speaking at the patient's level of understanding.*				
3	Assemble the crutches and be sure they are in good working order. Check the rubber, non-slip tips on the end of each crutch. Check the bar and hand rest to be sure they are covered with padding. If the padding is cracked or worn, replace them. Assure that the wing nuts are tightened appropriately.				
4	Measure for crutches. Place tape in the axillary area. Measure from there to a spot 2 inches before and 6 inches to the side of the foot. Adjust crutches to this measurement.				
5	Place the gait belt snugly around the patient's waist and tuck the excess belting under the belt to avoid tripping or entanglement.				
6	*Speaking at the patient's level of understanding,* instruct the patient to bear the weight of the body using the hands on the hand rests. Do not bear weight on the axillary area.				
7	Place both crutches at a comfortable distance in front of the patient's feet. Stand tall, looking forward rather than down at your feet.				
8	Move the affected leg up even with crutches. Transfer weight via the hands onto the crutches. Repeat the same sequence for the next step.				

No.	Step	Points	Check #1	Check #2	Check #3
9	Accurately document in the patient's chart or electronic medical record indicating the date, time, duration of ambulation, patient instruction, response of patient, vital signs if taken.				
	Student's Total Points				
	Points Possible				
	Final Score (Student's Total Points/Possible Points)				

Instructor's/Evaluator's Comments and Suggestions:

_____

_____

_____

_____

_____

_____

_____

CHECK #1	
Evaluator's Signature:	Date:

CHECK #2	
Evaluator's Signature:	Date:

CHECK #3	
Evaluator's Signature:	Date:

Work Documentation Form(s)

*Progress Note Template can be downloaded from the Premium Website

ABHES Competency: MA.A.1.9.1 Prepare patient for examinations and treatments

CAAHEP Competencies: I.A.2 Use language/verbal skills that enable patients' understanding; IV.P.6 Prepare a patient for procedures and/or treatments; IV.A.7 Demonstrate recognition of the patient's level of understanding; XI.P.11 Use proper body mechanics

Name _____ **Date** _____ **Score** _____

● COMPETENCY ASSESSMENT

Procedure 33-7:   Assisting a Patient to Ambulate with a Cane

Task: To teach patients how to walk safely with a cane.

Conditions: • Appropriate cane for the patient
  • Gait belt

Standards: Perform the Task within 15 minutes with a minimum score of _____ points, as determined by your instructor.

Time began: _____   **Time ended:** _____   **Total time:** _____

No.	Step	Points	Check #1	Check #2	Check #3
1	Wash hands.				
2	*Introduce yourself and identify patient.*				
3	Select the appropriate cane per the provider's orders.				
4	Examine the tip of the cane to assure that the rubber is not worn. If a quad cane or walk cane is to be used, be sure that all the legs have rubber tips.				
5	Assemble cane and gait belt.				
6	Place the gait belt snugly around the patient's waist and tuck the excess belting under the belt to avoid tripping or entanglement.				
7	Place the cane relatively close to the body to the side of the foot of the strong leg. Adjust the cane so the handle is level with the patient's hip joint.				
8	During weight bearing, the patient's elbow should be flexed 20° to 30°.				
9	The cane and the involved leg are advanced simultaneously.				
10	Have the patient move the weak leg forward while transferring the weight to the cane.				
11	Have the patient step forward with the unaffected leg past the cane.				
12	Repeat the procedure for the next step.				
13	Support the patient by grasping the gait belt in the back while standing slightly behind the patient.				

No.	Step	Points	Check #1	Check #2	Check #3
14	Follow along behind and on the patient's affected side.				
15	Wash hands.				
16	Accurately document in the patient's chart or electronic medical record indicating the date, time, duration of ambulation, patient instruction, response of patient, and vital signs if taken.				
Student's Total Points					
Points Possible					
Final Score (Student's Total Points/Possible Points)					

Instructor's/Evaluator's Comments and Suggestions:

_____

_____

_____

_____

_____

_____

CHECK #1	
Evaluator's Signature:	Date:

CHECK #2	
Evaluator's Signature:	Date:

CHECK #3	
Evaluator's Signature:	Date:

Work Documentation Form(s)

*Progress Note Template can be downloaded from the Premium Website

ABHES Competency: MA.A.1.9.1 Prepare patient for examinations and treatments

CAAHEP Competencies: I.A.2 Use language/verbal skills that enable patients' understanding; IV.P.6 Prepare a patient for procedures and/or treatments; IV.A.7 Demonstrate recognition of the patient's level of understanding; XI.P.11 Use proper body mechanics

Name _____ **Date** _____ **Score** _____

● COMPETENCY ASSESSMENT

Procedure 34-1: Provide Instruction for Health Maintenance and Disease Prevention

Task: To instruct patients about how to exercise more responsibility and take control of their health in order to extend their lives and enjoy healthy years.

Conditions:
- Discussion
- DVDs
- Videos
- Print material
- Authenticated web-based interactive information
- Community resources directories
- Seminars
- Classes (self-directed and self-paced)

Standards: Perform the Task within 20 minutes with a minimum score of _____ points, as determined by your instructor.

Time began: _____ **Time ended:** _____ **Total time:** _____

No.	Step	Points	Check #1	Check #2	Check #3
1	*Introduce yourself and identify patient.*				
2	Gather materials to be utilized during the educational session for health maintenance and disease prevention.				
3	Select a quiet and private area to begin the instruction.				
4	Assess patient's learning style and preference. *Involve the patient's support system.*				
5	*Speaking at the patient's level of understanding,* provide information to the patient regarding a specific illness, medical management, health maintenance, and/or disease prevention. Instruct patient to: • Schedule regular screenings for illness as is age appropriate, such as yearly physical examination, Pap smear, mammogram, occult blood testing, colonoscopy, urinalysis, electrocardiogram, chest X-ray, blood tests for anemia, chemistry profiles, hearing and vision tests. • Avoid tobacco. • Get regular exercise at least 30 minutes most days (walk dog, bicycle, rake leaves, do housework, swim). • Maintain a balanced diet (see ChooseMyPlate at http://www.choosemyplate.gov). • Practice safety to prevent injuries (make sure smoke detectors work, wear seat belts, do not drink and drive). • Control weight, blood pressure, and cholesterol.				

No.	Step	Points	Check #1	Check #2	Check #3
	• Watch sun exposure and use a sun block factor of at least SPF 30 all year. • Keep vaccine immunizations current. • Practice food safety by preparing food with clean hands and on clean surfaces.				
6	Educate patients who do not have a home computer regarding access at the public library.				
7	Accurately document in the patient's chart or electronic medical record indicating date, time, topic of education, demonstration of patient understanding and planned follow-up.				
Student's Total Points					
Points Possible					
Final Score (Student's Total Points/Possible Points)					

Instructor's/Evaluator's Comments and Suggestions:

_____

_____

_____

_____

_____

_____

CHECK #1	
Evaluator's Signature:	Date:

CHECK #2	
Evaluator's Signature:	Date:

CHECK #3	
Evaluator's Signature:	Date:

Work Documentation Form(s)

*Progress Note Template can be downloaded from the Premium Website

ABHES Competencies: MA.A.1.4.a Document accurately; MA.A.1.9.l Prepare patient for examinations and treatments

CAAHEP Competencies: IV.C.4 Identify techniques for overcoming communication barriers; IV.C.5 Recognize the elements of oral communication using sender-receiver process

Name _____ **Date** _____ **Score** _____

● COMPETENCY ASSESSMENT

Procedure 35-1:   Proper Disposal of Drugs

Task: To properly dispose of drugs that have reached their expiration dates.

Conditions: • Drugs (oral and parenteral) that have reached their expiration dates

Standards: Perform the Task within 10 minutes with a minimum score of ____ points, as determined by your instructor.

Competency Assessment Information

Use the following information to demonstrate the proper disposal of expired medications. Complete the Medication Disposal Log (Work Documentation).

Time began: _____ **Time ended:** _____ **Total time:** _____

No.	Step	Points	Check #1	Check #2	Check #3
1	Consult practice policy for disposal of expired medication.				
2	Access the drug closet or narcotics cabinet and evaluate the expiration date on all medications.				
3	Gather expired drugs, either prescription or over-the-counter.				
4	Medication take-back programs for disposal are a good way to remove expired medications. Consult your city or county government's household trash and recycling service to learn about any special rules regarding which medicines can be taken back. Explain the process.				
5	*Pay attention to detail.* Only if the label or accompanying patient information specifically instructs flushing drugs down the toilet or sink can you do so.				
6	Wash hands.				
7	Accurately document instructions in the medication log book or in the appropriate data collection area that the medications with expired dates were disposed of. Be sure to document the method of disposal. Have a co-worker co-sign the entry.				
Student's Total Points					
Points Possible					
Final Score (Student's Total Points/Possible Points)					

Instructor's/Evaluator's Comments and Suggestions:

_____

_____

_____

_____

_____

_____

_____

CHECK #1	
Evaluator's Signature:	Date:

CHECK #2	
Evaluator's Signature:	Date:

CHECK #3	
Evaluator's Signature:	Date:

ABHES Competencies: MA.A.1.4.a Document accurately; MA.A.1.4.c Follow established policies when initiating or terminating medical treatment

CAAHEP Competencies: I.P.11 Perform quality control measures; IX.P.8 Apply local, state, and federal health care legislation and regulation appropriate to the medical assisting practice setting

Work Documentation Form(s)

Disposal of Prescription and Nonprescription Medication Log

Date	Name	Medication	Disposal of Amt/Pill Count	Method of Disposal	Signature	Witness' Signature of the Count and Med. Disposal

Name_____ **Date**_____ **Score**_____

● COMPETENCY ASSESSMENT

Procedure 36-1: Administration of Oral Medications

Task: Correctly administer an oral medication after receiving the provider's order and assembling the necessary equipment and supplies.

Conditions:
- Medication order per provider
- Correct medication
- Medication card
- Medicine cup
- Fluid for swallowing the medication (water, juice, or milk)

Standards: Perform the Task within 10 minutes with a minimum score of _____ points, as determined by your instructor.

Competency Assessment Information

Tomas Meyers is being seen in Dr. Miller's office today for an allergic skin reaction. After the examination, Dr. Miller orders Benadryl 50 mg po now.

Time began: _____ **Time ended:** _____ **Total time:** _____

No.	Step	Points	Check #1	Check #2	Check #3
1	Perform medical asepsis handwashing procedure. Adhere to OSHA guidelines.				
2	Verify the provider's order and prepare a medication card.				
3	Follow the "Six Rights" of medication administration.				
4	Work in a well-lighted, quiet, clean area.				
5	*Paying attention to detail*, gather appropriate equipment and supplies.				
6	Review the medication card. Select the correct medication from the medication area.				
7	Compare the medication label with the medication card (first check).				
8	If unfamiliar with the medication, consult the PDR or other reputable reference.				
9	Check the expiration date.				
10	Carefully calculate the dosage based on medication order and medication available.				
11	Correctly prepare: • Multiple-dose solid medication • Unit dose medication • Liquid medication				

No.	Step	Points	Check #1	Check #2	Check #3
12	Compare the medication label with the medication card (second check).				
13	Discard any refuse generated during the preparation.				
14	Carefully transport the medication to the patient exam room. Bring the medication container with the prepared medication.				
15	***Introduce yourself and identify the patient. Explain the procedure and expectations to the patient, speaking at the patient's level of understanding.***				
16	Ask the patient about medication allergies.				
17	Assess the patient. Take vital signs if indicated.				
18	Assure the patient is in a comfortable, upright position.				
19	Review the medication card and the medication (third check).				
20	Administer the medication. Provide an adequate amount of fluid to assure ease of swallowing.				
21	Have the patient open his mouth and move his tongue around to assure that the patient has swallowed the medication.				
22	If it is the first time that the patient has received the medication, have the patient remain in the office setting per the provider's preference.				
23	***Being courteous, patient, and respectful,*** assess the patient every 5 minutes for signs of reaction.				
24	***Paying attention to detail,*** return the medication container to the appropriate place in the medication area.				
25	Accurately document in the patient's chart or electronic medical record the medication, dose, route, site of injection, and patient reaction. Sign and add date and time.				
Student's Total Points					
Points Possible					
Final Score (Student's Total Points/Possible Points)					

Instructor's/Evaluator's Comments and Suggestions:

_____

_____

_____

_____

_____

_____

_____

CHECK #1	
Evaluator's Signature:	Date:

CHECK #2	
Evaluator's Signature:	Date:

CHECK #3	
Evaluator's Signature:	Date:

Work Documentation Form(s)

*Progress Note Template can be downloaded from the Premium Website

ABHES Competencies: MA.A.1.4.a Document accurately; MA.A.1.6.a Demonstrate accurate occupational math and metric conversions for proper medication administration; MA.A.1.6.b Properly utilize PDR, drug handbook, and other drug references to identify a drug's classification, usual dosage, usual side effects, and contraindications; MA.A.1.9.b Apply principles of aseptic techniques and infection control; MA.A.1.9.d Recognize and understand various treatment protocols; MA.A.1.9.g Maintain medication and immunization records; MA.A.1.9.l Prepare patient for examinations and treatments

CAAHEP Competencies: I.P.8 Administration of oral medications; I.A.1 Apply critical thinking skills in performing patient assessment and care; I.A.2 Use language/verbal skills that enable patients' understanding; II.P.1 Prepare proper dosages of medication for administration; II.A.1 Verify ordered dose/dosages prior to administration; III.P.2 Practice standard precautions; III.P.4 Perform hand washing; III.A.2 Explain the rationale for performance of a procedure to a patient; IV.P. 8 Document patient care; IX.P.2 Perform within scope of practice

Name_____   **Date**_____   **Score**_____

● COMPETENCY ASSESSMENT

Procedure 36-2:   Withdrawing Medication from a Vial

Task: Correctly draw medication from a vial with 100% accuracy.

Conditions:
- Medication order per provider
- Medication card
- Appropriately sized syringe and needle of the correct gauge and length
- Correct medication
- Alcohol wipes
- Disposable nonsterile gloves
- Sharps container

Standards: Perform the Task within 5 minutes with a minimum score of _____ points, as determined by your instructor.

Time began: _____   **Time ended:** _____   **Total time:** _____

No.	Step	Points	Check #1	Check #2	Check #3
1	Perform medical asepsis handwashing procedure. Adhere to OSHA guidelines.				
2	Verify the provider's order and prepare a medication card. Follow the "Six Rights" of medication administration.				
3	Work in a well-lighted, quiet, clean area.				
4	*Paying attention to detail,* gather appropriate equipment and supplies.				
5	Review the medication card. Select the correct medication from the medication area.				
6	Compare the medication label with the medication card (first check).				
7	If unfamiliar with the medication, consult the PDR or other reputable reference.				
8	Check the expiration date.				
9	Carefully calculate the dosage based on medication order and medication available.				
10	Compare the medication label with the medication card (second check).				
11	Remove the metal or plastic cap from the vial. Clean the vial stopped with an alcohol wipe using a circular motion.				

No.	Step	Points	Check #1	Check #2	Check #3
12	Carefully remove the needle cover. Inject air into the vial as follows: • Hold the syringe pointed upward at eye level. Pull the plunger back to the level of the expected amount of medication to be withdrawn. • Leave vial on tabletop/countertop. • Insert the needle through the center of the rubber stopper of the vial. • Inject the air by pushing the plunger slowly.				
13	Invert the vial. Hold the vial and the syringe steady. Carefully and slowly pull back on the plunger to withdraw the correct amount of medication. Measure accurately. Keep the tip of the needle below the surface of the liquid; otherwise, air will enter the syringe. Keep the syringe at eye level.				
14	Check the syringe for air bubbles. Remove them by tapping sharply on the syringe. Push the air bubbles back into the vial. Check the measurement for accuracy, and draw out more medication if necessary.				
15	Remove the needle from the vial. Replace the sterile needle cover using the "scoop" technique.				
16	Check the label on the vial with the medication card (third check).				
17	If the medication is a tissue irritant, change the needle utilized to withdraw the medication.				
18	Carefully carry the syringe and medication vial to the patient's bedside.				
19	Refer to the appropriate procedure (subcutaneous, intradermal, or intramuscular injection).				
20	Activate the safety mechanism to cover the needle. Immediately dispose of the needle and syringe in the sharps container.				
21	Remove gloves and dispose of according to OSHA guidelines.				
22	Wash hands.				
23	*Paying attention to detail,* return the medication container to the appropriate place in the medication area.				
24	Accurately document in the patient's chart or electronic medical record the medication, dose, route, site of injection, and patient reaction. Sign and add date and time.				
25	Following clinic procedure, return the vial to the medication cabinet. Destroy the medication card.				
Student's Total Points					
Points Possible					
Final Score (Student's Total Points/Possible Points)					

Instructor's/Evaluator's Comments and Suggestions:

●
_____
_____
_____
_____
_____
_____
_____

CHECK #1 Evaluator's Signature:	Date:

CHECK #2 Evaluator's Signature:	Date:

CHECK #3 Evaluator's Signature:	Date:

Work Documentation Form(s)

*Progress Note Template can be downloaded from the Premium Website

ABHES Competencies: MA.A.1.4.a Document accurately; MA.A.1.6.a Demonstrate accurate occupational math and metric conversions for proper medication administration; MA.A.1.6.b Properly utilize PDR, drug handbook, and other drug references to identify a drug's classification, usual dosage, usual side effects, and contraindications; MA.A.1.9.b Apply principles of aseptic techniques and infection control; MA.A.1.9.d Recognize and understand various treatment protocols; MA.A.1.9.g Maintain medication and immunization records; MA.A.1.9.l Prepare patient for examinations and treatments

CAAHEP Competencies: I.P.7 Select proper sites for parenteral medication; I.P.9 Administer parenteral (excluding IV) medications; I.A.1 Apply critical thinking skills in performing patient assessment and care; I.A.2 Use language/verbal skills that enable patients' understanding; II.P.1 Prepare proper dosages of medication for administration; II.A.1 Verify ordered dose/dosages prior to administration; III.P.2 Practice standard precautions; III.P.4 Perform hand washing; III.A.2 Explain the rationale for performance of a procedure to a patient; IV.P. 8 Document patient care; IX.P.2 Perform within scope of practice

Name_____ **Date**_____ **Score**_____

● COMPETENCY ASSESSMENT

Procedure 36-3:   Withdrawing Medication from an Ampule

Task: Correctly draw a medication from an ampule with 100% accuracy.

Conditions:
- Medicine order per provider
- Medication card
- Ampule of correct medication
- Alcohol wipes
- Sterile gauze sponges
- Sharps container
- Sterile filter needle
- Disposable nonsterile gloves
- Appropriately sized syringe and needle of the correct gauge and length

Standards: Perform the Task within 5 minutes with a minimum score of _____ points, as determined by your instructor.

Time began: _____ **Time ended:** _____ **Total time:** _____

No.	Step	Points	Check #1	Check #2	Check #3
1	Perform medical asepsis handwashing procedure. Adhere to OSHA guidelines.				
2	Verify the provider's order and prepare a medication card.				
3	Follow the "Six Rights" of medication administration.				
4	Work in a well-lighted, quiet, clean area.				
5	*Paying attention to detail,* gather appropriate equipment and supplies.				
6	Review the medication card. Select the correct medication from the medication area.				
7	Compare the medication label with the medication card (first check).				
8	If unfamiliar with the medication, consult the PDR or other reputable reference.				
9	Check the expiration date.				
10	Carefully calculate the dosage based on medication order and medication available.				
11	Compare the medication label with the medication card (second check).				
12	Don nonsterile disposable gloves.				

No.	Step	Points	Check #1	Check #2	Check #3
13	Grasp the ampule of medication. The medication will often get "trapped" in the neck of the ampule. To return it to the body of the ampule, swirl the ampule in a circular motion by holding onto the upper end above the neck. The medication will return to the body of the vial.				
14	Thoroughly disinfect the neck of the ampule by wiping with an alcohol wipe.				
15	With a sterile gauze, wipe dry the neck of the ampule. Completely surround the ampule with the gauze and forcefully snap off the top of the ampule by pulling the top toward you.				
16	*Paying attention to detail,* carefully place the open ampule on the countertop.				
17	Check the provider's order, medication card and label on ampule (third check).				
18	With a sterile syringe and a filter needle, aspirate the required dose into the syringe. Cover needle with sheath using scoop method and transport it with medication ampule to patient on the medicine tray.				
19	Cover the filer needle with the cap using the "scoop" method.				
20	Remove the filter needle from the syringe and immediately discard in an appropriate sharps container.				
21	Select the appropriate needle gauge and length for injection.				
22	Place the new needle, using sterile technique, on the syringe with the medication.				
23	Follow the steps for appropriate administration of subcutaneous, intradermal, or intramuscular injection.				
Student's Total Points					
Points Possible					
Final Score (Student's Total Points/Possible Points)					

Instructor's/Evaluator's Comments and Suggestions:

CHECK #1	
Evaluator's Signature:	Date:

CHECK #2	
Evaluator's Signature:	Date:

CHECK #3	
Evaluator's Signature:	Date:

Work Documentation Form(s)

*Progress Note Template can be downloaded from the Premium Website

ABHES Competencies: MA.A.1.4.a Document accurately; MA.A.1.6.a Demonstrate accurate occupational math and metric conversions for proper medication administration; MA.A.1.6.b Properly utilize PDR, drug handbook, and other drug references to identify a drug's classification, usual dosage, usual side effects, and contraindications; MA.A.1.9.b Apply principles of aseptic techniques and infection control; MA.A.1.9.d Recognize and understand various treatment protocols; MA.A.1.9.g Maintain medication and immunization records; MA.A.1.9.j Prepare and administer oral and parenteral medications as directed by physician; MA.A.1.9.l Prepare patient for examinations and treatments

CAAHEP Competencies: I.P.7 Select proper sites for parenteral medication; I.P.9 Administer parenteral (excluding IV) medications; I.A.1 Apply critical thinking skills in performing patient assessment and care; I.A.2 Use language/verbal skills that enable patients' understanding; II.P.1 Prepare proper dosages of medication for administration; II.A.1 Verify ordered dose/dosages prior to administration; III.P.2 Practice standard precautions; III.P.4 Perform hand washing; III.A.2 Explain the rationale for performance of a procedure to a patient; IV.P.8 Document patient care; IX.P.2 Perform within scope of practice

Name _____ **Date** _____ **Score** _____

⬤ **COMPETENCY ASSESSMENT**

Procedure 36-4: Administration of Subcutaneous, Intramuscular, and Intradermal Injections

Task: Properly administer subcutaneous, intramuscular, and intradermal injections with 100% accuracy.

Conditions:
- Ampule of correct medication
- Medication order per provider and medication card
- Appropriately sized syringe and needle of the correct gauge and length
- Alcohol wipes
- Disposable nonsterile gloves

Standards: Perform the Task within 10 minutes with a minimum score of _____ points, as determined by your instructor.

Time began: _____   **Time ended:** _____   **Total time:** _____

No.	Step	Points	Check #1	Check #2	Check #3
1	Perform medical asepsis handwashing procedure. Adhere to OSHA guidelines.				
2	Verify the provider's order and prepare a medication card.				
3	Follow the "Six Rights" of medication administration.				
4	Work in a well-lighted, quiet, clean area.				
5	*Paying attention to detail,* gather appropriate equipment and supplies.				
6	Review the medication card. Select the correct medication from the medication area.				
7	Compare the medication label with the medication card (first check).				
8	If unfamiliar with the medication, consult the PDR or other reputable reference.				
9	Check the expiration date.				
10	Carefully calculate the dosage based on medication order and medication available.				
11	Compare the medication label with the medication card (second check).				
12	Don nonsterile disposable gloves.				
13	Withdraw medication from vial using correct syringe and needle.				
14	Check the provider's order, medication card, and label on ampule (third check).				

No.	Step	Points	Check #1	Check #2	Check #3
15	Keeping the syringe, medication, alcohol swab and medication card together, transport to the patient's bedside.				
16	*Introduce yourself and identify the patient. Explain the procedure and expectations to the patient, speaking at the patient's level of understanding.* State the name of the medication and the purpose of the injection. *Allay the patient's fears regarding the procedure being performed and help her feel safe and comfortable.*				
17	Ask the patient about medication allergies.				
18	*If you are beyond your comfort zone or experience, ask a more knowledgeable peer or the provider to assist you. Remember to work within your scope of practice.*				
19	Assess the patient to determine the most appropriate site to administer an injection. Rotate sites if appropriate.				
20	Don nonsterile disposable gloves.				
21	Prepare the patient for the injection (position, provide privacy, drape).				
22	Cleanse the injection site that has been chosen. Use an alcohol wipe using a circular motion, beginning at the site of injection and circling outward to a diameter of 2 inches.				
23	Allow the skin to dry.				
24	Carefully, remove the needle cover.				
25	Using the correct angle of injection, insert the needle into the proper anatomical area.				
26	Aspirate by holding the syringe steady and gently pulling back on the syringe plunger. Check for blood in the syringe. • If blood is evident, remove the needle from the skin • Discard syringe appropriately in hazardous waste needle box • Notify provider				
27	Remove the needle in the direction that it was inserted.				
28	Activate the safety mechanism to cover the needle.				
29	If indicated, massage the site using the alcohol wipe.				
30	Cover the site if indicated with an adhesive bandage.				

No.	Step	Points	Check #1	Check #2	Check #3
31	Remove gloves and dispose of according to OSHA guidelines.				
32	Wash hands.				
33	If it is the first time that the patient has received the medication, she must remain in the exam room for 20 minutes to assure there is no reaction.				
34	*Being courteous, patient, and respectful,* assess the patient every 5 minutes for signs of reaction.				
35	*Paying attention to detail,* return the medication container to the appropriate place in the medication area.				
36	Discard the medication card.				
37	Accurately document in the patient's chart or electronic medical record the medication, dose, route, site of injection, and patient reaction. Sign and add date and time.				
Student's Total Points					
Points Possible					
Final Score (Student's Total Points/Possible Points)					

Instructor's/Evaluator's Comments and Suggestions:

_____

_____

_____

_____

_____

_____

_____

CHECK #1	
Evaluator's Signature:	Date:

CHECK #2	
Evaluator's Signature:	Date:

CHECK #3	
Evaluator's Signature:	Date:

Work Documentation Form(s)

*Progress Note Template can be downloaded from the Premium Website

ABHES Competencies: MA.A.1.4.a Document accurately; MA.A.1.6.a Demonstrate accurate occupational math and metric conversions for proper medication administration; MA.A.1.6.b Properly utilize PDR, drug handbook, and other drug references to identify a drug's classification, usual dosage, usual side effects, and contraindications; MA.A.1.9.b Apply principles of aseptic techniques and infection control; MA.A.1.9.d Recognize and understand various treatment protocols; MA.A.1.9.g Maintain medication and immunization records; MA.A.1.9.j Prepare and administer oral and parenteral medications as directed by physician; MA.A.1.9.l Prepare patient for examinations and treatments

CAAHEP Competencies: I.P.7 Select proper sites for parenteral medication; I.P.9 Administer parenteral (excluding IV) medications; I.A.1 Apply critical thinking skills in performing patient assessment and care; I.A.2 Use language/verbal skills that enable patients' understanding; II.P.1 Prepare proper dosages of medication for administration; II.A.1 Verify ordered dose/dosages prior to administration; III.P.2 Practice standard precautions; III.P.4 Perform hand washing; III.A.2 Explain the rationale for performance of a procedure to a patient; IV.P.8 Document patient care; IX.P.2 Perform within scope of practice

Name _____   **Date** _____   **Score** _____

● COMPETENCY ASSESSMENT

Procedure 36-5:   Administering a Subcutaneous Injection

Task: Correctly administer a subcutaneous injection with 100% accuracy.

Conditions: • Medication ordered per provider
                 • Medication card
                 • Appropriate syringe size and needle gauge and length
                 • Alcohol wipes
                 • Nonsterile disposable gloves
                 • Sharps container
                 • Adhesive bandage

Standards: Perform the Task within 10 minutes with a minimum score of _____ points, as determined by your instructor.

Time began: _____   **Time ended:** _____   **Total time:** _____

No.	Step	Points	Check #1	Check #2	Check #3
1	Perform medical asepsis handwashing procedure. Adhere to OSHA guidelines.				
2	Verify the provider's order and prepare a medication card.				
3	Follow the "Six Rights" of medication administration.				
4	Work in a well-lighted, quiet, clean area.				
5	*Paying attention to detail*, gather appropriate equipment and supplies.				
6	Review the medication card. Select the correct medication from the medication area.				
7	Compare the medication label with the medication card (first check).				
8	If unfamiliar with the medication, consult the PDR or other reputable reference.				
9	Check the expiration date.				
10	Carefully calculate the dosage based on medication order and medication available.				
11	*Displaying sound judgment*, correctly prepare the parenteral medication.				
12	Compare the medication label with the medication card (second check).				
13	Withdraw the medication from the vial using proper technique.				

No.	Step	Points	Check #1	Check #2	Check #3
14	Discard any refuse generated during the preparation.				
15	Carefully transport the medication to the patient exam room. Bring the medication container (vial) with the prepared medication.				
16	*Introduce yourself and identify the patient. Explain the procedure and expectations to the patient, speaking at the patient's level of understanding.* State the name of the medication and the purpose of the injection. *Allay the patient's fears regarding the procedure being performed and help him feel safe and comfortable.*				
17	Ask the patient about medication allergies.				
18	*If you are beyond your comfort zone or experience, ask a more knowledgeable peer or the provider to assist you. Remember to work within your scope of practice.*				
19	Assess the patient to determine the most appropriate site to administer an intramuscular injection. Don gloves.				
20	Prepare the patient for the injection (position, provide privacy, drape).				
21	Review the medication card and the medication (third check).				
22	Cleanse the injection site that has been chosen. Use an alcohol wipe and using a circular motion, beginning at the site of injection and circling outward to a diameter of 2 inches.				
23	Allow the skin to dry.				
24	Carefully remove the needle guard.				
25	Using your non-dominant hand, grasp the skin and pinch upward to form a 1-inch fold.				
26	Instruct the patient to take a deep breath and slowly release it.				
27	Insert the needle quickly at a 45-degree angle.				
28	Aspirate by holding the syringe steady and gently pulling back on the syringe plunger. Check for blood in the syringe. • If blood is evident, remove the needle from the skin • Discard syringe appropriately in hazardous waste needle box • Notify provider				
29	Slowly and steadily inject the medication.				
30	Remove the needle in the direction that it was inserted.				

No.	Step	Points	Check #1	Check #2	Check #3
31	Activate the safety mechanism to cover the needle. Immediately dispose of the needle and syringe in the sharps container.				
32	If indicated, massage the site using the alcohol wipe. Cover the site, if indicated, with an adhesive bandage.				
33	Remove gloves and dispose of according to OSHA guidelines. Wash hands.				
34	If it is the first time that the patient has received the medication, he must remain in the exam room for 20 minutes to assure there is no reaction.				
35	*Being courteous, patient, and respectful,* assess the patient every 5 minutes for signs of reaction.				
36	*Paying attention to detail,* return the medication container to the appropriate place in the medication area.				
37	Accurately document in the patient's chart or electronic medical record the medication, dose, route, site of injection, and patient reaction. Sign and add date and time.				
Student's Total Points					
Points Possible					
Final Score (Student's Total Points/Possible Points)					

Instructor's/Evaluator's Comments and Suggestions:

_____

_____

_____

_____

_____

_____

_____

CHECK #1	
Evaluator's Signature:	Date:

CHECK #2	
Evaluator's Signature:	Date:

CHECK #3	
Evaluator's Signature:	Date:

Work Documentation Form(s)

*Progress Note Template can be downloaded from the Premium Website

ABHES Competencies: MA.A.1.4.a Document accurately; MA.A.1.6.a Demonstrate accurate occupational math and metric conversions for proper medication administration; MA.A.1.9.b Apply principles of aseptic techniques and infection control; MA.A.1.9.d Recognize and understand various treatment protocols; MA.A.1.9.g Maintain medication and immunization records; MA.A.1.9.j Prepare and administer oral and parenteral medications as directed by physician; MA.A.1.9.l Prepare patient for examinations and treatments

CAAHEP Competencies: I.P.7 Select proper sites for parenteral medication; I.P.9 Administer parenteral (excluding IV) medications; I.A.1 Apply critical thinking skills in performing patient assessment and care; I.A.2 Use language/verbal skills that enable patients' understanding; II.P.1 Prepare proper dosages of medication for administration; II.A.1 Verify ordered dose/dosages prior to administration; III.P.2 Practice standard precautions; III.P.4 Perform hand washing; III.A.2 Explain the rationale for performance of a procedure to a patient; IV.P.8 Document patient care; IX.P.2 Perform within scope of practice

Name _____ **Date** _____ **Score** _____

● **COMPETENCY ASSESSMENT**

Procedure 36-6: Administering an Intramuscular Injection

Task: Correctly administer an intramuscular injection with 100% accuracy.

Conditions:
- Medication order per provider with medication card
- Appropriate syringe size and needle gauge and length
- Alcohol wipes
- Nonsterile disposable gloves
- Sharps container
- Adhesive bandage

Standards: Perform the Task within 10 minutes with a minimum score of _____ points, as determined by your instructor.

Time began: _____   **Time ended:** _____   **Total time:** _____

No.	Step	Points	Check #1	Check #2	Check #3
1	Perform medical asepsis handwashing procedure. Adhere to OSHA guidelines.				
2	Verify the provider's order and prepare a medication card.				
3	Follow the "Six Rights" of medication administration.				
4	Work in a well-lighted, quiet, clean area.				
5	*Paying attention to detail*, gather appropriate equipment and supplies.				
6	Review the medication card. Select the correct medication from the medication area.				
7	Compare the medication label with the medication card (first check).				
8	If unfamiliar with the medication, consult the PDR or other reputable reference.				
9	Check the expiration date.				
10	Carefully calculate the dosage based on medication order and medication available.				
11	*Displaying sound judgment,* correctly prepare the parenteral medication.				
12	Compare the medication label with the medication card (second check).				
13	Withdraw the medication from the vial using proper technique.				
14	Discard any refuse generated during the preparation.				

No.	Step	Points	Check #1	Check #2	Check #3
15	Carefully transport the medication to the patient exam room. Bring the medication container (vial) with the prepared medication.				
16	*Introduce yourself and identify the patient. Explain the procedure and expectations to the patient, speaking at the patient's level of understanding.* State the name of the medication and the purpose of the injection. *Allay the patient's fears regarding the procedure being performed and help him feel safe and comfortable.*				
17	Ask the patient about medication allergies.				
18	*If you are beyond your comfort zone or experience, ask a more knowledgeable peer or the provider to assist you. Remember to work within your scope of practice.*				
19	Assess the patient to determine the most appropriate site to administer an intramuscular injection. Don gloves.				
20	Prepare the patient for the injection (position, provide privacy, drape).				
21	Review the medication card and the medication (third check).				
22	Cleanse the injection site that has been chosen. Use an alcohol wipe using a circular motion, beginning at the site of injection and circling outward to a diameter of 2 inches. Allow the skin to dry.				
23	Carefully remove the needle cover.				
24	Using your non-dominant hand, stretch the skin taut in the area that has been cleansed and is dry.				
25	Instruct the patient to take a deep breath and slowly release it.				
26	Using a dartlike motion, insert needle to the hub at a 90-degree angle.				
27	Release the skin.				
28	Aspirate by holding the syringe steady and gently pulling back on the syringe plunger. Check for blood in the syringe. • If blood is evident, remove the needle from the skin • Discard syringe appropriately in hazardous waste needle box • Notify provider				
29	Steadily and slowly inject the medication.				

No.	Step	Points	Check #1	Check #2	Check #3
30	Remove the needle in the direction that it was inserted. Activate the safety mechanism to cover the needle. Immediately dispose of the needle and syringe in the sharps container.				
31	If indicated, massage the site using the alcohol wipe.				
32	Cover the site if indicated with an adhesive bandage.				
33	Remove gloves and dispose of according to OSHA guidelines.				
34	Wash hands.				
35	If it is the first time that the patient has received the medication, he must remain in the exam room for 20 minutes to assure there is no reaction.				
36	*Being courteous, patient, and respectful,* assess the patient every 5 minutes for signs of reaction.				
37	*Paying attention to detail,* return the medication container to the appropriate place in the medication area.				
38	Accurately document in the patient's chart or electronic medical record the medication, dose, route, site of injection and patient reaction. Sign and add date and time.				
Student's Total Points					
Points Possible					
Final Score (Student's Total Points/Possible Points)					

Instructor's/Evaluator's Comments and Suggestions:

_____

_____

_____

_____

_____

_____

_____

CHECK #1	
Evaluator's Signature:	Date:

CHECK #2	
Evaluator's Signature:	Date:

CHECK #3	
Evaluator's Signature:	Date:

Work Documentation Form(s)

*Progress Note Template can be downloaded from the Premium Website

ABHES Competencies: MA.A.1.4.a Document accurately; MA.A.1.6.a Demonstrate accurate occupational math and metric conversions for proper medication administration; MA.A.1.9.b Apply principles of aseptic techniques and infection control; MA.A.1.9.d Recognize and understand various treatment protocols; MA.A.1.9.g Maintain medication and immunization records; MA.A.1.9.j Prepare and administer oral and parenteral medications as directed by physician; MA.A.1.9.l Prepare patient for examinations and treatments

CAAHEP Competencies: I.P.7 Select proper sites for parenteral medication; I.P.9 Administer parenteral (excluding IV) medications; I.A.1 Apply critical thinking skills in performing patient assessment and care; I.A.2 Use language/verbal skills that enable patients' understanding; II.P.1 Prepare proper dosages of medication for administration; II.A.1 Verify ordered dose/dosages prior to administration; III.P.2 Practice standard precautions; III.P.4 Perform hand washing; III.A.2 Explain the rationale for performance of a procedure to a patient; IV.P.8 Document patient care; IX.P.2 Perform within scope of practice

Name_____ **Date**_____ **Score**_____

● **COMPETENCY ASSESSMENT**

Procedure 36-7: Administering an Intradermal Injection of Purified Protein Derivative (PPD)

Task: Demonstrate the correct administration of an intradermal injection of PPD with 100% accuracy.

Conditions:
- Medication order per provider with medication card
- Appropriate syringe and needle gauge and length
- Alcohol wipes
- Nonsterile disposable gloves
- Sharps container
- Adhesive bandage

Standards: Perform the Task within 15 minutes with a minimum score of _____ points, as determined by your instructor.

Time began: _____ **Time ended:** _____ **Total time:** _____

No.	Step	Points	Check #1	Check #2	Check #3
1	Perform medical asepsis handwashing procedure. Adhere to OSHA guidelines.				
2	Verify the provider's order and prepare a medication card.				
3	Follow the "Six Rights" of medication administration.				
4	Work in a well-lighted, quiet, clean area.				
5	*Paying attention to detail*, gather appropriate equipment and supplies.				
6	Review the medication card. Select the correct medication from the medication area.				
7	Compare the medication label with the medication card (first check).				
8	If unfamiliar with the medication, consult the PDR or other reputable reference.				
9	Check the expiration date.				
10	Carefully calculate the dosage based on the medication order and available medication.				
11	*Displaying sound judgment*, correctly prepare the parenteral medication.				
12	Compare the medication label with the medication card (second check).				
13	Withdraw the medication from the vial using proper technique.				

No.	Step	Points	Check #1	Check #2	Check #3
14	Discard any refuse generated during the preparation.				
15	Carefully transport the medication to the patient exam room. Bring the medication (vial/container) with the prepared medication.				
16	*Introduce yourself and identify the patient. Explain the procedure and expectations to the patient, speaking at the patient's level of understanding. Allay the patient's fears regarding the procedure being performed and help her feel safe and comfortable.*				
17	Ask the patient about medication allergies.				
18	*If you are beyond your comfort zone or experience, ask a more knowledgeable peer or the provider to assist you. Remember to work within your scope of practice.*				
19	Assess the patient to determine the most appropriate site to administer an intradermal injection. Don gloves.				
20	Prepare the patient for the injection (position for injection, provide privacy, drape).				
21	Review the medication card and the medication (third check).				
22	Cleanse the injection site that has been chosen. Use an alcohol wipe in a circular motion, starting at the injection site and circling outward to a diameter of 2 inches. Allow the skin to dry.				
23	Carefully remove the needle cover.				
24	Using your nondominant hand, pull the skin taut.				
25	Instruct the patient to take a deep breath and slowly release it.				
26	Carefully insert the needle at a 10- to 15-degree angle, bevel upward, to a depth of ⅛ inch. Do not aspirate. Release skin.				
27	Steadily inject PPD to form a wheal or bleb.				
28	Carefully remove the needle in the direction that it was inserted.				
29	Activate the safety mechanism to cover the needle.				
30	Immediately dispose of the needle and syringe in the sharps container.				
31	Blot site of injection. Do not massage.				

No.	Step	Points	Check #1	Check #2	Check #3
32	Instruct the patient not to rub wheal.				
33	Remove gloves and discard in appropriate waste container.				
34	Wash hands.				
35	If this is the first time that the patient has received a PPD injection, the patient must be observed for 20 minutes to assure no reaction.				
36	*Being courteous, patient, and respectful,* assess the patient every 5 minutes for signs of reaction.				
37	*Paying attention to detail,* return the medication vial to the appropriate area for storage.				
38	Discard the medication card.				
39	Accurately document in the patient's chart or electronic medical record indicating the medication, dose, route, site of injection, and any patient reaction. Sign and date.				
Student's Total Points					
Points Possible					
Final Score (Student's Total Points/Possible Points)					

Instructor's/Evaluator's Comments and Suggestions:

_____

_____

_____

_____

_____

_____

_____

_____

CHECK #1	
Evaluator's Signature:	Date:

CHECK #2	
Evaluator's Signature:	Date:

CHECK #3	
Evaluator's Signature:	Date:

Work Documentation Form(s)

*Progress Note Template can be downloaded from the Premium Website

ABHES Competencies: MA.A.1.4.a Document accurately; MA.A.1.6.a Demonstrate accurate occupational math and metric conversions for proper medication administration; MA.A.1.9.b Apply principles of aseptic techniques and infection control; MA.A.1.9.d Recognize and understand various treatment protocols; MA.A.1.9.g Maintain medication and immunization records; MA.A.1.9.j Prepare and administer oral and parenteral medications as directed by physician; MA.A.1.9.l Prepare patient for examinations and treatments

CAAHEP Competencies: I.P.7 Select proper sites for parenteral medication; I.P.9 Administer parenteral (excluding IV) medications; I.A.1 Apply critical thinking skills in performing patient assessment and care; I.A.2 Use language/verbal skills that enable patients' understanding; II.P.1 Prepare proper dosages of medication for administration; II.A.1 Verify ordered dose/dosages prior to administration; III.P.2 Practice standard precautions; III.P.4 Perform hand washing; III.A.2 Explain the rationale for performance of a procedure to a patient; IV.P.8 Document patient care; IX.P.2 Perform within scope of practice

Name _____ **Date** _____ **Score** _____

● COMPETENCY ASSESSMENT

Procedure 36-8: Reconstituting a Powdered Medication for Administration

Task: Correctly reconstitute a powder medication and calculate correct dosage with 100% accuracy.

Conditions: • Medication order per provider and medication card
              • Diluent
              • Powdered medication
              • Appropriate syringe and needle gauge and length
              • Alcohol wipes
              • Nonsterile disposable gloves
              • Sharps container

Standards: Perform the Task within 10 minutes with a minimum score of _____ points, as determined by your instructor.

Time began: _____ **Time ended:** _____ **Total time:** _____

No.	Step	Points	Check #1	Check #2	Check #3
1	Perform medical asepsis handwashing procedure. Adhere to OSHA guidelines.				
2	Verify the provider's order and prepare a medication card.				
3	Follow the "Six Rights" of medication administration.				
4	Work in a well-lighted, quiet, clean area.				
5	*Paying attention to detail*, gather appropriate equipment and supplies. If unfamiliar with the medication, consult the PDR or other reputable reference.				
6	Check the expiration date.				
7	Prepare the needle–syringe unit in preparation for reconstituting powdered medication.				
8	Remove tops from diluent and powdered medication containers and wipe with alcohol swabs.				
9	Fill the syringe with air equal to the amount of diluent that is to be added to the medication.				
10	Carefully insert the needle through the rubber stopper on the vial of diluent.				
11	Withdraw the appropriate amount of diluent to be added to the powdered medication.				
12	Inject the diluents slowly and carefully into the powdered medication.				
13	Remove the needle and syringe appropriately in a biohazard sharps container.				

No.	Step	Points	Check #1	Check #2	Check #3
14	DO NOT SHAKE THE VIAL. Roll the vial between the palms of the hands to completely mix together the powder and the diluents.				
15	If the medication is contained in a multidose vial, label the vial with the name of the medication and the strength after dilution, the date and time, your initials, and the expiration date.				
16	With a second sterile needle and syringe, withdraw the desired amount of medication.				
17	Flick away any air bubbles that cling to side of syringe.				
18	The medicine tray with reconstituted medication and medication card are ready for transport to the patient.				
Student's Total Points					
Points Possible					
Final Score (Student's Total Points/Possible Points)					

Instructor's/Evaluator's Comments and Suggestions:

CHECK #1	
Evaluator's Signature:	Date:

CHECK #2	
Evaluator's Signature:	Date:

CHECK #3	
Evaluator's Signature:	Date:

ABHES Competencies: MA.A.1.9.b Apply principles of aseptic techniques and infection control; MA.A.1.9.d Recognize and understand various treatment protocols; MA.A.1.9.g Maintain medication and immunization records; MA.A.1.9.j Prepare and administer oral and parenteral medications as directed by physician

CAAHEP Competencies: II.P.1 Prepare proper dosages of medication for administration; II.A.1 Verify ordered dose/dosages prior to administration; III.P.2 Practice standard precautions; III.P.4 Perform hand washing

Name _____ **Date** _____ **Score** _____

● **COMPETENCY ASSESSMENT**

Procedure 36-9:   Z-Track Intramuscular Injection Technique

Task: Correctly administer a Z-track intramuscular injection with 100% accuracy.

Conditions: • Medication order per provider and medication card
                 • Appropriately sized syringe and needle with correct guage and length
                 • Alcohol wipes
                 • Disposable nonsterile gloves
                 • Sharps container
                 • Adhesive bandage

Standards: Perform the Task within 10 minutes with a minimum score of _____ points, as determined by
                 your instructor.

Time began: _____   **Time ended:** _____   **Total time:** _____

No.	Step	Points	Check #1	Check #2	Check #3
1	Perform medical asepsis handwashing procedure. Adhere to OSHA guidelines.				
2	Verify the provider's order and prepare a medication card.				
3	Follow the "Six Rights" of medication administration.				
4	Work in a well-lighted, quiet, clean area.				
5	*Paying attention to detail*, gather appropriate equipment and supplies.				
6	Select the correct medication from the medication storage area.				
7	Check the expiration date.				
8	Compare label information to provider's order (first check).				
9	If unfamiliar with the medication, consult the PDR or other reputable reference.				
10	Calculate the correct dose based on provider's order and medication on hand.				
11	*Displaying sound judgment*, Correctly prepare the parenteral medication.				
12	Compare medication label with the medication card (second check).				
13	Withdraw the medication from the vial using proper technique.				

No.	Step	Points	Check #1	Check #2	Check #3
14	Change the needle after aspirating the medication from the vial to avoid irritation of the tissues.				
15	Discard any refuse generated during the preparation.				
16	Carefully transport the medication to the patient exam room. Bring the medication container (vial) with the prepared medication.				
17	*Introduce yourself and identify the patient. Explain the procedure and expectations to the patient, speaking at the patient's level of understanding.* State the name of the medication and the purpose of the injection. *Allay the patient's fears regarding the procedure being performed and help him feel safe and comfortable.*				
18	Ask the patient about medication allergies.				
19	*If you are beyond your comfort zone or experience, ask a more knowledgeable peer or the provider to assist you. Remember to work within your scope of practice.*				
20	Assess the patient to determine the most appropriate site to administer an intramuscular injection. Don gloves.				
21	Prepare the patient for the injection (position, provide privacy, drape).				
22	Review the medication card and the medication (third check).				
23	Cleanse the injection site that has been chosen. Use an alcohol wipe using a circular motion, beginning at the site of injection and circling outward to a diameter of 3–4 inches. Allow the skin to dry.				
24	Carefully remove the needle cover.				
25	Using your nondominant hand, and placing fingers outside of the prepped area, gently pull the skin laterally 1½ inches away from the chosen injection site.				
26	Instruct the patient to take a deep breath and slowly release it.				
27	Keeping the skin pulled laterally and using a dart-like motion, insert the needle at a 90-degree angle.				

No.	Step	Points	Check #1	Check #2	Check #3
28	Aspirate by holding the syringe steady and gently pulling back on the syringe plunger. Check for blood in the syringe. • If blood is evident, remove the needle from the skin • Discard syringe appropriately in hazardous waste needle box • Notify provider				
29	Slowly and steadily inject the medication.				
30	Remove the needle in the direction that it was inserted.				
31	Immediately release the traction of the Z position to seal off the needle track.				
32	Activate the safety mechanism to cover the needle. Immediately dispose of the needle and syringe in the sharps container.				
33	Cover the site. Do not massage.				
34	Cover the site if indicated with an adhesive bandage.				
35	Remove gloves and dispose of according to OSHA guidelines. Wash hands.				
36	If it is the first time that the patient has received the medication, he must remain in the exam room for 20 minutes to ensure there is no reaction.				
37	*Being courteous, patient, and respectful,* assess the patient every 5 minutes for signs of reaction.				
38	*Paying attention to detail,* return the medication container to the appropriate place in the medication area.				
39	Accurately document in the patient's chart or electronic medical record the medication, dose, route, site of injection, and patient reaction. Sign and add date and time.				
Student's Total Points					
Points Possible					
Final Score (Student's Total Points/Possible Points)					

Instructor's/Evaluator's Comments and Suggestions:

_____

_____

_____

_____

_____

_____

_____

CHECK #1	
Evaluator's Signature:	Date:

CHECK #2	
Evaluator's Signature:	Date:

CHECK #3	
Evaluator's Signature:	Date:

Work Documentation Form(s)

*Progress Note Template can be downloaded from the Premium Website

ABHES Competencies: MA.A.1.4.a Document accurately; MA.A.1.6.a Demonstrate accurate occupational math and metric conversions for proper medication administration; MA.A.1.9.b Apply principles of aseptic techniques and infection control; MA.A.1.9.d Recognize and understand various treatment protocols; MA.A.1.9.g Maintain medication and immunization records; MA.A.1.9.j Prepare and administer oral and parenteral medications as directed by physician; MA.A.1.9.l Prepare patient for examinations and treatments

CAAHEP Competencies: I.P.7 Select proper sites for parenteral medication; I.P.9 Administer parenteral (excluding IV) medications; I.A.1 Apply critical thinking skills in performing patient assessment and care; I.A.2 Use language/verbal skills that enable patients' understanding; II.P.1 Prepare proper dosages of medication for administration; II.A.1 Verify ordered dose/dosages prior to administration; III.P.2 Practice standard precautions; III.P.4 Perform hand washing; III.A.2 Explain the rationale for performance of a procedure to a patient; IV.P.8 Document patient care; IX.P.2 Perform within scope of practice

Name_____   **Date**_____   **Score**_____

⬤ COMPETENCY ASSESSMENT

Procedure 37-1: Perform Single-Channel or Multichannel Electrocardiogram

Task: To obtain an accurate, graphic, artifact-free reading of the electrical activity of the heart for diagnostic purposes.

Conditions:
- Examination or ECG table with pillow and sheet or blanket
- Patient gown (open in the front)
- Automated electrocardiograph with patient cable wires
- Alligator clips
- Electropads (sensors)
- ECG paper
- Alcohol wipes
- Gauze squares
- Mounting form/card
- Razor

Standards: Perform the Task within 20 minutes with a minimum score of ___ points, as determined by your instructor.

Competency Assessment Information

Mr. Rutledge is a 61-year-old male with a history of a myocardial infarction at age 45. Treatment at the time of the MI was stenting of the proximal Right Coronary Artery. He is being seen in the office for his annual exam by his cardiologist. An ECG is ordered.

Time began: _____   **Time ended:** _____   **Total time:** _____

No.	Step	Points	Check #1	Check #2	Check #3
1	Perform tracing in a quiet, warm, and comfortable room away from electrical equipment that may cause artifacts.				
2	Wash hands, gather equipment, *identify the patient, and explain the procedure to patient, speaking at the patient's level of understanding.*				
3	Have the patient remove clothing from the waist up and uncover lower legs; nylon stockings must be removed; socks can be worn.				
4	Explain that the procedure is painless and why it is necessary not to move or talk during the procedure.				
5	Place the electrocardiograph with the power cord pointing away from the patient. Do not allow the cord to go underneath the table.				
6	Apply the limb electropads (sensors) first. Apply the sensors to the fleshy parts of the four limbs. If the sensor does not adhere well, use an alcohol wipe on the skin, let it dry, and apply a new sensor. Shave sites if necessary. Place sensors on a nonbony, nonmuscular (fleshy) area of the upper arms and lower legs. Arm sensors should have tab pointing down, leg sensors point upward.				

No.	Step	Points	Check #1	Check #2	Check #3
7	Place the sensors on the appropriate intercostal spaces with sensors pointing downward. Shave chest sites if necessary.				
8	Attach the lead wires from the ECG machine to each sensor using alligator clips, special clips applied to the ends of the lead wires. Be sure to connect lead wires to the correct sensors. Lead wire are labeled with abbreviations and are color-coded. The lead wires should follow the patient's body contour.				
9	The patient cable is supported either on the table or on the patient's abdomen. Plug the patient cable into the electrocardiograph.				
10	Turn the instrument ON.				
11	Enter information (patient name, date of birth, age, height, weight, sex, identification number, and cardiac medications the patient is presently taking).				
12	Remind the patient not to talk and to try not to move.				
13	Press AUTO and the machine will automatically record and standardize the tracing.				
14	The single-channel machine prints each lead sequentially on a strip of RCG paper. A multichannel machine prints the tracing on an 8½ × 11 inch sheet of paper.				
15	Check the quality of the tracing before disconnecting the lead wires. If it is necessary to repeat the tracing, first correct the problem that is causing a poor quality tracing.				
16	Disconnect the lead wires and remove the electropad sensor from the patient.				
17	Assist patient as needed.				
18	Be certain the patient information is on the tracing before giving it to the provider to read.				
19	If the tracing is a single-channel tracing, cut and mount it, remembering to handle it carefully. Place in patient's record.				
20	Accurately document the procedure in the patient's chart or electronic medical record.				
Student's Total Points					
Points Possible					
Final Score (Student's Total Points/Possible Points)					

Instructor's/Evaluator's Comments and Suggestions:

_____
_____
_____
_____
_____
_____
_____
_____

CHECK #1	
Evaluator's Signature:	Date:

CHECK #2	
Evaluator's Signature:	Date:

CHECK #3	
Evaluator's Signature:	Date:

Work Documentation Form(s)

*Progress Note Template can be downloaded from the Premium Website

ABHES Competencies: MA.A.1.2.d Common diseases, diagnoses, and treatments; MA.A.1.4.a Documentation; MA.A.1.9.d Treatment protocols; MA.A.1.9.f Test results; MA.A.1.9.l Patient preparation; MA.A.1.9.o Electrocardiograms, respiratory testing, screening, sterilization, first aid, and CPR; MA.A.1.9.p Patient instructions

CAAHEP Competencies: I.C.5 Describe the normal function of each body system; I.P.5 Perform electrocardiography; I.A.1 Apply critical thinking skills in performing patient assessment and care; I.A.2 Use language/verbal skills that enable patient's understanding; IV.P.2 Report relevant information to others succinctly and accurately; IV.P.3 Use medical terminology, pronouncing medical terms, correctly, to communicate information, patient history, data, and observations; IV.P.6 Prepare a patient for procedures and/or treatments; IV.P.8 Document patient care; IV.A.7 Demonstrate recognition of the patient's level of understanding in communications

Name _____ **Date** _____ **Score** _____

● **COMPETENCY ASSESSMENT**

Procedure 37-2: Holter Monitor Application (Cassette and Digital)

Task: To apply a monitoring device that allows recording of sporadic cardiac arrhythmias, evaluate chest pain and cardiac status after pacemaker implantation or after acute myocardial infarction.

Conditions:
- Holter monitor
- Patient activity diary
- Blank magnetic tape or flash memory card
- Disposable electrodes
- Razor
- Alcohol wipes
- Gauze
- Carrying case
- Belt or shoulder strap

Standards: Perform the Task within 20 minutes with a minimum score of ___ points, as determined by your instructor.

Competency Assessment Information

Ms. Jarreau, age 42, is seen in the office today with a history of syncope and chest pain with exertion. Your provider has ordered a Holter monitor to be placed for continuous monitoring for 72 hours. You are instructed to place the Holter monitor and explain the procedure to Ms. Jarreau.

Time began: _____ **Time ended:** _____ **Total time:** _____

No.	Step	Points	Check #1	Check #2	Check #3
1	Wash hands and assemble equipment.				
2	Prepare the equipment by removing old (used) battery from the monitor and replacing it with a new battery. Insert a blank magnetic tape or flash card into the monitor.				
3	Wash hands.				
4	*Identify the patient and explain the procedure, speaking at the patient's level of understanding.*				
5	Have the patient remove clothing from the waist up.				
6	Have the patient sit on the examination table or chair.				
7	Locate the correct electrode placement sites. The skin must be prepared in the following way: • Dry shave patient's chest at each electrode site if chest is hairy. • Cleanse the shaved area with an alcohol wipe. Let area dry. • Abrade the skin slightly with a dry 4 × 4 gauze. Areas should be red.				

No.	Step	Points	Check #1	Check #2	Check #3
8	Take the electrodes from the package and peel away the backing from one of them (electrode should be moist). Continue to remove electrodes one by one and attach as in Step 9.				
9	Apply adhesive-backed electrode to the appropriate sites by applying firm pressure at the center of the electrode and moving outward toward the edges. Run your fingers along the outer rim to ensure firm attachment. Avoid moving from one side of electrode to the other. Gel could be forced out and could cause interference.				
10	Attach the lead wires to the electrodes. Connect them to the patient cable.				
11	Plug the monitor into the electrocardiograph with the test cable. Run a baseline tracing (not necessary with digital monitor).				
12	Place the electrode cable so that it extends from between the buttons of the patient's shirt or from below the bottom of the shirt.				
13	Place the recorder into its carrying case and either attach it to the patient's belt or over the patient's shoulder. Be certain there is no pulling on the lead wires.				
14	Plug the electrode cable into the monitor. Record the starting time in the patient activity log (diary). These data will already be recorded in a digital monitor.				
15	Record the starting time in the patient activity log.				
16	Help patient get dressed.				
17	Give the activity log to the patient, being certain that the patient information is completed.				
18	Inform patient what time the following day the monitor will be removed. Remind the patient to bring along the activity log/diary.				
19	Wash hands.				
20	Document the procedure in patient's chart or electronic medical record.				
21	Upon the patient's return 24 hours later, take the patient's electrodes off, remove flash memory card, accept cassette, remove battery.				
22	Document patient returned with equipment.				
Student's Total Points					
Points Possible					
Final Score (Student's Total Points/Possible Points)					

Instructor's/Evaluator's Comments and Suggestions:

_____

_____

_____

_____

_____

_____

_____

CHECK #1	
Evaluator's Signature:	Date:

CHECK #2	
Evaluator's Signature:	Date:

CHECK #3	
Evaluator's Signature:	Date:

Work Documentation Form(s)

*Progress Note Template can be downloaded from the Premium Website

ABHES Competencies: MA.A.1.2.d Common diseases, diagnoses, and treatments; MA.A.1.4.a Documentation; MA.A.1.9.d Treatment protocols; MA.A.1.9.f Test results; MA.A.1.9.l Patient preparation; MA.A.1.9.o Electrocardiograms, respiratory testing, screening, sterilization, first aid, and CPR; MA.A.1.9.p Patient instructions

CAAHEP Competencies: I.C.5 Describe the normal function of each body system; I.P.5 Perform electrocardiography; I.A.1 Apply critical thinking skills in performing patient assessment and care; I.A.2 Use language/verbal skills that enable patient's understanding; IV.P.2 Report relevant information to others succinctly and accurately; IV.P.3 Use medical terminology, pronouncing medical terms, correctly, to communicate information, patient history, data, and observations; IV.P.6 Prepare a patient for procedures and/or treatments; IV.P.8 Document patient care; IV.A.7 Demonstrate recognition of the patient's level of understanding in communications

Name_____ **Date**_____ **Score**_____

● COMPETENCY ASSESSMENT

Procedure 39-1:   Using the Microscope

Task: Properly use a microscope to view microscopic organisms using the coarse and fine adjustments, as well as the low- and high-power and oil-immersion objectives.

Conditions:
- Hand disinfectant
- Microscope, compound
- Manufacturer's manual
- Lens cleaner and paper
- Prepared slides (commercially available)
- Immersion oil
- Surface disinfectant, biohazard and sharps waste containers

Standards: Perform the Task within 15 minutes with a minimum score of ___ points, as determined by your instructor.

Competency Assessment Information

Use the prepared slides to properly use the microscope. This procedure will vary slightly according to the microscope being used. If more than one type of microscope is available, try to use different models to become efficient in a variety of microscopes. Consult the operating instructions with each microscope.

Time began: _____   **Time ended:** _____   **Total time:** _____

No.	Step	Points	Check #1	Check #2	Check #3
1	Wash hands.				
2	Assemble equipment and materials.				
3	Clean the ocular(s) and objectives with lens paper.				
4	Use the coarse adjustment to raise the eyepiece or lens unit.				
5	Rotate the 10x, or low-power, objective into position so that it is directly over the opening in the stage.				
6	Turn on the microscope light. Open the diaphragm until maximum light comes up through the condenser.				
7	Place the slide on the stage (specimen side up).				
8	Locate the coarse adjustment. Look directly at the stage and 10x objective and turn the coarse adjustment until the objective is as close to the slide as it will go.				

No.	Step	Points	Check #1	Check #2	Check #3
9	Look into the ocular(s) and slowly turn the coarse adjustment in the opposite direction to raise the objective (or lower the stage) until the object on the slide comes into view.				
10	Locate the fine adjustment. Turn the fine adjustment to sharpen the image.				
11	Scan the slide.				
12	Rotate the high-power (40x) objective into position while observing the objective and the slide to see that the objective does not strike the slide.				
13	Look through the ocular(s) to view the object on the slide; it should almost be in focus.				
14	Locate the fine adjustment. Look through the ocular(s) and turn the fine adjustment until the object is in focus. Do not use the coarse adjustment.				
15	Adjust the amount of light.				
16	Scan the slide as in Step 11, using the fine adjustment if necessary to keep the object in focus.				
17	Rotate the oil-immersion objective to the side slightly (so that no objective is in position). Place one drop of immersion oil on the portion of the slide that is directly over the condenser.				
18	Rotate the oil-immersion objective into position, being careful not to rotate the 40x objective through the oil. Look to see that the oil-immersion objective is touching the drop of oil.				
19	Look through the ocular(s) and slowly turn the fine adjustment until the image is clear. Use only the fine adjustment to focus the oil-immersion objective.				
20	Adjust the amount of light. Scan the slide.				
21	Rotate the 10x objective into position (do not allow the 40x objective to touch the oil).				
22	Remove the slide from the microscope stage and gently clean the oil from the slide with lens paper.				
23	Clean objectives and oculars with clean lens paper and lens cleaner. Clean any oil from the microscope stage and condenser.				
24	Turn off the microscope light and disconnect.				

No.	Step	Points	Check #1	Check #2	Check #3
25	Position the eyepiece in the lowest position using the coarse adjustment. Center the stage so that it does not project from either side of the microscope.				
26	Cover the microscope and return it to storage. Clean the work area; return slides to storage.				
27	Wash hands.				
Student's Total Points					
Points Possible					
Final Score					
(Student's Total Points/Possible Points)					

Instructor's/Evaluator's Comments and Suggestions:

_____

_____

_____

_____

_____

_____

_____

CHECK #1	
Evaluator's Signature:	Date:

CHECK #2	
Evaluator's Signature:	Date:

CHECK #3	
Evaluator's Signature:	Date:

ABHES Competencies: MA.A.1.9.i. Use standard precautions; MA.A.1.10.c. Dispose of biohazardous materials

CAAHEP Competencies: III.P.2 Practice standard precautions; III.P.3 Select appropriate barrier/personal protection equipment (PPE) for potentially infectious situations

Name_____   **Date**_____   **Score**_____

● COMPETENCY ASSESSMENT

Procedure 40-1:   Palpating a Vein and Preparing a Patient for Venipuncture

Task: Palpate a vein and assess patient preparation prior to performing venipuncture.

Conditions: • Gloves
                 • Tourniquet

Standards: Perform the Task within 5 minutes with a minimum score of ___ points.

Time began: _____   **Time ended:** _____   **Total time:** _____

No.	Step	Points	Check #1	Check #2	Check #3
1	*Introduce yourself by name and credential. Identify the patient and explain the procedure.* Ask the patient's name and verify it with the computer label or identification number. If a fasting specimen is required, verify that the patient has not had anything to eat or drink except water for 12 hours.				
2	Wash hands. Put on gloves.				
3	Apply tourniquet 2 to 3 inches above the venipuncture site. Apply tightly enough to slow venous blood flow but not so tight that blood flow in arteries is stopped.				
4	Have the patient close the hand and place the patient's arm in a downward position. Do not allow the patient to pump his or her hand.				
5	Palpate the antecubital space of the arm, feeling for the basilic or cephalic vein with the tip of your middle or ring finger. Feel for a soft bounce and a roundness to the vein.				
6	After locating an acceptable vein, mentally map the location. Visualize the puncture site. Follow the direction of the vein with your finger tip, making a mental note of any turns, dips, and twists.				
7	If a vein cannot be found in the antecubital space of either arm, then the hand veins must be checked following the same procedure. The butterfly technique is more successful for hand venipuncture.				
Student's Total Points					
Points Possible					
Final Score (Student's Total Points/Possible Points)					

Instructor's/Evaluator's Comments and Suggestions:

_____

_____

_____

_____

_____

_____

_____

CHECK #1	
Evaluator's Signature:	Date:

CHECK #2	
Evaluator's Signature:	Date:

CHECK #3	
Evaluator's Signature:	Date:

ABHES Competency: MA.A.1.8.cc Communicate on the recipient's level of comprehension

CAAHEP Competency: I.A.2 Use language/verbal skills that enable patients' understanding

Name_____ **Date**_____ **Score**_____

● COMPETENCY ASSESSMENT

Procedure 40-2: Venipuncture by Syringe

Task: Obtain venous blood acceptable for laboratory testing as requested by the provider.

Conditions: • PPE: gloves, goggles, and mask
                 • 10-mL syringe, 21-gauge safety needle
                 • Vacuum tube(s) or special collection tube(s)
                 • Tourniquet
                 • 70% isopropyl alcohol swab, cotton balls
                 • Adhesive bandage or tape
                 • Sharps container and biohazard red bag
                 • Test tube rack
                 • Biohazard transport bag
                 • Lab requisition*

Standards: Perform the Task within 15 minutes with a minimum score of ___ points, as determined by your instructor.

Competency Assessment Information

Use the following information to complete the Lab Requisition (Work Documentation).

Use today's date and time. Patient's name is Sharon Kruml. Her address is 5678 Color Way, River City, NY 23230. She is female and has Medicare (444-55-6621A). Her chart/medical record number is 99882. Her birthdate is January 16, 1950. She will be fasting for 12 hours.

Dr. King has requested that blood be collected and sent to the lab for a CBC, ESR, and a coagulation study.

Time began: _____   **Time ended:** _____   **Total time:** _____

No.	Step	Points	Check #1	Check #2	Check #3
1	Assemble the supplies.				
2	*Introduce yourself by name and credential.* Position and identify the patient. *Ask the patient's name and verify it* with the tests ordered and the computer label or identification number. If a fasting specimen is required, verify that the patient has not had anything to eat or drink except water for 12 hours.				
3	*Explain the procedure and expectations to the patient. Allay the patient's fears regarding the procedure to help her feel safe and comfortable.*				
4	Wash hands and apply gloves and goggles/mask.				
5	Open the sterile needle and sterile syringe packages and assemble if necessary. Pull the plunger halfway out and push it all the way in again.				

No.	Step	Points	Check #1	Check #2	Check #3
6	Select the proper vacuum tubes for later transfer of the specimen; tap all tubes containing anticoagulants and check the expiration dates. Arrange them in a holding rack in proper order.				
7	Apply the tourniquet and select a site. See Procedure 40-1.				
8	Ask the patient to close the hand. The patient must not pump the hand. Place the hand in a downward position.				
9	Select a vein, noting the location and direction of the vein.				
10	Cleanse the site with an alcohol swab with one firm swipe. Avoid touching the site after cleansing.				
11	Draw the skin taut with your thumb by placing it 1 to 2 inches below the puncture site.				
12	With the bevel up, line up the needle with the direction of the vein and perform the puncture. The point of the needle should enter the skin about ¼ inch below where the vein was palpated. With experience, a sensation of entering the vein can be felt. Once the vein has been entered, do not move the needle from side to side. Do not push down or pull up the needle. The needle can be moved in or out gently if needed to locate the vein.				
13	Let go of the skin and use that hand to pull back on the plunger. Pull gently and only as fast as the syringe fills. If the vein collapses, stop pulling on the plunger and let the vein refill.				
14	When the syringe is full, have the patient open the hand. Remove the tourniquet.				
15	Lightly place a cotton ball above the puncture site and remove the needle in the same direction as inserted.				
16	Apply pressure to the site for 2 to 3 minutes, or longer if the patient is taking prescribed anticoagulants (blood thinners) such as warfarin (Coumadin) or is taking aspirin or an herbal blood thinner such as ginkgo biloba. Let the patient assist by holding the pressure if desired. The patient can elevate the arm but should be instructed not to bend the elbow.				
17	Aliquot blood into the appropriate tubes in the rack in the proper order. During transfer, hold each tube at the base only.				
18	Puncture the vacuum tube through the rubber stopper with the syringe needle and allow the blood to enter the tube until the flow stops. Never push on the plunger or force blood into the tube.				
19	Implement safety mechanism or devices on the needle immediately.				

No.	Step	Points	Check #1	Check #2	Check #3
20	Mix any anticoagulant tubes immediately.				
21	Discard the syringe and needle into a sharps container and the contaminated cotton ball and other contaminated waste into a red biohazard bag.				
22	Label all tubes before leaving the room. If any special treatment is required for the specimens, institute the handling protocol right away.				
23	Check the patient. Observe her for signs of stress.				
24	When sufficient pressure has been applied to stop the bleeding, apply a small pressure bandage by pulling a cotton ball in half, applying it to the puncture site, and placing an adhesive bandage or tape over it. Instruct the patient to remove the bandage in 20 minutes. If the patient is sensitive or allergic to latex be sure to use non-latex paper tape. If the bleeding has not stopped after 2 to 3 minutes, have the patient continue to hold direct pressure on the site for another 5 minutes with her arm elevated above the heart. She can do this by lying down with her arm on a pillow. Recheck after 5 minutes.				
25	Disinfect tray and supplies and dispose of all contaminated items properly. Remove gloves using proper technique.				
26	Wash hands, record the procedure, and complete the laboratory requisition in the presence of the patient.				
27	Place specimen and requisition into biohazard transport bag and notify the laboratory that the specimen is ready for pickup.				
Student's Total Points					
Points Possible					
Final Score (Student's Total Points/Possible Points)					

Instructor's/Evaluator's Comments and Suggestions:

_____

_____

_____

_____

_____

_____

_____

CHECK #1	
Evaluator's Signature:	Date:

CHECK #2	
Evaluator's Signature:	Date:

CHECK #3	
Evaluator's Signature:	Date:

Work Documentation Form(s)

*Lab Requisition Form can be downloaded from the Premium Website

ABHES Competencies: MA.A.1.8.cc Communicate on the recipient's level of comprehension; MA.A.1.9.i.i Use standard precautions; MA.A.1.10.d.d (1) Perform venipuncture

CAAHEP Competencies: I.A.2 Use language/verbal skills that enable patients' understanding; I.P.2 Perform venipuncture; III.P.2 Practice Standard Precautions

Name_____ **Date**_____ **Score**_____

⬤ COMPETENCY ASSESSMENT

Procedure 40-3:   Venipuncture by Vacuum Tube System

Task: Obtain venous blood acceptable for laboratory testing as requested by a provider.

Conditions:
- PPE: gloves, goggles, and mask
- Vacuum tube(s) adapter/holder
- Lab requisition*
- 70% isopropyl alcohol swab, cotton balls, 2 × 2 gauze
- 21-gauge multidraw needle
- Vacuum tube(s) or special collection tube(s)
- Tourniquet
- Adhesive bandage or tape
- Sharps container and biohazard red bag
- Biohazard transport bag

Standards: Perform the Task within 15 minutes with a minimum score of ___ points, as determined by your instructor.

Competency Assessment Information

Use the following information to complete the Lab Requisition (Work Documentation).

Use today's date and time. Patient's name is Elaine Hardin. Her address is 1234 10th Street, River City, NY 98765. She is female and has no insurance. Her chart/medical record number is 55443. Her birthdate is 9/27/1950. She will be fasting for 12 hours.

Dr. Lewis has requested that blood be collected and sent to the lab for a CBC and a basic metabolic panel (chemistry).

Time began: _____ **Time ended:** _____ **Total time:** _____

No.	Step	Points	Check #1	Check #2	Check #3
1	*Introduce yourself by name and credential. Explain the procedure and expectations to the patient. Allay the patient's fears regarding the procedure to help her feel safe and comfortable.*				
2	Position and identify the patient. *Ask the patient's name and verify it* with the tests ordered and the computer label or identification number. If a fasting specimen is required, verify that the patient has not had anything to eat or drink except water for 12 hours.				
3	Wash hands and apply gloves and goggles/mask.				
4	Break the seal on the shorter needle; thread the shorter needle into the holder/adapter. Select the first tube and gently place it into the holder/adapter (do not puncture the tube yet).				
5	Tap all tubes containing anticoagulants and check the expiration dates.				
6	Select a site and apply the tourniquet (see Procedure 40-1).				

No.	Step	Points	Check #1	Check #2	Check #3
7	Ask the patient to close the hand. The patient must not pump the hand. Place the hand in a downward position.				
8	Select a vein, noting the location and direction of the vein.				
9	Cleanse the site with an alcohol swab with one firm swipe.				
10	Avoid touching the site after cleansing.				
11	Draw the skin taut with your thumb by placing it 1 to 2 inches below the puncture site.				
12	With the bevel up, line up the needle with the direction of the vein and perform the puncture. The point of the needle should enter the skin about ¼ inch below where the vein was palpated. With experience, a sensation of entering the vein can be felt. Once the vein has been entered, do not move the needle.				
13	Let go of the skin and use that hand to grasp the flange of the vacuum tube holder and push the tube forward until the needle has completely entered the tube. Do not change hands while performing venipuncture. The hand performing the venipuncture is the hand that is holding the vacuum tube holder. The other hand is free for tube insertion and removal.				
14	Fill the tube until the vacuum is exhausted and the blood flow stops. For better visibility, rotate tubes so the label is down.				
15	When the blood ceases, gently remove the vacuum tube from the needle and holder. Do this by grasping the tube with the fingers and palm of your spare hand and using your thumb to push off from the flange of the holder.				
16	Immediately mix the blood in the anticoagulant tubes by gently inverting them several times.				
17	Insert the second tube onto the needle by using the same motion as the first tube. Let it fill; then remove it with the same motion as the first tube. Invert it several times if it contains anticoagulants.				
18	When the last tube has filled, remove it from the needle. Ask the patient to open her hand and release the tourniquet.				
19	Lightly place the cotton ball above the puncture site and smoothly remove the needle from the arm in the same direction of insertion.				
20	Immediately activate the safety device.				
21	Apply pressure on the site for 2 to 3 minutes. Let the patient assist by holding the pressure. Ask her not to bend her arm, but she can elevate her arm while applying pressure.				

No.	Step	Points	Check #1	Check #2	Check #3
22	Dispose of the needle into a sharps container and the contaminated cotton ball and other contaminated waste into a biohazard red bag.				
23	Label all the tubes before leaving the patient. If any special treatment is required for the specimens, institute the handling protocol right away.				
24	Check the patient. Observe her for signs of stress. She should stop bleeding within 2 to 3 minutes. If the bleeding has stopped, apply a small pressure bandage by pulling a cotton ball in half, applying it to the site, and placing an adhesive bandage or tape over it. The patient should be instructed to remove the bandage in about 20 minutes. If the patient is sensitive to latex, be sure to use a non-latex paper tape. If the bleeding has not stopped, have the patient continue to hold direct pressure another 5 minutes with her arm elevated above her heart level. Have her lie down with her arm up on a pillow. Recheck the site after 5 minutes of additional direct pressure.				
25	Disinfect all surfaces and supplies/equipment. Remove gloves using proper technique. Dispose of contaminated items appropriately.				
26	Wash hands, record the procedure, and complete the laboratory requisition in the presence of the patient. Place specimen and requisition into biohazard transport bag and notify the laboratory that the specimen is ready for pickup.				
Student's Total Points					
Points Possible					
Final Score (Student's Total Points/Possible Points)					

Instructor's/Evaluator's Comments and Suggestions:

_____

_____

_____

_____

_____

_____

_____

CHECK #1	
Evaluator's Signature:	Date:

CHECK #2	
Evaluator's Signature:	Date:

CHECK #3	
Evaluator's Signature:	Date:

Work Documentation Form(s)

*Lab Requisition Form can be downloaded from the Premium Website

ABHES Competencies: MA.A.1.8.cc Communicate on the recipient's level of comprehension; MA.A.1.9.i Use standard precautions; MA.A.1.10.d (1) Perform venipuncture

CAAHEP Competencies: I.A.2 Use language/verbal skills that enable patients' understanding; I.P.2 Perform venipuncture; III.P.2 Practice Standard Precautions

Name_____ Date_____ Score_____

⬤ COMPETENCY ASSESSMENT

Procedure 40-4:   Venipuncture by Butterfly Needle System

Task: Obtain venous blood acceptable for laboratory testing as requested by a provider.

Conditions:
- PPE: gloves, goggles, and mask
- Vacuum tube holder if using a vacuum tube connection
- A 10- to 15-mL/cc syringe if using a syringe connection
- Butterfly needle system with a 21-gauge needle (use a multisample needle system with a Luer-lok adapter for attaching to the vacuum tube and a hypodermic needle for the syringe attachment)
- Vacuum tubes if appropriate
- Tourniquet
- 70% isopropyl alcohol swab, 2 × 2 gauze
- Adhesive bandage or tape
- Sharps container and biohazard red bag
- Lab requisition*

Standards: Perform the Task within 15 minutes with a minimum score of ___ points, as determined by your instructor.

Competency Assessment Information

Use the following information to complete the Lab Requisition (Work Documentation).

Use today's date and time. Patient's name is Terri Smith. Her address is 24 Domino Street, River City, NY 98765. She is female and has Regence insurance (#6452). Her chart/medical record number is 55443. Her birthdate is 9/27/1950. She will be fasting for 12 hours.

Dr. Rice has requested that blood be collected and sent to the lab for a CBC and a blood type test.

Time began: _____   Time ended: _____   Total time: _____

No.	Step	Points	Check #1	Check #2	Check #3
1	Assemble the supplies.				
2	*Introduce yourself by name and credential.*				
3	Position and identify the patient. *Ask the patient's name and verify it* with the computer label or identification number. If a fasting specimen is required, verify that the patient has not had anything to eat or drink except water for 12 hours.				
4	*Explain the procedure and expectations to the patient. Allay the patient's fears regarding the procedure to help her feel safe and comfortable.*				
5	Wash hands. Put on gloves, as well as goggles and mask if there is a potential for blood splatter.				
6	Open the package of butterfly needle system. If using the multi sample needle, connect the needle to the vacuum tube holder/adapter. If using the hypodermic needle and syringe, connect the needle to the syringe. If using a syringe, set the vacuum tubes in a rack for later use.				

No.	Step	Points	Check #1	Check #2	Check #3
7	Tap the vacuum tubes to be sure any additive is dislodged from the stopper and sides of the tube. Check the expiration dates.				
8	Apply the tourniquet. Select a vein.				
9	Ask the patient to close her hand. The patient should not pump her hand. If possible, place the arm in a downward position.				
10	Select the vein, noting the direction and location of the vein.				
11	Cleanse the site with an alcohol swab using one firm swipe and allow to dry.				
12	Avoid touching the site after cleansing.				
13	Draw the skin taut by placing your thumb 1 to 2 inches below the site and pulling down firmly.				
14	Hold the wings of the butterfly together with the bevel up, line up the needle with the vein, and smoothly insert it into the vein at about a 5- to 10-degree angle.				
15	Remove your hand from holding the skin taut.				
16	If you are connected to a vacuum tube holder, grasp the flange of the vacuum tube holder and push the tube forward until the needle has completely entered the tube.				
17	If you are connected to a syringe, pull gently on the syringe.				
18	Do not change hands while performing venipuncture. The hand performing the venipuncture is the hand that is holding the vacuum tube holder. The other hand is for inserting and removing the vacuum tubes.				
19	If you are collecting directly into vacuum tubes, remove and replace the vacuum tubes as explained in Procedure 40-3 until you have drawn the necessary amounts. If you are drawing into a syringe, you will be limited to the size of the syringe being used.				
20	When the syringe is filled, ask the patient to open her hand. Release the tourniquet.				
21	Lightly place a cotton ball above the puncture site and smoothly remove the needle from the arm in the same direction of insertion.				
22	Activate the safety device of the butterfly needle immediately.				
23	Apply pressure on the site. Let the patient assist by holding the pressure. Ask her not to bend her arm. She can elevate her arm while applying pressure though.				
24	If using a syringe, aliquot blood into the appropriate tubes as outlined in Procedure 40-2.				
25	Dispose of the needle into a sharps container.				

No.	Step	Points	Check #1	Check #2	Check #3
26	Label all the tubes.				
27	Check the patient. Observe her for signs of stress.				
28	The patient should stop bleeding within 2 to 3 minutes. If the bleeding has stopped, apply a small pressure bandage by pulling a cotton ball in half, applying it to the site, and placing an adhesive bandage or tape over it. The patient should be instructed to remove the bandage in about 20 minutes. If the patient is sensitive to latex, be sure to use a non-latex paper tape. If the bleeding has not stopped, have the patient continue to hold pressure another 5 minutes with her arm elevated above her heart level, then recheck.				
29	Clean up tray and supplies; dispose of contaminated cotton ball. Remove gloves using proper technique. Discard gloves into biohazard container and disinfect goggles.				
30	Wash hands, record the procedure, and complete the laboratory requisition. Place specimen and requisition into biohazard transfer bag in the presence of the patient and notify the laboratory that the specimen is ready for pickup.				
Student's Total Points					
Points Possible					
Final Score (Student's Total Points/Possible Points)					

Instructor's/Evaluator's Comments and Suggestions:

_____

_____

_____

_____

_____

_____

_____

CHECK #1	
Evaluator's Signature:	Date:

CHECK #2	
Evaluator's Signature:	Date:

CHECK #3	
Evaluator's Signature:	Date:

Work Documentation Form(s)

*Lab Requisition Form can be downloaded from the Premium Website

ABHES Competencies: MA.A.1.8.cc Communicate on the recipient's level of comprehension; MA.A.1.9.i. Use standard precautions; 10.d.(1) Perform venipuncture

CAAHEP Competencies: I.A.2 Use language/verbal skills that enable patients' understanding; I.P.2 Perform venipuncture; III.P.2 Practice Standard Precautions

Name _____   **Date** _____   **Score** _____

● **COMPETENCY ASSESSMENT**

Procedure 40-5:   Capillary Puncture

Task: Obtain capillary blood acceptable for laboratory testing as required by a provider.

Conditions:
- Gloves
- 70% isopropyl alcohol swab, cotton balls, gauze 2×2
- Microcollection tubes or capillary tubes
- Safety lancet
- Adhesive bandage or tape
- Sharps container
- Biohazard red bag
- Lab requisition*
- Biohazard transport bag (optional)

Standards: Perform the Task within 5 minutes with a minimum score of ___ points, as determined by your instructor.

Competency Assessment Information

Use the following information to complete the Lab Requisition (Work Documentation).

Use today's date and time. Patient's name is Linda Sterns. Her address is 3232 Camano Lane, River City, NY 23230. She is female and has Regence insurance (ID number ZLF 987654321). Her chart/medical record number is 86541. Her birthdate is January 23, 1950. She will be fasting for 12 hours.

Dr. King has requested that blood be collected and sent to the lab for a hemoglobin, hematocrit, and Hgl A1c.

Time began: _____   **Time ended:** _____   **Total time:** _____

No.	Step	Points	Check #1	Check #2	Check #3
1	Assemble the supplies.				
2	*Identify the patient, introduce yourself by name and credential* and recheck the provider's orders.				
3	*Explain the procedure and expectations to the patient. Allay the patient's fears regarding the procedure to help her feel safe and comfortable.*				
4	Wash hands and apply gloves.				
5	Select the puncture site on the fleshy part of the ring or middle finger, avoiding the very tip and the extreme sides.				
6	Have the patient wash her hands in very warm water; if necessary, apply a warming pack to the fingertip, encourage the patient to relax, and provide a comfortable, professional atmosphere.				
7	Clean the selected puncture site with an alcohol swab and allow it to air dry or dry it with a gauze pad.				
8	Holding the distal phalange firmly, perform the puncture across the lines of the fingerprint rather than along the lines.				

No.	Step	Points	Check #1	Check #2	Check #3
9	Using a gauze pad, wipe away the first drop.				
10	Collect the specimen according to the test being performed.				
11	Have patient hold firm, direct pressure on the site with a cotton ball for at least 2 minutes. If the bleeding has stopped, an adhesive strip can be applied. If the bleeding has not stopped yet, hold firm, direct pressure on the site for another 5 minutes and then recheck. Adhesive strips are not recommended for patients younger than 2 years.				
12	Disinfect the area and equipment, remove gloves, and dispose of them into a biohazard waste container/red bag. Wash hands.				
13	Record the procedure. If the test is being sent to an outside laboratory, complete the requisition in the presence of the patient, insert both into the biohazard transport bag, and alert the laboratory to pick up the specimen. If the test is to be performed in your POL, proceed with the completion of the test immediately, record the results, and *notify the provider of the results*.				
Student's Total Points					
Points Possible					
Final Score (Student's Total Points/Possible Points)					

Instructor's/Evaluator's Comments and Suggestions:

_____

_____

_____

_____

_____

_____

_____

CHECK #1 Evaluator's Signature:	Date:

CHECK #2 Evaluator's Signature:	Date:

CHECK #3 Evaluator's Signature:	Date:

Work Documentation Form(s)

*The Lab Requisition Form can be downloaded from the Premium Website

ABHES Competencies: MA.A.1.8.cc Communicate on the recipient's level of comprehension; MA.A.1.9.i Use standard precautions; 10.d (2) Perform capillary puncture

CAAHEP Competencies: I.A.2 Use language/verbal skills that enable patients' understanding; I.P.3 Perform capillary puncture; III.P.2 Practice Standard Precautions

Name _____ **Date** _____ **Score** _____

● COMPETENCY ASSESSMENT

Procedure 40-6: Obtaining a Capillary Specimen for Transport Using a Microtainer Transport Unit

Task: Obtain a specimen of capillary blood for transport to a laboratory for testing, using a Microtainer.

Conditions:
- Gloves (goggles and mask are optional)
- 70% isopropyl alcohol swab, cotton balls, gauze
- Safety lancet
- Adhesive bandage
- Sharps container and biohazard waste receptacle
- Microtainer transport unit
- Laboratory requisition*
- Small sturdy container with a tightly fitting lid (such as a urine specimen cup or red top vacuum tube)
- Biohazard specimen transport bag

Standards: Perform the Task within 20 minutes with a minimum score of ___ points, as determined by your instructor.

Competency Assessment Information

Use the following information to complete the Lab Requisition (Work Documentation).

Use today's date and time. Patient's name is Todd Pike. His address is 5959 Atomic Bay Drive, River City, NY 98765. He is male and has Blue Cross insurance (54789). His chart/medical record number is 102030. His birthdate is January 22, 1980.

Dr. Rice has requested that a capillary sample be sent to the lab for a hemoglobin/hematocrit.

Time began: _____   **Time ended:** _____   **Total time:** _____

No.	Step	Points	Check #1	Check #2	Check #3
1	Determine the appropriateness of submitting a capillary specimen for the specific test you are performing.				
2	Assemble the supplies.				
3	*Identify the patient, introduce yourself by name and credential* and recheck the provider's orders.				
4	*Explain the procedure and expectations to the patient. Allay the patient's fears regarding the procedure to help him feel safe and comfortable.*				
5	Wash hands, apply gloves, and perform the capillary puncture according to Procedure 40-5.				
6	Discard the first drop of blood. Wipe it away with a gauze square. Allow a good size drop to form.				

No.	Step	Points	Check #1	Check #2	Check #3
7	Scoop the drop into the Microtainer.				
8	Tip the Microtainer, allowing the drop to slide into the tube.				
9	Gently agitate the tube.				
10	Continue collection of blood until the tube is filled.				
11	Provide the patient with a cotton ball and ask him to hold pressure on the puncture site.				
12	Remove the scoop from the Microtainer and discard the scoop into the sharps container.				
13	Remove the colored cap from the back of the Microtainer and place it securely onto the opening.				
14	Place the capped Microtainer into a small sturdy container with a tight-fitting lid. Label the container.				
15	Fill out the laboratory requisition while the patient is present. Place the specimen and the requisition into the biohazard transport bag in their separate compartments.				
16	Check the patient's puncture site. If bleeding has stopped, apply an adhesive strip, answer any questions the patient has, and release the patient.				
17	Document procedure in patient's chart or electronic medical record and notify the laboratory that the specimen is ready for pickup.				
Student's Total Points					
Points Possible					
Final Score (Student's Total Points/Possible Points)					

Instructor's/Evaluator's Comments and Suggestions:

_____

_____

_____

_____

_____

_____

CHECK #1	
Evaluator's Signature:	Date:

CHECK #2	
Evaluator's Signature:	Date:

CHECK #3	
Evaluator's Signature:	Date:

Work Documentation Form(s)

*Lab Requisition Form can be downloaded from the Premium Website

ABHES Competencies: MA.A.1.8.cc Communicate on the recipient's level of comprehension; MA.A.1.9.i. Use standard precautions; 10.d (2) Perform capillary puncture

CAAHEP Competencies: I.A.2 Use language/verbal skills that enable patients' understanding; I.P.3 Perform capillary puncture; III.P.2 Practice Standard Precautions

Name_____ Date_____ Score_____

● COMPETENCY ASSESSMENT

Procedure 40-7:   Obtaining Blood for Blood Culture

Task: While performing venipuncture from two separate sites, prepare two culture bottles of blood from each site for culture (four total).

Conditions: • Nonsterile gloves for use with povidine-iodine solution
                • Sterile gloves
                • Laboratory requisition*
                • Blood culture bottles, anaerobic and aerobic
                • 70% isopropyl alcohol
                • Povidone-iodine solution swabs or towelettes
                • Venipuncture supplies (according to method used) for two separate sites
                • Biohazard red bag
                • Sharps container
                • Labeling pen
                • Biohazard transport bag

Standards: Perform the Task within 30 minutes with a minimum score of ___ points, as determined by your instructor.

Competency Assessment Information

Use the following information to complete the Lab Requisition (Work Documentation).

● Use today's date and time. Patient's name is C. J. Jackson. Her address is 992 Golden Girl Circle, River City, NY 23230. She is female and has Group Health insurance (#896625). Her chart/medical record number is 2145. Her birthdate is April 10, 1956.

Dr. King has requested that blood be collected and sent to the lab for a blood culture.

Time began: _____   Time ended: _____   Total time: _____

No.	Step	Points	Check #1	Check #2	Check #3
1	*Identify the patient, and introduce yourself by name and credential.*				
2	*Explain the procedure and expectations to the patient. Allay the patient's fears regarding the procedure to help her feel safe and comfortable.*				
3	Ensure that the patient has not initiated antimicrobial therapy.				
4	Wash hands and put on gloves.				
5	Assemble equipment and supplies according to the venipuncture procedure being used and the laboratory requirements. Check expiration dates on all collection and culture supplies.				
6	Place the culture bottles on a flat surface within reach during the procedure. Mark the correct fill line on both bottles at 10 mL per bottle (1–3 mL per bottle for pediatric patients).				

No.	Step	Points	Check #1	Check #2	Check #3
7	Prepare the venipuncture site with isopropyl alcohol and allow to dry, then apply povidone-iodine in progressively larger concentric circles from the inside outward. The iodine must remain on the skin for 1 full minute and be allowed to dry naturally. The venipuncture site should not be touched after the skin is disinfected.				
8	Cleanse the bottle tops with alcohol and povidone-iodine solution.				
9	Remove the preparation gloves and apply the sterile gloves using sterile procedure.				
10	Perform venipuncture according to method used. Insert the aerobic culture bottle onto the needle. Fill to the appropriate line, usually 10 mL per bottle (1–3 mL for pediatric patients). Remove the first bottle, invert 8 to 10 times, and apply the second (anaerobic) bottle. Fill. Remove the second bottle and invert 8 to 10 times.				
11	Complete the venipuncture procedure as determined by the method used. Remove the remaining iodine from the skin with isopropyl alcohol.				
12	Perform venipuncture at the second site, repeating the process as stated above. The second and subsequent culture bottles must be collected within 30 minutes of the first.				
13	The culture bottles should be stored at room temperature and not refrigerated.				
14	Label the bottles with the patient's name, date, time, and other required information.				
15	Dispose of all contaminated supplies, disinfect all surfaces, remove gloves, and wash hands.				
16	Complete the laboratory requisition in the presence of the patient, including the date and time of each specimen collected, any antibiotic therapy the patient is on, the name and strength of the antibiotic, as well as the dosage, duration, and the last dose taken. Include the clinical diagnosis and any special organisms suspected or to rule out. The laboratory requisition must indicate if the culture is for *brucella* or *francisella*. The information on the laboratory requisition should match exactly the information given on the bottles.				
17	Place the specimen and the requisition in the biohazard transport bag in their separate compartments and notify the laboratory that the specimen is ready for pickup.				
18	Document the procedure in the laboratory section of the patient's chart or electronic medical record.				
Student's Total Points					
Points Possible					
Final Score (Student's Total Points/Possible Points)					

Instructor's/Evaluator's Comments and Suggestions:

_____

_____

_____

_____

_____

_____

CHECK #1	
Evaluator's Signature:	Date:

CHECK #2	
Evaluator's Signature:	Date:

CHECK #3	
Evaluator's Signature:	Date:

Work Documentation Form(s)

*The Lab Requisition Form can be downloaded from the Premium Website

ABHES Competencies: MA.A.1.8.cc Communicate on the recipient's level of comprehension; MA.A.1.9.i Use standard precautions; MA.A.1.10.d (1) Perform venipuncture

CAAHEP Competencies: I.A.2 Use language/verbal skills that enable patients' understanding; I.P.2 Perform venipuncture; III.P.2 Practice Standard Precautions

Name_____ **Date**_____ **Score**_____

● COMPETENCY ASSESSMENT

Procedure 41-1:   Hemoglobin Determination Using a CLIA Waived Hemoglobin Analyzer

Task: Properly and safely perform an automated hemoglobin determination to evaluate the oxygen-carrying capacity of the blood.

Conditions:
- Gloves
- Biohazard container
- Sharps container
- Capillary puncture equipment:
  - 70% isopropyl alcohol
  - Safety lancet
  - Cotton ball
  - Gauze 2 × 2
  - Adhesive bandage
- CLIA waived hemoglobin analyzer with test slides
- Lab report form

Standards: Perform the Task within 15 minutes with a minimum score of ___ points, as determined by your instructor.

Competency Assessment Information

Use the following information to complete the Lab Report (Work Documentation):

Use today's date and time. Patient's name is Shirley Miller. Her chart/medical record number is 98563.

Dr. Lewis has requested that you obtain a blood sample and run a hemoglobin level.

Time began: _____   **Time ended:** _____   **Total time:** _____

No.	Step	Points	Check #1	Check #2	Check #3
1	Assemble and organize equipment and supplies.				
2	Wash hands and put on gloves.				
3	Turn on the analyzer and calibrate or standardize according to the manufacturer's instructions.				
4	*Introduce yourself by name and credential, identify the patient,* and recheck the provider's orders.				
5	*Explain the procedure and expectations to the patient. Allay the patient's fears regarding the procedure to help her feel safe and comfortable.*				
6	Select the site, prepare the site, and perform the capillary puncture. Wipe away the first drop with gauze.				
7	Apply the second drop of blood into the slide reservoir using the appropriate technique for the analyzer.				

No.	Step	Points	Check #1	Check #2	Check #3
8	Apply a cotton ball to the puncture site and ask the patient to hold pressure for 2 minutes.				
9	Place the slide into the analyzer and perform appropriate steps as required by the manufacturer's instructions.				
10	Read and make a note of the test results.				
11	Assess the patient and apply a bandage strip to the puncture site.				
12	Disinfect analyzer according to manufacturer's instructions. Discard all contaminated equipment and supplies into appropriate biohazard waste receptacles. Disinfect counter space.				
13	Discard note, remove gloves and discard into biohazard container, and wash hands.				
14	Document the procedure in the patient's medical record in the progress notes charting section and complete a lab report. File the lab report in the lab section of the patient record. Notify the provider of the results.				
Student's Total Points					
Points Possible					
Final Score (Student's Total Points/Possible Points)					

Instructor's/Evaluator's Comments and Suggestions:

_____

_____

_____

_____

_____

_____

_____

_____

CHECK #1	
Evaluator's Signature:	Date:

CHECK #2	
Evaluator's Signature:	Date:

CHECK #3	
Evaluator's Signature:	Date:

Work Documentation Form(s)

*Lab Report form can be downloaded from the Premium Website

ABHES Competencies: MA.A.1.8.cc Communicate on the recipient's level of comprehension; MA.A.1.9.i Use standard precautions; MA.A.1.10.d (2) Perform capillary puncture; MA.A.1.10.b (2) Hematology testing

CAAHEP Competencies: I.A.2 Use language/verbal skills that enable patients' understanding; I.P.3 Perform capillary puncture; I.P.12 Perform hematology testing; III.P.2 Practice Standard Precautions

Name _____ **Date** _____ **Score** _____

● **COMPETENCY ASSESSMENT**

Procedure 41-2:   Microhematocrit Determination

Task: Properly and safely perform a microhematocrit determination.

Conditions:
- Gloves
- Biohazard container
- Sharps container
- Capillary puncture equipment:
  - 70% isopropyl alcohol
  - Safety lancet
  - Cotton ball
  - Gauze 2 × 2
  - Adhesive bandage
- Microhematocrit tubes (heparinized, plastic, self-sealing or use sealing clay)
- Microhematocrit centrifuge and reader

Standards: Perform the Task within 15 minutes with a minimum score of ___ points, as determined by your instructor.

Competency Assessment Information

Use the following information to complete the Lab Report (Work Documentation):

Use today's date and time. Patient's name is Roger Carter. His chart/medical record number is 445521.

● Dr. Rice has requested that you perform a hematocrit level.

Time began: _____   **Time ended:** _____   **Total time:** _____

No.	Step	Points	Check #1	Check #2	Check #3
1	Assemble and organize equipment and supplies.				
2	Wash hands and put on gloves.				
3	*Introduce yourself by name and credential, identify the patient,* and recheck the provider's orders.				
4	*Explain the procedure and expectations to the patient. Allay the patient's fears regarding the procedure to help him feel safe and comfortable.*				
5	Select the site, prepare the site, and perform the capillary puncture. Wipe away the first drop with gauze.				
6	Allow the second drop of blood to form on the patient's finger. Holding the microhematocrit tube horizontally, touch the end onto the top of the blood drop and let the tube fill by capillary action until the tube is approximately 3/4 full.				
7	With a 2 × 2 gauze, wipe off the end of the tube. Gently place the tube into clay until a plug is formed or use a self-sealing tube.				
8	Repeat the procedure with one more tube.				

No.	Step	Points	Check #1	Check #2	Check #3
9	Apply a cotton ball to the puncture site and ask the patient to hold pressure for 2 minutes.				
10	Place the tubes into the centrifuge with sealed ends outward against the gasket. Make certain the tubes balance each other across the centrifuge. Fasten the lid securely, lock into place, and turn the centrifuge on. Set the timer and spin for the appropriate amount of time as required by the manufacturer's instructions.				
11	Assess the patient and apply a bandage strip to the puncture site.				
12	Allow the centrifuge to come to a complete stop before touching it. Remove the tubes. Using a reader or accompanying graph, determine the hematocrit level. Read and make a note of the test results.				
13	Discard all contaminated equipment and supplies into appropriate biohazard waste receptacles. Disinfect counter space and centrifuge according to manufacturer's instructions.				
14	Discard note, remove gloves and discard into biohazard container, and wash hands.				
15	Document the procedure in the patient's medical record in the progress notes charting section and complete a lab report. Notify the provider of the results and file the lab report in the lab section of the patient record.				
Student's Total Points					
Points Possible					
Final Score (Student's Total Points/Possible Points)					

Instructor's/Evaluator's Comments and Suggestions:

_____

_____

_____

_____

_____

_____

_____

CHECK #1	
Evaluator's Signature:	Date:

CHECK #2	
Evaluator's Signature:	Date:

CHECK #3	
Evaluator's Signature:	Date:

Work Documentation Form(s)

*Lab Report form can be downloaded from the Premium Website

ABHES Competencies: MA.A.1.8.cc Communicate on the recipient's level of comprehension; MA.A.1.9.i Use standard precautions; MA.A.1.10.d (2) Perform capillary puncture; MA.A.1.10.b (2) Hematology testing

CAAHEP Competencies: I.A.2 Use language/verbal skills that enable patients' understanding; I.P.3 Perform capillary puncture; I.P.12 Perform hematology testing; III.P.2 Practice Standard Precautions

Name _____ **Date** _____ **Score** _____

● **COMPETENCY ASSESSMENT**

Procedure 41-3:   Erythrocyte Sedimentation Rate

Task: Properly and safely examine a blood sample by using either the Sediplast® (Westergren) or Wintrobe method to record the ESR.

Conditions:
- Gloves
- Samples of venous blood collected in EDTA (purple top tube)
- Sediplast® kit (or other ESR kit): sedivial and sedirack, Sediplast® autozeroing pipette, pipette capable of delivering up to 1.0 mL
- Wintrobe method: Wintrobe sedimentation tube (disposable or reusable), Wintrobe sedimentation rack, long-stem Pasteur-type pipette with rubber bulb
- Timer
- Disinfectant
- Biohazard disposal container
- Acrylic face shield or goggles and mask
- Sharps container
- Lab report form

Standards: Perform the Task within 75 minutes with a minimum score of ___ points, as determined by your instructor.

Competency Assessment Information

Use the following information to complete the Lab Report (Work Documentation):

Use today's date and time. The patient's name is Charlotte Furchert. She has no insurance. Her medical record number is 66773.

Dr. Rice has requested that you perform a sed rate test.

Time began: _____   **Time ended:** _____   **Total time:** _____

No.	Step	Points	Check #1	Check #2	Check #3
1	Wash hands and put on gloves.				
2	Assemble equipment and materials.				
3	Gently mix blood sample for 2 minutes.				
4	Perform Sediplast® ESR procedure: • Remove stopper on sedivial and fill to the indicated mark with 0.8 mL blood. Replace stopper and invert vial several times to mix (or mix using pipette). • Place sedivial in Sediplast® rack on a level surface. • Gently insert the disposable Sediplast® pipette through the pierceable stopper with a twisting motion and push down until the pipette rests on the bottom of the vial. The pipette will autozero the blood and any excess will flow into the sealed reservoir compartment.				

No.	Step	Points	Check #1	Check #2	Check #3
	• Set timer for 1 hour. • Return blood sample to proper storage. (If no laboratory work will be performed during the incubation, remove gloves, discard appropriately, and wash hands. Reglove before handling test materials.) • Let the pipette stand undisturbed for exactly 1 hour, and then read the results of the ESR: Use the scale on the tube to measure the distance from the top of the plasma to the top of the RBCs. • Record the sedimentation rate: ESR (Mod. Westergren, 1 hr) = ___ mm. • Dispose of tube and vial in appropriate biohazard container.				
5	Perform Wintrobe ESR procedure: • Place tube in Wintrobe sedimentation rack. • Check the leveling bubble to ensure that the Wintrobe rack is level. • Fill Wintrobe tube to the zero mark with well-mixed blood using the Pasteur pipette and being careful not to overfill. • Set timer for 1 hour. Be certain the tube is vertical and left undisturbed for the entire hour. • Return blood sample to proper storage. (If no other laboratory work is scheduled, remove gloves, discard appropriately, and wash hands. Reglove before handling test materials.) • Measure the distance the erythrocytes have fallen (in mm): after exactly 1 hour, use the scale on the tube to measure the distance from the top of the plasma to the top of the RBCs. • Record the sedimentation rate: ESR (Wintrobe, 1 hr) = ___ mm. • Disinfect and clean equipment and return to storage.				
6	Clean work area with surface disinfectant.				
7	Remove gloves and discard into biohazard container.				
8	Wash hands.				
9	Document the procedure in the patient's medical record in the progress notes charting section and complete a lab report. Notify the provider of the results and file the lab report in the lab section of the patient record.				
Student's Total Points					
Points Possible					
Final Score (Student's Total Points/Possible Points)					

Instructor's/Evaluator's Comments and Suggestions:

CHECK #1	
Evaluator's Signature:	Date:

CHECK #2	
Evaluator's Signature:	Date:

CHECK #3	
Evaluator's Signature:	Date:

Work Documentation Form(s)

*Progress Note Template and Lab Report form can be downloaded from the Premium Website

ABHES Competencies: MA.A.1.10.b (2) Hematology testing; MA.A.1.9.i Use standard precautions

CAAHEP Competencies: I.P.12 Perform hematology testing; III.P.2 Practice Standard Precautions

Name _____ **Date** _____ **Score** _____

● **COMPETENCY ASSESSMENT**

Procedure 41-4:   Prothrombin Time (Using CLIA Waived ProTime Analyzer)

Task: Properly and safely perform an automated prothrombin time determination to evaluate the clotting time of a drop of blood.

Conditions:
- Gloves
- Biohazard container
- Sharps container
- Capillary puncture equipment:
  - 70% isopropyl alcohol
  - Tenderlett safety lancet
  - Cotton ball
  - Gauze 2 × 2
  - Adhesive bandage
- CLIA Waived ProTime Analyzer (ITC ProTime-3) with accessories
- Lab report form

Standards: Perform the Task within 15 minutes with a minimum score of ___ points, as determined by your instructor.

Competency Assessment Information

Use the following information to complete the Lab Report (Work Documentation):

Use today's date and time. Patient's name is Sharyn Erickson. Her chart/medical record number is 98882.

Dr. Lewis has asked you to perform a prothrombin time test.

Time began: _____   **Time ended:** _____   **Total time:** _____

No.	Step	Points	Check #1	Check #2	Check #3
1	Assemble and organize equipment and supplies. Check expiration dates.				
2	Wash hands and put on gloves.				
3	Turn on the ProTime-3 and follow the prompts. Insert the test cuvette into the analyzer.				
4	*Introduce yourself by name and credential, identify the patient,* and recheck the provider's orders.				
5	*Explain the procedure and expectations to the patient. Allay the patient's fears regarding the procedure to help her feel safe and comfortable.*				
6	Select the site, prepare the site, and perform the capillary puncture using the Tenderlett lancet. Remember to use gauze to wipe away the first drop.				

No.	Step	Points	Check #1	Check #2	Check #3
7	Fill the Tenderlett lancet cup to the fill line and then place it onto the cuvette, which was placed into the machine in Step 3. Be sure it is snapped into place. Press the start button.				
8	Apply a cotton ball and ask the patient to hold pressure for 3 to 5 minutes. Assess that the bleeding has stopped and apply bandage.				
9	Stay by the analyzer and await a prompt to remove the Tenderlett lancet device. When prompted, immediately remove the device and discard it into a nearby sharps container.				
10	Read the clotting time in seconds and the INR. Record the results.				
11	*Notify the provider* immediately if the results fall within a critical range.				
12	Disinfect analyzer according to manufacturer's instructions, discard all contaminated equipment and supplies into appropriate biohazard waste receptacles, and disinfect counter space. Remove gloves and wash hands.				
13	Document the procedure in the patient's medical record in the progress notes charting section and complete a lab report. File the lab report in the lab section of the patient record.				
Student's Total Points					
Points Possible					
Final Score (Student's Total Points/Possible Points)					

Instructor's/Evaluator's Comments and Suggestions:

_____

_____

_____

_____

_____

_____

_____

CHECK #1	
Evaluator's Signature:	Date:

CHECK #2	
Evaluator's Signature:	Date:

CHECK #3	
Evaluator's Signature:	Date:

Work Documentation Form(s)

*Progress Note Template and Lab Report form can be downloaded from the Premium Website

ABHES Competencies: MA.A.1.8.cc Communicate on the recipient's level of comprehension; MA.A.1.9.i Use standard precautions; MA.A.1.10.b (2) Perform hematology testing

CAAHEP Competencies: I.A.2 Use language/verbal skills that enable patients' understanding; I.P.12 Perform hematology testing; III.P.2 Practice Standard Precautions

Name _____ **Date** _____ **Score** _____

● COMPETENCY ASSESSMENT

Procedure 42-1: Assessing Urine Volume, Color, and Clarity (Physical Urinalysis)

Task: Determine and document the volume, color, and clarity of a urine sample.

Conditions:
- Gloves
- Urine container
- Biohazard container
- Disinfectant cleaner
- Urinalysis Report form

Standards: Perform the Task within 10 minutes with a minimum score of ___ points, as determined by your instructor.

Competency Assessment Information

Use the following patient information on the Urinalysis Report Form (Work Documentation).

Use today's date and time. The patient's name is Wanda Hinds. She has Medicare coverage, and her identification number is 900-89-7890.

Dr. Rice has requested a physical examination of her urine.

Urine volume, color, and clarity are not performed outside of a complete urinalysis (or chemical urine test). This procedure is offered as a separate procedure only for lab practice options.

● Time began: _____ Time ended: _____ Total time: _____

No.	Step	Points	Check #1	Check #2	Check #3
1	Wash hands and put on gloves.				
2	Assemble equipment and supplies.				
3	Follow all safety guidelines, being careful not to splash the urine specimen. Wipe up all spills immediately with disinfectant cleaner.				
4	Examine the specimen for proper labeling, *paying attention to detail*. Any unlabeled specimen cannot be identified and the patient should be notified to submit a new specimen. The provider ordering the test should be notified of the delay. The specimen should be labeled on the cup, not the lid.				
5	Ensure the lid is securely tightened and mix the urine thoroughly.				
6	Measure and note the amount of urine in the specimen if it is less than 10 mL. The amount of the specimen does not have to be noted if it is more than 10 mL.				
7	Note and assess the urine color.				

No.	Step	Points	Check #1	Check #2	Check #3
8	After the volume and color have been assessed and recorded, assess the clarity of the urine. Holding the urine against a white background with good lighting, observe it for cloudiness. If the urine appears cloudy, it is said to be slightly cloudy, cloudy, or very cloudy/turbid. Record the description on the report form.				
9	If a complete urinalysis is being performed, proceed to the chemical analysis of the urine.				
10	Dispose of the specimen into the toilet or designated sink and all supplies into appropriate biohazard containers. Disinfect all reusable equipment and all surfaces.				
11	Remove gloves. Wash hands.				
12	Document procedure in patient's chart or electronic medical record.				
Student's Total Points					
Points Possible					
Final Score (Student's Total Points/Possible Points)					

Instructor's/Evaluator's Comments and Suggestions:

_____

_____

_____

_____

_____

_____

CHECK #1	
Evaluator's Signature:	Date:

CHECK #2	
Evaluator's Signature:	Date:

CHECK #3	
Evaluator's Signature:	Date:

ABHES Competency: MA.A.1.9.i Use Standard Precautions

CAAHEP Competency: III.P.2 Practice Standard Precautions

Work Documentation Form(s)

Urinalysis Report Form

Patient Name: _____

Age: _____ M _____ F _____

Physician's Name: _____

Collection Date: _____ Test Date: _____ MA's Initials: _____

Physical Examination

Color: ☐ colorless ☐ yellow ☐ amber ☐ _____

Appearance: ☐ clear ☐ hazy ☐ cloudy ☐ turbid

Chemical Examination (circle one)

specific gravity	1.000	1.005	1.010	1.015	1.020	1.025	1.030
pH		5	6	7	8	9	
leukocytes		neg	trace	+	++		
nitrite		neg	pos	(any pink color is considered positive)			
protein (mg/dL)		neg	trace	+/30	++/100	+++/500	
glucose (mg/dL)		normal	50	100	250	500	1000
ketones		neg	+small	++mod	+++large		
urobilinogen (mg/dL)		normal	1	4	8	12	
bilirubin		neg	+	++	+++		
blood (ery/µl)		neg	trace	50	250		
hemoglobin (ery/µl)			10	50	250		

Comments: _____

_____

_____

_____

_____

Name _____ **Date** _____ **Score** _____

● COMPETENCY ASSESSMENT

Procedure 42-2: Using the Refractometer to Measure Specific Gravity (Physical Urinalysis, Continued)

Task: Measure and record the specific gravity of a urine specimen.

Conditions:
- Refractometer
- Urine sample
- Gloves
- Pipettes
- Distilled water
- Lint-free tissues
- Biohazard container
- Disinfectant cleaners
- Urinalysis report form

Standards: Perform the Task within 5 minutes with a minimum score of ___ points, as determined by your instructor.

Competency Assessment Information

Use the following patient information for the Urinalysis Report Form (Work Documentation).

Use today's date and time. The patient's name is Cindy Urie. She has Regence coverage, and her identification number is 51-58459.

Dr. Rice has requested a test of the specific gravity of her urine.

Urine specific gravity is not performed outside of a complete urinalysis (or chemical urine test). This procedure is offered as a separate procedure only for lab practice options.

Time began: _____ **Time ended:** _____ **Total time:** _____

No.	Step	Points	Check #1	Check #2	Check #3
1	Wash hands and put on gloves.				
2	Assemble equipment and supplies.				
3	Follow all safety guidelines, being careful not to splash the urine specimen. Wipe up all spills immediately with disinfectant cleaner.				
4	Perform quality control on the refractometer before every use by checking the specific gravity of a drop of distilled water: • Clean the surface of the prism and the cover with lint-free tissue and distilled water. Wipe dry. • Depending on the type of refractometer used, you may either apply the drop and then close the cover, or close the cover and apply the drop of distilled water to the notched portion of the cover so it flows over the prism.				

No.	Step	Points	Check #1	Check #2	Check #3
	• With the instrument tilted to allow light to enter, view the scale and read the specific gravity number. It should be exactly 1.000. • If the quality control test shows the refractometer is calibrated properly, record the results and proceed to test the urine specimen. If the quality control test shows the refractometer to be inaccurate, the instrument is not calibrated properly. Use the small screwdriver to adjust the calibration. Do this adjustment using distilled water until the gauge reads 1.000.				
5	Test the urine specimen exactly as the distilled water was tested and record the specific gravity on the urinalysis report form.				
6	If a complete urinalysis was being performed, you would proceed to the chemical analysis of urine.				
7	Dispose of the specimen into the toilet or designated sink and all supplies into appropriate biohazard containers. Disinfect all reusable equipment and all surfaces.				
8	Remove gloves. Wash hands.				
9	Document procedure in patient's chart or electronic medical record.				
Student's Total Points					
Points Possible					
Final Score (Student's Total Points/Possible Points)					

Instructor's/Evaluator's Comments and Suggestions:

_____

_____

_____

_____

_____

_____

_____

CHECK #1	
Evaluator's Signature:	Date:

CHECK #2	
Evaluator's Signature:	Date:

CHECK #3	
Evaluator's Signature:	Date:

ABHES Competency: MA.A.1.9.i Use Standard Precautions

CAAHEP Competency: III.P.2 Practice Standard Precautions

Work Documentation Form(s)

Urinalysis Report Form

Patient Name: _____

Age: _____M_____F_____

Physician's Name: _____

Collection Date: _____ Test Date: _____MA's Initials: _____

Physical Examination

Color: ☐ colorless   ☐ yellow   ☐ amber   ☐ _____

Appearance: ☐ clear   ☐ hazy   ☐ cloudy ☐ turbid

Chemical Examination (circle one)

specific gravity	1.000	1.005	1.010	1.015	1.020	1.025	1.030
pH		5	6	7	8	9	
leukocytes		neg	trace	+	++		
nitrite		neg	pos	(any pink color is considered positive)			
protein (mg/dL)		neg	trace	+/30	++/100	+++/500	
glucose (mg/dL)		normal	50	100	250	500	1000
ketones		neg	+small	++mod	+++large		
urobilinogen (mg/dL)		normal	1	4	8	12	
bilirubin		neg	+	++	+++		
blood (ery/µl)		neg	trace	50	250		
hemoglobin (ery/µl)			10	50	250		

Comments: _____

_____

_____

_____

_____

Name_____ **Date**_____ **Score**_____

● COMPETENCY ASSESSMENT

Procedure 42-3: Performing a Chemical Urinalysis

Task: Detect any abnormal chemical constituents of a urine specimen.

Conditions: • Gloves
                 • Urine test strips
                 • Urine specimen in a properly labeled urine cup with a tightly fitted lid
                 • Biohazard container
                 • Disinfectant cleaner
                 • Urinalysis report form

Standards: Perform the Task within 5 minutes with a minimum score of ___ points, as determined by your instructor.

Competency Assessment Information

Use the following information to complete the Urinalysis Report Form (Work Documentation):

Use today's date and time. Patient's name is Heather Rogers. Her chart/medical record number is 75213.

Dr. Rice has requested a chemical test on urine.

Time began: _____   **Time ended:** _____   **Total time:** _____

No.	Step	Points	Check #1	Check #2	Check #3
1	Wash hands and put on gloves.				
2	Assemble equipment and supplies.				
3	Follow all safety guidelines, being careful not to splash the urine specimen. Wipe up all spills immediately with disinfectant cleaner.				
4	Examine the specimen for proper labeling, *paying attention to detail.* Any unlabeled specimen is not to be tested. If the missing, unlabeled specimen cannot be identified, the patient should be notified to submit a new specimen. The provider ordering the test should be notified of the delay. The specimen should be labeled on the cup, not the lid.				
5	Ensure the lid is securely tightened and mix the urine thoroughly.				
6	If you are planning to perform a complete urinalysis, label a urine centrifuge tube with the patient's name and pour 10 mL into the tube for the microscopic examination. Set aside in the centrifuge.				
7	Read and follow the manufacturer's instructions, *paying attention to detail.*				
8	Remove a test strip from the container and replace the cap tightly.				
9	Immerse the test strip completely in the well-mixed urine and remove it immediately. While removing the test strip from the cup, tap it gently onto a paper towel to remove excess urine.				

No.	Step	Points	Check #1	Check #2	Check #3
10	Properly time the test for each test pad.				
11	Holding the test strip close to the container (or chart) but not touching it, compare the color of the pads on the test strip with the color guides on the container (or chart).				
12	Record the results on the laboratory report form.				
13	If a complete urinalysis is ordered, proceed with setting up for the microscopic examination of the urine.				
14	Dispose of the specimen into the toilet or designated sink and all supplies into appropriate biohazard containers. Disinfect all reusable equipment and all surfaces.				
15	Remove gloves. Wash hands.				
16	Document procedure in patient's chart or electronic medical record.				
Student's Total Points					
Points Possible					
Final Score (Student's Total Points/Possible Points)					

Instructor's/Evaluator's Comments and Suggestions:

_____

_____

_____

_____

_____

_____

_____

CHECK #1	
Evaluator's Signature:	Date:

CHECK #2	
Evaluator's Signature:	Date:

CHECK #3	
Evaluator's Signature:	Date:

ABHES Competency: MA.A.1.9.i Use Standard Precautions

CAAHEP Competency: III.P.2 Practice Standard Precautions

Work Documentation Form(s)

Urinalysis Report Form

Patient Name: _____

Age: _____M_____F_____

Physician's Name: _____

Collection Date: _____ Test Date: _____MA's Initials: _____

Physical Examination

Color: ☐ colorless   ☐ yellow   ☐ amber   ☐ _____

Appearance: ☐ clear   ☐ hazy   ☐ cloudy ☐ turbid

Chemical Examination (circle one)

specific gravity	1.000	1.005	1.010	1.015	1.020	1.025	1.030
pH		5	6	7	8	9	
leukocytes		neg	trace	+	++		
nitrite		neg	pos	(any pink color is considered positive)			
protein (mg/dL)		neg	trace	+/30	++/100	+++/500	
glucose (mg/dL)		normal	50	100	250	500	1000
ketones		neg	+small	++mod	+++large		
urobilinogen (mg/dL)		normal	1	4	8	12	
bilirubin		neg	+	++	+++		
blood (ery/µl)		neg	trace	50	250		
hemoglobin (ery/µl)			10	50	250		

Comments: _____

_____

_____

_____

_____

Name _____ **Date** _____ **Score** _____

● **COMPETENCY ASSESSMENT**

Procedure 42-4:   Preparing Slide for Microscopic Examination of Urine Sediment

Task: Prepare a slide for a microscopic examination of urine sediment.

Conditions:
- Gloves
- Microscope
- Centrifuge
- Microscope slides
- Coverslips
- Disposable pipettes
- Sharps container
- Centrifuge tubes and holder
- Urine atlas guide
- Disinfectant cleaner
- Biohazard container
- Sedi-Stain® (optional)

Standards: Perform the Task within 5 minutes with a minimum score of ___ points, as determined by your instructor.

Time began: _____   **Time ended:** _____   **Total time:** _____

No.	Step	Points	Check #1	Check #2	Check #3
1	Wash hands and put on gloves.				
2	Assemble equipment and supplies.				
3	Follow all safety guidelines, being careful not to splash the urine specimen. Wipe up all spills immediately with disinfectant cleaner.				
4	Examine the specimen for proper labeling, *paying attention to detail*. Any unlabeled specimen is not to be tested. If the missing, unlabeled specimen cannot be identified, the patient should be notified to submit a new specimen. The provider ordering the test should be notified of the delay. The specimen should be labeled on the cup, not the lid.				
5	Ensure the lid is securely tightened and mix the urine thoroughly.				
6	Label a urine centrifuge tube with the patient's name and pour 10 mL into the tube. Set into the centrifuge. Balance the centrifuge, securely close and lock the lid, and spin at 1,500 *g* (revolutions per minute) for 5 minutes.				
7	After centrifugation, pour off the supernatant, leaving about 1 mL in the bottom of the tube. Add two drops of Sedi-Stain® if desired. Remix the sediment by tapping gently on the counter or with your fingernail.				

No.	Step	Points	Check #1	Check #2	Check #3
8	Place a drop of the well-mixed sediment onto a clean microscope slide. Cover with a coverslip by holding the coverslip at an angle to the drop, bringing the edge close to the drop until the urine spreads along the edge of the coverslip, and then gently lower the coverslip onto the drop. Keep the tube.				
9	Place the slide onto the microscope stage but do not leave the light on.				
10	Alert the provider that the slide is ready for viewing.				
11	After the provider is finished with the specimen and the patient has left the clinic, dispose of the specimen into the toilet or designated sink and all used supplies into appropriate biohazard containers. Disinfect all reusable equipment and all surfaces. Remove gloves and wash hands.				
Student's Total Points					
Points Possible					
Final Score (Student's Total Points/Possible Points)					

Instructor's/Evaluator's Comments and Suggestions:

_____

_____

_____

_____

_____

_____

CHECK #1	
Evaluator's Signature:	Date:

CHECK #2	
Evaluator's Signature:	Date:

CHECK #3	
Evaluator's Signature:	Date:

ABHES Competency: MA.A.1.9.i Use Standard Precautions

CAAHEP Competency: III.P.2 Practice Standard Precautions

Name _____ **Date** _____ **Score** _____

● **COMPETENCY ASSESSMENT**

Procedure 42-5: Performing a Complete Urinalysis

Task: Perform a complete urinalysis, including the physical and chemical, and microscopic examination within 30 minutes of obtaining the specimen.

Conditions:
- Gloves
- Urine specimen
- Pipettes
- Centrifuge tube
- Centrifuge
- Microscope
- Microscope slides
- Coverslip
- Permanent marker
- Sedi-Stain® (optional)
- Reagent test strips
- Urine atlas
- Refractometer
- Distilled water
- Lint-free tissues
- Biohazard container
- Sharps container
- Disinfectant cleaner
- Urinalysis report form

Standards: Perform the Task within 15 minutes with a minimum score of ___ points, as determined by your instructor.

Competency Assessment Information

Use the following information to complete the Urinalysis Report Form (Work Documentation).

Use today's date and time. Patient's name is Charlie Woo. His chart/medical record number is 10224.

Dr. King has requested a complete urinalysis.

Time began: _____   **Time ended:** _____   **Total time:** _____

No.	Step	Points	Check #1	Check #2	Check #3
1	Wash hands and put on gloves.				
2	Assemble equipment and supplies.				
3	Follow all safety guidelines.				
4	Examine the specimen for proper labeling, *paying attention to detail.*				
5	Ensure the lid is securely tightened and mix the urine thoroughly.				

No.	Step	Points	Check #1	Check #2	Check #3
6	Label a urine centrifuge tube with the patient's name, pour 10 mL into the tube, and set it into the centrifuge. Balance the centrifuge, securely close and lock the lid, and spin at 1,500 *g* (revolutions per minute) for 5 minutes.				
7	While the sample is being centrifuged, assess and record the color and clarity.				
8	Perform the specific gravity test using a refractometer if specific gravity is not included in the chemical test strip.				
9	Perform the chemical examination following the manufacturer's instructions. Record the results.				
10	After centrifugation, pour off the supernatant, leaving about 1 mL in the bottom of the tube. Add two drops of Sedi-Stain® if desired. Remix the sediment by tapping gently on the counter or with your fingernail.				
11	Place a drop of the well-mixed sediment onto a clean microscope slide. Cover with a coverslip.				
12	Place the slide onto the microscope stage and alert the provider that the slide is ready for viewing.				
13	Dispose of the specimen into the toilet or designated sink and all supplies into appropriate biohazard containers. Disinfect all reusable equipment and all surfaces. Remember that microscopic slides and coverslips are glass and should be placed into an appropriate biohazard sharps container. Remove gloves and wash hands.				
14	File the completed laboratory report form into the laboratory section of the patient's chart or electronic medical record and document the procedure.				
Student's Total Points					
Points Possible					
Final Score (Student's Total Points/Possible Points)					

Instructor's/Evaluator's Comments and Suggestions:

_____

_____

_____

_____

_____

_____

_____

CHECK #1	
Evaluator's Signature:	Date:

CHECK #2	
Evaluator's Signature:	Date:

CHECK #3	
Evaluator's Signature:	Date:

ABHES Competencies: MA.A.1.8.cc Communicate on the recipient's level of comprehension; MA.A.1.9.i Use standard precautions; MA.A.1.10.b (1) Perform urinalysis

CAAHEP Competencies: I.A.2 Use language/verbal skills that enable patients' understanding; I.P.14 Perform urinalysis; III.P.2 Practice Standard Precautions

Work Documentation Form(s)

Urinalysis Report Form

Patient Name: _____

Age: _____M_____F_____

Physician's Name: _____

Collection Date: _____ Test Date: _____ MA's Initials: _____

Physical Examination

Color: ☐ colorless   ☐ yellow   ☐ amber   ☐ ——

Appearance: ☐ clear   ☐ hazy   ☐ cloudy   ☐ turbid

Chemical Examination (circle one)

specific gravity	1.000	1.005	1.010	1.015	1.020	1.025	1.030
pH		5	6	7	8	9	
leukocytes		neg	trace	+	++		
nitrite		neg	pos	(any pink color is considered positive)			
protein (mg/dL)		neg	trace	+/30	++/100	+++/500	
glucose (mg/dL)		normal	50	100	250	500	1000
ketones		neg	+small	++mod	+++large		
urobilinogen (mg/dL)		normal	1	4	8	12	
bilirubin		neg	+	++	+++		
blood (ery/µl)		neg	trace	50	250		
hemoglobin (ery/µl)			10	50	250		

Comments: _____

_____

_____

_____

_____

Name _____ **Date** _____ **Score** _____

● COMPETENCY ASSESSMENT

Procedure 42-6: Utilizing a Urine Transport System for C&S

Task: Prepare a urine specimen for transport using a culture and sensitivity transport kit.

Conditions:
- Gloves
- Sterile urine cup and specimen
- Urine culture and sensitivity transport kit
- Paper towel
- Laboratory requisition form

Standards: Perform the task within 15 minutes with a minimum score of ___ points, as determined by your instructor.

Competency Assessment Information

Use the following information to complete the Laboratory Requisition Form (Work Documentation).

Use today's date and time. Patient's name is James Bouloumpas. His address is 118 Heaven's Way, River City, NY 98765. He is male, and has Medicaid (345-99-9087). His chart/medical record number is 10224. His birthdate is August 2, 1965.

Dr. King has requested that you transfer a sample of urine to the lab for culture and sensitivity testing.

Time began: _____ **Time ended:** _____ **Total time:** _____

No.	Step	Points	Check #1	Check #2	Check #3
1	Wash hands and put on gloves.				
2	Assemble equipment and supplies.				
3	Follow all safety guidelines, being careful not to splash the urine specimen. Wipe up all spills immediately with disinfectant cleaner.				
4	Examine the specimen for proper labeling, *paying attention to detail*.				
5	Check the urine C&S transport kit expiration date.				
6	Open the urine C&S transport kit package. Remove the cap from the specimen cup, placing the lid upside down on the paper towel.				
7	Follow the manufacturer's instructions exactly: • Place the urine tube in the tube adapter and the specimen straw into the urine within the specimen cup. • Advance urine tube into the adapter, pushing the tube onto the needle while keeping the specimen straw submerged in the urine. • Allow the vacuum in the urine tube to draw up the urine. Fill to the exhaustion of the vacuum within the tube. • Remove the tube and the specimen straw/adapter unit and dispose of it into a biohazard container. • Gently invert the tube 8 to 10 times to mix the preservative within the tube.				

No.	Step	Points	Check #1	Check #2	Check #3
8	Label the tube with patient's name, date, time, and other required information.				
9	Dispose of all contaminated supplies, disinfect all surfaces, remove gloves, and wash hands.				
10	Complete the laboratory requisition and document the procedure in patient's chart or electronic medical record.				
Student's Total Points					
Points Possible					
Final Score (Student's Total Points/Possible Points)					

Instructor's/Evaluator's Comments and Suggestions:

_____

_____

_____

_____

_____

_____

_____

CHECK #1 Evaluator's Signature:	Date:

CHECK #2 Evaluator's Signature:	Date:

CHECK #3 Evaluator's Signature:	Date:

Work Documentation Form(s)

*The Laboratory Requisition form can be downloaded from the Premium Website

ABHES Competencies: MA.A.1.9.i Use Standard Precautions; MA.A.1.10.d Collect, label and process specimens
CAAHEP Competency: III.P.2 Practice Standard Precautions

Name _____ **Date** _____ **Score** _____

COMPETENCY ASSESSMENT

Procedure 42-7: Instructing a Patient in the Collection of a Clean-Catch, Midstream Urine Specimen

Task: To instruct a patient in the proper technique of collecting a urine specimen suitable for urinalysis testing.

Conditions:
- Gloves
- Urine cup with a secure lid
- Cleansing towelettes (two for males, three for females)
- Marking pen
- Written instructions posted appropriately in the restroom

Standards: Perform the Task within 15 minutes with a minimum score of ___ points, as determined by your instructor.

Time began: _____ **Time ended:** _____ **Total time:** _____

No.	Step	Points	Check #1	Check #2	Check #3
1	Wash hands and assemble the supplies.				
2	*Introduce yourself by name and credential. Identify the patient,* and provide for a private area free from distractions.				
3	Provide the patient with a capped urine cup labeled with his/her name, a pair of gloves, and the cleansing towelettes.				
4	Show the patient the written instructions posted in the bathroom.				
5	*Speaking to the patient's level of understanding,* explain why the urine sample should be a clean-catch midstream sample and what that means.				
6	Ask the patient to first wash his or her hands and apply the gloves.				
7	*Demonstrate professionalism and courtesy to the patient* while you explain the cleansing process for a clean-catch.				
8	*Explain the process* of obtaining the midstream specimen.				
9	Explain to the patient that he or she should secure the cap onto the cup.				
10	The patient may rinse the outside of the capped cup if needed and towel dry it.				

No.	Step	Points	Check #1	Check #2	Check #3
11	The patient is to then remove the gloves, dispose of them into the red bag waste receptacle, and wash his or her hands.				
12	*Ask the patient if he or she has any questions and provide appropriate responses.*				
13	Using a paper towel as a barrier, the cup may be returned to the medical assistant or placed in the lab receptacle as directed.				
Student's Total Points					
Points Possible					
Final Score (Student's Total Points/Possible Points)					

Instructor's/Evaluator's Comments and Suggestions:

_____

_____

_____

_____

_____

_____

_____

CHECK #1	
Evaluator's Signature:	Date:

CHECK #2	
Evaluator's Signature:	Date:

CHECK #3	
Evaluator's Signature:	Date:

ABHES Competencies: MA.A.1.8.cc Communicate on the recipient's level of comprehension; MA.A.1.9.i Use standard precautions; MA.A.1.10.e Instruct patient in the collection of a clean-catch, mid-stream urine specimen

CAAHEP Competencies: I.A.2 Use language/verbal skills that enable patients' understanding; III.P.2 Practice Standard Precautions

Name _____ **Date** _____ **Score** _____

COMPETENCY ASSESSMENT

Procedure 43-1:   Obtaining a Throat Specimen for Culture

Task: Obtain secretions from the nasopharnyx and tonsillar area as a means of identifying pathogenic microorganisms.

Conditions:
- Tongue depressor
- Culture tube with applicator stick or commercially prepared culture collection system (culturette)
- Label and requisition form
- Gloves and face shield
- Good light source
- Biohazard transport bag

Standards: Perform the Task within 15 minutes with a minimum score of ___ points, as determined by your instructor.

Competency Assessment Information

Use the following information to complete the Lab Requisition form (Work Documentation).

Use today's date and time. Patient's name is Jud Johnson. His address is 3667 Frog Creek, River City, NY 97455. He is male, and has no insurance. His chart/medical record number is 10224. His birth date is 12/25/1972.

Dr. King has requested a complete throat culture be obtained and sent to the lab for testing.

Time began: _____   **Time ended:** _____   **Total time:** _____

No.	Step	Points	Check #1	Check #2	Check #3
1	*Introduce yourself by name and credential and identify the patient.*				
2	*Explain the procedure and expectations to the patient. Allay the patient's fears regarding the procedure to help him feel safe and comfortable.*				
3	Have an emesis basin and tissues ready.				
4	Have the patient in a sitting position.				
5	Wash hands, gather supplies, and apply gloves and face shield.				
6	Ask the patient to open his or her mouth wide and then adjust the light source.				
7	Remove the swab from the culturette using sterile technique.				

No.	Step	Points	Check #1	Check #2	Check #3
8	Ask the patient to say "ah." Depress the tongue with the tongue depressor and swab the back of the throat and tonsillar area. Concentrate primarily on any red, raw areas and pustules. Take care to not touch the swab on the inside of the cheeks or on the tongue.				
9	Place the swab back into the culturette using sterile technique and crush the glass capsule containing the culture media.				
10	*Paying attention to detail,* label the culturette according to the POL policy and requirements.				
11	Ensure patient comfort and answer any questions related to the testing. *Provide appropriate responses and feedback.*				
12	Discard contaminated supplies into a biohazard waste container. Disinfect all work surfaces. Remove gloves and face shield and discard appropriately.				
13	Wash hands.				
14	Complete the laboratory requisition in the presence of the patient, then record the procedure in the patient's chart or electronic medical record.				
15	Place the specimen and the requisition in the biohazard transport bag in their separate compartments and notify the laboratory that the specimen is ready for pickup.				
Student's Total Points					
Points Possible					
Final Score (Student's Total Points/Possible Points)					

Instructor's/Evaluator's Comments and Suggestions:

_____

_____

_____

_____

_____

_____

_____

_____

CHECK #1	
Evaluator's Signature:	Date:

CHECK #2	
Evaluator's Signature:	Date:

CHECK #3	
Evaluator's Signature:	Date:

Work Documentation Form(s)

*Lab Requisition form can be downloaded from the Premium Website

ABHES Competencies: MA.A.1.8.cc Communicate on the recipient's level of comprehension; MA.A.1.9.i Use standard precautions; MA.A.1.10.d (4) Obtain throat specimen for microbiological testing

CAAHEP Competencies: I.A.2 Use language/verbal skills that enable patients' understanding; III.P.2 Practice Standard Precautions; III.P.7 Obtain specimen for microbiological testing

Name _____ **Date** _____ **Score** _____

COMPETENCY ASSESSMENT

Procedure 43-2: Wet-Mount and Hanging Drop Slide Preparations

Task: Prepare a slide for viewing live microorganisms for motility and identifying characteristics.

Conditions:
- Gloves
- Laboratory coat
- Clean glass slide
- Glass slide with concave well
- Coverslips
- Petroleum jelly
- Dropper
- Bacterial suspension

Standards: Perform the Task within 10 minutes with a minimum score of ___ points, as determined by your instructor.

Time began: _____   **Time ended:** _____   **Total time:** _____

No.	Step	Points	Check #1	Check #2	Check #3
1	Wash hands and apply gloves.				
2	Assemble equipment and supplies.				
3	For wet-mount slide preparation: • Place a drop of the bacterial suspension onto a clean glass slide. • Place petroleum jelly around the edges of the coverslip and place the coverslip on top of the bacterial suspension.				
4	For hanging drop slide preparation: • Place the bacterial specimen (in suspension) in the center of the coverslip with petroleum jelly around the edges. • Invert the slide and place the concave well of the slide over the specimen drop on the coverslip. • The slide is then carefully turned right side up for microscopic examination.				
5	Set the slides up for the microscopic examination, alert the provider that the slide is ready.				
6	Clean and disinfect the area, dispose of waste according to standards, remove gloves, wash hands.				
Student's Total Points					
Points Possible					
Final Score (Student's Total Points/Possible Points)					

Instructor's/Evaluator's Comments and Suggestions:

_____

_____

_____

_____

_____

_____

_____

CHECK #1	
Evaluator's Signature:	Date:

CHECK #2	
Evaluator's Signature:	Date:

CHECK #3	
Evaluator's Signature:	Date:

ABHES Competency: MA.A.1.9.i Use Standard Precautions

CAAHEP Competency: III.P.2 Practice Standard Precautions

Name _____ Date _____ Score _____

● **COMPETENCY ASSESSMENT**

Procedure 43-3:   Performing Strep Throat Testing

Task: Test for *Streptococcus* infection of the throat for diagnostic purposes.

Conditions:
- Gloves
- Commercial (CLIA waived) strep test kit including controls and reagents, sterile cotton-tipped swabs, test tubes and holder or receptacles
- Tongue blade
- Adjustable light source
- Lab report form

Standards: Perform the Task within 15 minutes with a minimum score of ___ points, as determined by your instructor.

Competency Assessment Information

The procedure steps are intentionally general, so a variety of kits can be used. Use the following information to complete the Lab Report form (Work Documentation).

Use today's date and time. Patient's name is Juanita Lopez. Her address is 1455 16th Avenue, River City, NY 98765. She is female, and has Blue Cross insurance. Her chart/medical record number is 45210. Her birth date is 6-19-2002.

Dr. King has requested a strep throat test be performed.

● **Time began: _____   Time ended: _____   Total time: _____**

No.	Step	Points	Check #1	Check #2	Check #3
1	Wash hands and apply personal protective equipment (PPE).				
2	Assemble and organize equipment and supplies.				
3	*Introduce yourself by name and credential, identify the patient.*				
4	*Explain the procedure and expectations to the patient. Allay the patient's fears regarding the procedure to help her feel safe and comfortable.*				
5	Using the tongue blade and light source, obtain the specimen from the patient's throat on the cotton-tipped applicator.				
6	*Ask the patient if she has any questions and provide appropriate responses.*				
7	*Paying attention to detail,* follow the manufacturer's instructions exactly to perform the strep throat test. Be sure to also run the controls tests.				
8	Properly dispose of all waste in biohazard container. Disinfect the equipment and the area.				

No.	Step	Points	Check #1	Check #2	Check #3
9	Complete the laboratory report form and notify the provider of the results.				
10	Document procedure in patient's chart or electronic medical record.				
Student's Total Points					
Points Possible					
Final Score (Student's Total Points/Possible Points)					

Instructor's/Evaluator's Comments and Suggestions:

_____

_____

_____

_____

_____

_____

_____

CHECK #1

Evaluator's Signature: Date:

CHECK #2

Evaluator's Signature: Date:

CHECK #3

Evaluator's Signature: Date:

Work Documentation Form(s)

*Lab Report form can be downloaded from the Premium Website

ABHES Competencies: MA.A.1.8.cc Communicate on the recipient's level of comprehension; MA.A.1.9.i.i Use Standard Precautions; MA.A.1.10.b (6)(b)Perform selected CLIA-waived tests that assist with diagnosis and treatment: Quick strep

CAAHEP Competencies: I.A.2 Use language/verbal skills that enable patients' understanding: III.P.7 Obtain specimens for microbiological testing; III.P.2 Practice Standard Precautions

Name _____ **Date** _____ **Score** _____

COMPETENCY ASSESSMENT

Procedure 43-4: Instructing a Patient on Obtaining a Fecal Specimen

Task: Instruct a patient in the correct collection of a fecal sample.

Conditions:
- Gloves
- Biohazard container
- Sturdy, opaque waterproof specimen container with a securely fitting lid
- Special laboratory manual instructions if needed
- Laboratory requisition form

Standards: Perform the Task within 15 minutes with a minimum score of ___ points, as determined by your instructor.

Competency Assessment Information

Use the following information to complete the Lab Requisition form (Work Documentation).

Use today's date and time. Patient's name is Amate Judilum. His address is 815 Pinewood Street, River City, NY 98765. He is male, and has no insurance. His chart/medical record number is 67699. His birth date is April 27, 1989.

Dr. King has requested a stool sample be sent to the lab for culture and sensitivity, and ova and parasite testing.

Time began: _____   **Time ended:** _____   **Total time:** _____

No.	Step	Points	Check #1	Check #2	Check #3
1	Assemble and organize equipment and supplies.				
2	*Introduce yourself by name and credential and identify the patient.*				
3	*Speaking to the patient's level of understanding, explain the procedure.* Provide written instructions as well. *Demonstrate professionalism and courtesy while you explain.*				
4	Hand the patient the labeled specimen container, instructing him to deposit a sample of stool into the cup then securely set the lid onto it.				
5	Caution the patient to avoid contaminating the stool specimen with urine.				
6	Give the patient a biohazard transport bag and instructions on which pocket to put the specimen into and how to secure the bag. The medical assistant can place the laboratory requisition into the other pocket.				
7	The patient should be prepared to transport the specimen to the laboratory as soon as possible while keeping the specimen at or just below body temperature.				

No.	Step	Points	Check #1	Check #2	Check #3
8	*Ask the patient if he has any questions and provide appropriate responses. Demonstrate professionalism and courtesy while answering questions.*				
9	Document that the instructions were given to the patient, both orally and written.				
Student's Total Points					
Points Possible					
Final Score (Student's Total Points/Possible Points)					

Instructor's/Evaluator's Comments and Suggestions:

_____

_____

_____

_____

_____

_____

_____

_____

CHECK #1 Evaluator's Signature:	Date:

CHECK #2 Evaluator's Signature:	Date:

CHECK #3 Evaluator's Signature:	Date:

Work Documentation Form(s)

*Lab Report form can be downloaded from the Premium Website

ABHES Competencies: MA.A.1.8.cc Communicate on the recipient's level of comprehension; MA.A.1.10.f Instruct patients in the collection of a fecal specimen

CAAHEP Competency: I.A.2 Use language/verbal skills that enable patients' understanding

Name _____ **Date** _____ **Score** _____

COMPETENCY ASSESSMENT

Procedure 44-1: Pregnancy Test

Task: Perform the waived category visual determination test to detect human chorionic gonadotropin (hCG) in urine to determine positive or negative pregnancy results.

Conditions:
- Gloves
- Urine specimen
- Stopwatch
- Disinfectant
- Biohazard container
- hCG negative and positive urine controls
- Pregnancy test kit

Standards: Perform the Task within 15 minutes with a minimum score of ___ points, as determined by your instructor.

Competency Assessment Information

Use the following information to complete the Lab Report (Work Documentation).

Use today's date and time. Patient's name is Sandra Whimsy. Her address is 100 Rocky Road, River City, NY 98765. She is female and has no insurance. Her chart/medical record number is 77845. Her birth date is 11-12-1982.

Dr. Lewis has requested a urine pregnancy test be performed.

Time began: _____ **Time ended:** _____ **Total time:** _____

No.	Step	Points	Check #1	Check #2	Check #3
1	Wash hands and put on gloves.				
2	Assemble all equipment and supplies.				
3	*Paying attention to detail,* perform the test following the manufacturer's instructions: • Determine materials are at room temperature. • Apply urine to the test unit using the dispenser provided. • Wait appropriate time interval. • Apply first reagent/antibody to test unit using dispenser provided. • Observe color development after appropriate time interval. • Stop reaction. • Consult manufacturer's package insert to interpret test results.				
4	Record the results of the test on a laboratory report form following laboratory policy.				
5	Repeat steps with both positive and negative urine controls.				

No.	Step	Points	Check #1	Check #2	Check #3
6	Disinfect reusable equipment. Discard disposable supplies into biohazard container. Dispose of specimen per laboratory policy. Clean work area with disinfectant.				
7	Remove gloves and discard into biohazard container. Wash hands.				
8	Document procedure in patient's chart or electronic medical record. Complete a lab report. After the provider has initialed the report, it should be filed in the lab section of the patient's chart.				
Student's Total Points					
Points Possible					
Final Score (Student's Total Points/Possible Points)					

Instructor's/Evaluator's Comments and Suggestions:

_____

_____

_____

_____

_____

_____

_____

_____

CHECK #1	
Evaluator's Signature:	Date:

CHECK #2	
Evaluator's Signature:	Date:

CHECK #3	
Evaluator's Signature:	Date:

Work Documentation Form(s)

Lab Report form can be downloaded from the Premium Website

ABHES Competencies: MA.A.1.8.cc Communicate on the recipient's level of comprehension; MA.A.1.9.i Use Standard Precautions; MA.A.1.10.b (6)(a) Perform selected CLIA-waived tests that assist with diagnosis and treatment (kit testing such as pregnancy)

CAAHEP Competencies: I.A.2 Use language/verbal skills that enable patients' understanding; III.P.2 Practice Standard Precautions

Name _____ **Date** _____ **Score** _____

COMPETENCY ASSESSMENT

Procedure 44-2:   Performing Infectious Mononucleosis Test

Task: Perform an accurate test of serum or plasma to detect the presence or absence of antibodies of infectious mononucleosis.

Conditions:
- Gloves
- Serum or plasma specimen
- Stopwatch or lab timer
- Surface disinfectant
- CLIA waived test kit for infectious mononucleosis
- Biohazard container

Standards: Perform the Task within 15 minutes with a minimum score of ___ points, as determined by your instructor.

Time began: _____   **Time ended:** _____   **Total time:** _____

No.	Step	Points	Check #1	Check #2	Check #3
1	Wash hands and put on gloves.				
2	Assemble all equipment and supplies.				
3	*Paying attention to detail,* perform the test according to the manufacturer's instructions exactly.				
4	Record the results on a laboratory report form following laboratory policy.				
5	Repeat the test procedure using positive and negative controls.				
6	Discard contaminated materials into biohazard container. Dispose of specimen appropriately and disinfect reusable materials. Clean work area with disinfectant.				
7	Remove gloves and discard into biohazard container. Wash hands.				
8	Document results in the patient chart or electronic medical record. Complete a lab report. After the provider has initialed the report, it should be filed in the lab section of patient's chart.				
Student's Total Points					
Points Possible					
Final Score (Student's Total Points/Possible Points)					

Instructor's/Evaluator's Comments and Suggestions:

_____

_____

_____

_____

_____

_____

_____

_____

_____

CHECK #1	
Evaluator's Signature:	Date:

CHECK #2	
Evaluator's Signature:	Date:

CHECK #3	
Evaluator's Signature:	Date:

Work Documentation Form(s)

Lab Report form can be downloaded from the Premium Website

ABHES Competencies: MA.A.1.8.cc Communicate on the recipient's level of comprehension; MA.A.1.9.i Use standard precautions; MA.A.1.10.b (6) Perform selected CLIA-waived tests that assist with diagnosis and treatment (kit testing)

CAAHEP Competencies: I.A.2 Use language/verbal skills that enable patients' understanding; III.P.2 Practice Standard Precautions

Name _____ **Date** _____ **Score** _____

COMPETENCY ASSESSMENT

Procedure 44-3:   Obtaining Blood Specimen for Phenylketonuria (PKU) Test

Task: Obtain a blood specimen using a PKU test card or "filter paper" to determine phenylalanine levels in newborns who are at least 3 days old.

Conditions:
- Gloves
- PKU filter paper test card and mailing envelope
- Alcohol swabs
- Cotton balls/gauze pads
- Sterile pediatric-sized lancet
- Biohazard waste container
- Official information pamphlet

Standards: Perform the Task within 20 minutes with a minimum score of ___ points, as determined by your instructor.

Competency Assessment Information

Use the following information to complete the test card and complete the Lab Requisition form (Work Documentation).

Use today's date and time. Patient's name is Mortimer Sloan. His address is 41012 Enchanted Garden Place, River City, NY 98765. He is male, and has Blue Cross insurance (71909). His chart/medical record number is 051410. He is 2 weeks old.

Dr. Rice has requested that you perform a heel stick for PKU testing.

Time began: _____   **Time ended:** _____   **Total time:** _____

No.	Step	Points	Check #1	Check #2	Check #3
1	Wash hands and put on gloves.				
2	*Introduce yourself by name and credential and identify the patient and his parents.*				
3	*Speaking to the parents' level of understanding, explain the procedure.* Provide written information as well. *Demonstrate professionalism and courtesy while you explain.*				
4	Select and clean an appropriate puncture site. Allow the alcohol to dry before the puncture.				
5	Grasp the infant's foot, taking care not to touch the cleansed area. Make a puncture approximately 1 to 2 mm deep in the infant's heel, making sure the infant's lateral, or side, portion of the heel pad is used. A pediatric-sized lancet, which limits the depth of puncture, should be used. If possible, recent puncture sites should always be avoided.				
6	Wipe away the first drop of blood with a gauze pad.				

No.	Step	Points	Check #1	Check #2	Check #3
7	To collect blood for the test, press the back side of the filter paper test card against the infant's heel while exerting gentle pressure on the heel. The drop of blood should be large enough to completely fill and soak through the circle. *Do not* layer the multiple blood drops within a single circle. Completely fill all of the circles on the test card.				
8	Hold a cotton ball over the puncture and apply gentle pressure until the bleeding stops. Do not apply a bandage.				
9	Properly dispose of all waste in biohazard container.				
10	Remove the gloves and wash hands.				
11	*Ask the parents if they have any questions and provide appropriate responses.*				
12	Allow the PKU test card to completely dry on a nonabsorbent surface at room temperature.				
13	After the test card is dry, complete the PKU test card with all patient and provider information.				
14	Place the test card in the mailer envelope and send it to the laboratory within 2 days.				
15	Document the procedure in patient's chart. When test results are returned, they should be initialed by the provider and be placed in the lab section of patient's chart.				
Student's Total Points					
Points Possible					
Final Score (Student's Total Points/Possible Points)					

Instructor's/Evaluator's Comments and Suggestions:

_____
_____
_____
_____
_____
_____
_____

CHECK #1	
Evaluator's Signature:	Date:

CHECK #2	
Evaluator's Signature:	Date:

CHECK #3	
Evaluator's Signature:	Date:

Work Documentation Form(s)

Lab Requisition form can be downloaded from the Premium Website

ABHES Competencies: MA.A.1.8.cc Communicate on the recipient's level of comprehension; MA.A.1.9.i Use Standard Precautions; MA.A.1.10.d (2) Collect, label, and process specimens: Perform capillary puncture

CAAHEP Competencies: I.A.2 Use language/verbal skills that enable patients' understanding; I.P.3 Perform capillary puncture; III.P.2 Practice Standard Precautions

Name _____ **Date** _____ **Score** _____

COMPETENCY ASSESSMENT

Procedure 44-4: Measurement of Blood Glucose Using an Automated Analyzer

Task: Measure blood glucose level.

Conditions:
- Gloves
- Goggles
- Safety lancet
- Alcohol swabs
- Glucose analyzer
- Adhesive strip
- Gauze 2 × 2
- Control solutions for glucose analyzer
- Test strips for glucose analyzer
- Laboratory tissues
- Cotton balls

Standards: Perform Task within 15 minutes with a minimum score of ___ points, as determined by your instructor.

Competency Assessment Information

Use the following information for blood to be drawn and complete the Lab Report form (Work Documentation).

Use today's date and time. Patient's name is Carol Ogren. Her address is 7246 Maple Valley Road, River City, NY 98765. She is female, and has no insurance. Her chart/medical record number is 65214. Her birth date is 8/6/1950. She last ate 3 hours ago.

Dr. King has requested a capillary glucose check.

Time began: _____   **Time ended:** _____   **Total time:** _____

No.	Step	Points	Check #1	Check #2	Check #3
1	*Paying attention to detail,* review the manufacturer's manual for the specific glucose analyzer being used. Turn on the analyzer.				
2	Clean the work area and assemble all materials and supplies.				
3	Wash hands. Put on gloves and goggles.				
4	Record the control ranges, control lot number, and test strip lot number.				
5	Perform the check test and the control test according to the manufacturer's instructions. If both tests are within range, proceed to the glucose test. Repeat both tests if either is out of acceptable range.				

No.	Step	Points	Check #1	Check #2	Check #3
To perform the glucose test:					
6	Remove a test strip from the bottle and replace the lid.				
7	Insert the test strip into the test chamber.				
8	Perform a capillary puncture. Wipe first drop with gauze.				
9	Apply a large drop of blood to the test strip.				
10	While the test is running, check the puncture site. If the bleeding has stopped, apply an adhesive strip.				
11	After the appropriate time interval has passed, read the glucose concentration.				
12	Properly dispose of all waste in a biohazard waste container.				
13	Remove gloves and wash hands.				
14	Document the procedure in the progress notes. Complete a lab report. After the provider has initialed the report, it should be filed in the lab section of patient's chart.				
Student's Total Points					
Points Possible					
Final Score (Student's Total Points/Possible Points)					

Instructor's/Evaluator's Comments and Suggestions:

_____

_____

_____

_____

_____

_____

_____

CHECK #1	
Evaluator's Signature:	Date:

CHECK #2	
Evaluator's Signature:	Date:

CHECK #3	
Evaluator's Signature:	Date:

Work Documentation Form(s)

*Lab Report form can be downloaded from the Premium Website

ABHES Competencies: MA.A.1.8.cc Communicate on the recipient's level of comprehension; MA.A.1.9.i Use Standard Precautions; MA.A.1.10.b (6) Perform selected CLIA-waived tests that assist with diagnosis and treatment: Kit testing; MA.A.1.10.d (2) Collect, label and process specimens: Perform capillary puncture

CAAHEP Competencies: I.A.2 Use language/verbal skills that enable patients' understanding; I.P.3 Perform capillary puncture; III.P.2 Practice Standard Precautions

Name_____ **Date**_____ **Score**_____

● COMPETENCY ASSESSMENT

Procedure 44-5:   Cholesterol Testing

Task:　　　　Measure cholesterol and triglyceride for monitoring purposes.

Conditions:
- Gloves
- Blood-collecting equipment
- Pipettes with disposable tips
- Disinfectant
- CLIA waived commercial kit for manual determination of cholesterol
- Controls and standards
- Marking pen
- Biohazard container

Standards:　Perform the Task within 15 minutes with a minimum score of ___ points, as determined by your instructor.

Competency Assessment Information

Use the following information to complete the Lab Report form (Work Documentation).

Use today's date and time. Patient's name is Lee Thimbles. Her address is 1805 Cornwall Avenue, River City, NY 98765. She is female, and has Regence insurance (71516). Her chart/medical record number is 925247. Her birth date is April 30, 1955. She has not eaten for 10 hours.

Dr. Lewis has requested a cholesterol screening check be performed.

Time began: _____ **Time ended:** _____ **Total time:** _____

No.	Step	Points	Check #1	Check #2	Check #3
1	Assemble all necessary equipment and materials.				
2	Wash hands; apply gloves.				
3	Obtain a blood sample from the patient, either by fingerstick or venipuncture, depending on the manufacturer's instructions.				
4	*Paying attention to detail,* follow the manufacturer's instructions to perform the cholesterol test. Be sure to run the controls also.				
5	Properly dispose of all waste in biohazard container.				
6	Record the results of the test on a laboratory report form and document the procedure in the patient's chart. After the provider has initialed the report, file it in the patient's chart.				
Student's Total Points					
Points Possible					
Final Score (Student's Total Points/Possible Points)					

Instructor's/Evaluator's Comments and Suggestions:

_____
_____
_____
_____
_____
_____
_____

CHECK #1	
Evaluator's Signature:	Date:

CHECK #2	
Evaluator's Signature:	Date:

CHECK #3	
Evaluator's Signature:	Date:

Work Documentation Form(s)

*Lab Report form can be downloaded from the Premium Website

ABHES Competencies: MA.A.1.8.cc Communicate on the recipient's level of comprehension; MA.A.1.9.i.i Use Standard Precautions

CAAHEP Competencies: I.A.2 Use language/verbal skills that enable patients' understanding; III.P.2 Practice Standard Precautions

Name_____ **Date**_____ **Score**_____

● **COMPETENCY ASSESSMENT**

Procedure 45-1: Completing a Medical Incident Report

Task: To complete an accurate medical incident report providing all legally required information and to submit it in a timely manner.

Conditions: • Appropriate medical incident report form or computer with Incident Report Software
• Notes taken regarding incident

Standards: Perform the Task within 15 minutes with a minimum score of ___ points, as determined by your instructor.

Time began: _____   **Time ended:** _____   **Total time:** _____

No.	Step	Points	Check #1	Check #2	Check #3
1	*Report the situations that were harmful* by discussing the incident with the employee(s) involved and read notes of pertinent information. Ask those who witnessed the incident to log when, where, and what they saw in their own words.				
2	*Paying attention to detail,* complete the clinic-approved Medical Incident Report form. A single-sheet, multiple-copy form is best. The form should contain basic patient identification data, a checklist of different incidents, and a space for written comments.				
3	The person completing the incident report form should be the individual who witnessed the incident, first discovered the incident, or is most familiar with the incident.				
4	Each section of the form must be completed. The incident description should be a brief narrative consisting of an objective description of the facts but should not draw any conclusions. Quotes should be used when appropriate with any unwitnessed incidents (e.g., "Patient states . . ."). The name(s) of any witnesses should be included on the report as well as employees directly involved in the incident.				
5	*Implement time management principles.* Incident reports must be submitted in a timely manner to the appropriate administrator or office following protocol identified in the Procedure Manual for the clinic. *Display sound judgment.*				
	Student's Total Points				
	Points Possible				
	Final Score (Student's Total Points/Possible Points)				

Instructor's/Evaluator's Comments and Suggestions:

_____

_____

_____

_____

_____

_____

CHECK #1	
Evaluator's Signature:	Date:

CHECK #2	
Evaluator's Signature:	Date:

CHECK #3	
Evaluator's Signature:	Date:

ABHES Competency: MA.A.1.4.e Perform risk management procedures

CAAHEP Competency: IX.P.6 Complete an incident report

Work Documentation Form(s)

U.S. Department of Labor
Occupational Safety and Health Administration

Form approved OMB no. 1218-0176

OSHA's Form 301
Injury and Illness Incident Report

This *Injury and Illness Incident Report* is one of the first forms you must fill out when a recordable work-related injury or illness has occurred. Together with the *Log of Work-Related Injuries and Illnesses* and the accompanying *Summary*, these forms help the employer and OSHA develop a picture of the extent and severity of work-related incidents.

Within 7 calendar days after you receive information that a recordable work-related injury or illness has occurred, you must fill out this form or an equivalent form. Some state workers' compensation, insurance, or other reports may be acceptable substitutes. To be considered an equivalent form, any substitute must contain all the information asked for on this form.

According to Public Law 91-596 and 29 CFR 1904, OSHA's recordkeeping rule, you must keep this form on file for 5 years following the year to which it pertains.

If you need additional copies of this form, you may photocopy and use as many as you need.

Attention: This form contains information relating to employee health and must be used in a manner that protects the confidentiality of employees to the extent possible while the information is being used for occupational safety and health purposes.

Information about the employee

1) Full name _____

2) Street _____
   City _____ State _____ ZIP _____

3) Date of birth ___ / ___ / ___

4) Date hired ___ / ___ / ___

5) ☐ Male
   ☐ Female

Information about the physician or other health care professional

6) Name of physician or other health care professional _____

7) If treatment was given away from the worksite, where was it given?
   Facility _____
   Street _____
   City _____ State _____ ZIP _____

8) Was employee treated in an emergency room?
   ☐ Yes
   ☐ No

9) Was employee hospitalized overnight as an in-patient?
   ☐ Yes
   ☐ No

Information about the case

10) Case number from the Log _____ *(Transfer the case number from the Log after you record the case.)*

11) Date of injury or illness ___ / ___ / ___

12) Time employee began work _____ AM / PM

13) Time of event _____ AM / PM ☐ Check if time cannot be determined

14) **What was the employee doing just before the incident occurred?** Describe the activity, as well as the tools, equipment, or material the employee was using. Be specific. *Examples:* "climbing a ladder while carrying roofing materials"; "spraying chlorine from hand sprayer"; "daily computer key-entry."

15) **What happened?** Tell us how the injury occurred. *Examples:* "When ladder slipped on wet floor, worker fell 20 feet"; "Worker was sprayed with chlorine when gasket broke during replacement"; "Worker developed soreness in wrist over time."

16) **What was the injury or illness?** Tell us the part of the body that was affected and how it was affected; be more specific than "hurt," "pain," or sore." *Examples:* "strained back"; "chemical burn, hand"; "carpal tunnel syndrome."

17) **What object or substance directly harmed the employee?** *Examples:* "concrete floor"; "chlorine"; "radial arm saw." *If this question does not apply to the incident, leave it blank.*

18) **If the employee died, when did death occur?** Date of death ___ / ___ / ___

Completed by _____

Title _____

Phone (____) ____ - ____   Date ___ / ___ / ___

Public reporting burden for this collection of information is estimated to average 22 minutes per response, including time for reviewing instructions, searching existing data sources, gathering and maintaining the data needed, and completing and reviewing the collection of information. Persons are not required to respond to the collection of information unless it displays a current valid OMB control number. If you have any comments about this estimate or any other aspects of this data collection, including suggestions for reducing this burden, contact: US Department of Labor, OSHA Office of Statistical Analysis, Room N-3644, 200 Constitution Avenue, NW, Washington, DC 20210. Do not send the completed forms to this office.

Courtesy of the U.S. Department of Labor, Occupational Safety and Health Administration

Name _____ **Date** _____ **Score** _____

COMPETENCY ASSESSMENT

Procedure 45-2: Preparing a Meeting Agenda

Task: To prepare a meeting agenda, a list of specific items to be discussed or acted on, and to maintain the focus of the group and allow business to be transacted in a timely fashion.

Conditions:
- List of participants
- Order of business
- Names of individuals giving reports
- Names of any guest speakers
- A computer and paper on which to print agendas

Standards: Perform the Task within 20 minutes with a minimum score of ___ points, as determined by your instructor.

Time began: _____ **Time ended:** _____ **Total time:** _____

No.	Step	Points	Check #1	Check #2	Check #3
1	*Pay attention to detail.* Reserve proposed date, time, and place of meeting.				
2	*Pay attention to detail.* Collect information for meeting agenda by previewing the previous meeting's minutes for old business items, checking with others for report items, and determining any new business items.				
3	Prepare a hard copy of the agenda and have it approved by the chair of the meeting.				
4	*Implement time management principles.* Send agenda to meeting participants a few days in advance of the meeting.				
Student's Total Points					
Points Possible					
Final Score (Student's Total Points/Possible Points)					

Instructor's/Evaluator's Comments and Suggestions:

_____

_____

_____

_____

_____

_____

CHECK #1 Evaluator's Signature:	Date:

CHECK #2 Evaluator's Signature:	Date:

CHECK #3 Evaluator's Signature:	Date:

ABHES Competency: MA.A.1.8.jj Perform fundamental writing skills including correct grammar, spelling, and formatting techniques when writing prescriptions, documenting medical records, etc.

CAAHEP Competency: IV.P.2 Report relevant information to others succinctly and accurately

Name_____ **Date**_____ **Score**_____

COMPETENCY ASSESSMENT

Procedure 45-3:   Supervising a Student Practicum

Task: To prepare a training path for a student extern being assigned to the clinic, make the involved personnel aware of their responsibilities, preplan the jobs the student will perform and in what sequence they will be assigned, and try to make the practicum successful by providing as much supervision and assistance as necessary.

Conditions:
- A schedule log, calendar
- Office procedures manual
- Any criteria presented by the program director.

Standards: Perform the Task within 30 minutes with a minimum score of ___ points, as determined by your instructor.

Time began: _____ **Time ended:** _____ **Total time:** _____

No.	Step	Points	Check #1	Check #2	Check #3
1	*Pay attention to detail.* Review the clinical practicum contract between your agency and the educational institution.				
2	Determine the amount of supervision the student will require.				
3	Identify the supervisor who will be immediately responsible for the student.				
4	*Working within your scope of practice,* plan which tasks the student will be allowed or encouraged to perform.				
5	Create a schedule outlining the time the student will be assigned to each unit.				
6	*Develop a strategic, realistic plan to achieve your goals by* orientating the student as soon as he or she arrives at the office. Include a tour of the office and introduction to the staff.				
7	Give the student a copy of the Clinic Policy Manual and the work schedule for the entire practicum. Answer any questions the student might have.				
8	*Pay attention to detail* by maintaining an accurate record of the hours the student works. Also log the date and reason for any missed days, late arrivals, or early dismissals.				
9	Check with the student frequently to be sure the student is receiving meaningful training from the work experience.				
10	Consult providers and staff members with whom the student has worked for their opinion of the student's capabilities. Follow up on any problems that might be identified.				

No.	Step	Points	Check #1	Check #2	Check #3
11	Report the student's progress to the medical assisting supervisor from the educational institution. This person usually visits once or twice each rotation.				
12	Prepare the student evaluation report from comments provided by the supervisor assigned and each employee who worked with the student.				
Student's Total Points					
Points Possible					
Final Score (Student's Total Points/Possible Points)					

Instructor's/Evaluator's Comments and Suggestions:

_____

_____

_____

_____

_____

_____

CHECK #1	
Evaluator's Signature:	Date:

CHECK #2	
Evaluator's Signature:	Date:

CHECK #3	
Evaluator's Signature:	Date:

ABHES Competency: MA.A.1.8.kk Adapt to individualized needs

CAAHEP Competency: IV.P.4 Explain general office policies

Name _____   **Date** _____   **Score** _____

COMPETENCY ASSESSMENT

Procedure 45-4:   Developing and Maintaining a Procedure Manual

Task: To develop and maintain a comprehensive, up-to-date procedure manual covering each medical, technical, and administrative procedure in the office with step-by-step directions and rationales for performing each task.

Conditions:
- A computer
- Three-ring binder
- Paper
- Standard procedure manual format

Standards: Perform the Task within 20 minutes with a minimum score of ___ points, as determined by your instructor.

Time began: _____   **Time ended:** _____   **Total time:** _____

No.	Step	Points	Check #1	Check #2	Check #3
1	*Pay attention to detail* by writing detailed, step-by-step procedures and rationales for each medical, technical, and administrative function. Each procedure is written by experienced employees close to the function and then reviewed by a supervisor or clinic manager.				
2	Include regular maintenance instructions and flow sheets for the cleaning, servicing, and calibrating of all clinic equipment, both in the clinical area and in the office/business areas.				
3	Include step-by-step instructions on how to accomplish each task in the office/clinic in both the clinical and in the administrative areas.				
4	Include local and out-of-the-area resources for clinical and administrative staff, providers, and patients. Provide a listing in each area with contact information and services provided.				
5	*Recognize the importance of local, state, and federal legislation and regulations* that are related to processes performed in both clinical and administrative areas.				
6	Include the clinic procedures and flow sheets for taking inventory in each of the areas, and instructions on ordering procedures.				
7	Collect the procedures into the Clinic Procedure Manual.				
8	Store one complete manual in a common library area. Provide a completed copy to the provider–employer and the clinic manager. Distribute appropriate sections to the various departments.				

No.	Step	Points	Check #1	Check #2	Check #3
9	Review the procedure manual annually and add any new procedures, delete or modify as necessary, and indicate the revision date (e.g., Rev. 10/12/XX).				
	Student's Total Points				
	Points Possible				
	Final Score (Student's Total Points/Possible Points)				

Instructor's/Evaluator's Comments and Suggestions:

_____

_____

_____

_____

_____

_____

CHECK #1	
Evaluator's Signature:	Date:

CHECK #2	
Evaluator's Signature:	Date:

CHECK #3	
Evaluator's Signature:	Date:

ABHES Competency: MA.A.1.8.d Apply concepts for office procedures

CAAHEP Competencies: IX.P.5 Incorporate the Patient's Bill of Rights into personal practice and medical office policies and procedures; IX.P.8 Apply local, state, and federal health care legislation and regulation appropriate to the medical assisting practice setting

Name _____ **Date** _____ **Score** _____

COMPETENCY ASSESSMENT

Procedure 45-5: Making Travel Arrangements with a Travel Agent

Task: To make travel arrangements for the provider.

Conditions:
- Travel plan/preferences
- Telephone and telephone directory
- Computer
- Provider's or clinic credit card to pay for reservations.

Standards: Perform the Task within 20 minutes with a minimum score of ___ points, as determined by your instructor.

Time began: _____   **Time ended:** _____   **Total time:** _____

No.	Step	Points	Check #1	Check #2	Check #3
1	*Pay attention to detail* by confirming the trip dates, time, and place for departure and arrival; preferred mode of transportation (plane, train, bus, car); number of travelers; preferred lodging type and price range; and whether travelers checks are required.				
2	Make travel and lodging reservations by calling travel agent or using the computer for online ticket services.				
3	Pick up tickets or arrange for their delivery.				
4	Check to see that ticket arrangements are accurate (dates, times, places).				
5	Check to see that car rental and lodging accommodations are accurate and confirmed.				
6	Make additional copies of the itinerary or create the itinerary if making arrangements via computer. The itinerary should list date and time of departures and arrivals, including flight numbers and seat assignments. Note mode of transportation to lodging (shuttle, bus, car, taxi). Include name, address, and telephone number of lodgings and meeting places.				
7	Maintain one copy of the itinerary in the clinic file.				
8	Give several copies of the itinerary to the provider.				
	Student's Total Points				
	Points Possible				
	Final Score (Student's Total Points/Possible Points)				

Instructor's/Evaluator's Comments and Suggestions:

_____

_____

_____

_____

_____

_____

CHECK #1	
Evaluator's Signature:	Date:

CHECK #2	
Evaluator's Signature:	Date:

CHECK #3	
Evaluator's Signature:	Date:

Name _____ **Date** _____ **Score** _____

● COMPETENCY ASSESSMENT

Procedure 45-6: Making Travel Arrangements via the Internet

Task: To make travel arrangements for the provider using the Internet.

Conditions:
- A travel plan/preferences
- Computer
- Provider's or clinic credit card to pay for reservations

Standards: Perform the Task within 20 minutes with a minimum score of ___ points, as determined by your instructor.

Time began: _____   **Time ended:** _____   **Total time:** _____

No.	Step	Points	Check #1	Check #2	Check #3
1	*Pay attention to detail* by confirming the planned trip dates, time, and place for departure and arrival; preferred mode of transportation (plane, train, bus, car); number of travelers; preferred lodging type and price range; and whether travelers checks are required.				
2	Go to the computer and access the Internet.				
3	*Show initiative* by selecting a search engine to locate Web pages using the key term "air fares." Web pages may provide links to air fares, auto reservations, and hotel/motel reservations. Follow Web page instructions for making arrangements. Review and copy confirmation of your transaction.				
4	Pick up tickets or arrange for their delivery, if necessary. Tickets purchased on the Internet can be mailed or picked up at an airport, or they can be electronic tickets.				
5	Make additional copies of the itinerary or create the itinerary. The itinerary should list date and time of departures and arrivals, including flight numbers and seat assignments. Note the mode of transportation to lodging (shuttle, bus, car, taxi). Include name, address, and telephone number of lodgings and meeting places.				
6	Maintain one copy of the itinerary in the clinic file.				
7	Give several copies of the itinerary to the provider.				
Student's Total Points					
Points Possible					
Final Score (Student's Total Points/Possible Points)					

Instructor's/Evaluator's Comments and Suggestions:

_____

_____

_____

_____

_____

_____

CHECK #1 Evaluator's Signature:	Date:

CHECK #2 Evaluator's Signature:	Date:

CHECK #3 Evaluator's Signature:	Date:

CAAHEP Competency: V.P.7 Use Internet to access information related to the medical office

Name _____ **Date** _____ **Score** _____

COMPETENCY ASSESSMENT

Procedure 45-7:   Processing Employee Payroll

Task: To process payroll compensating employees, calculating all deductions accurately.

Conditions: • Computer and payroll software or checkbook
                  • Tax withholding tables
                  • Federal Employers Tax Guide

Standards: Perform the Task within 45 minutes with a minimum score of ___ points, as determined by your instructor.

Time began: _____   **Time ended:** _____   **Total time:** _____

No.	Step	Points	Check #1	Check #2	Check #3
1	Verify that copies of the employee's Social Security card and current I-9 and W-4 forms are in each employee file.				
2	Review time cards looking for any tardiness, early dismissals, or absences.				
3	Calculate the salary or hourly wages due the employee for the work period.				
4	*Pay attention to detail* by calculating any deductions that must be withheld from the paycheck. These may include federal, state, and local taxes; Social Security withholdings; Medicare withholdings; insurance; savings; or donations.				
5	Use computer and payroll software or hand write the payroll check and explanation of deductions.				
6	Distribute individual payroll checks in envelopes according to clinic protocol.				
Student's Total Points					
Points Possible					
Final Score (Student's Total Points/Possible Points)					

Instructor's/Evaluator's Comments and Suggestions:

_____

_____

_____

_____

_____

_____

CHECK #1	
Evaluator's Signature:	Date:

CHECK #2	
Evaluator's Signature:	Date:

CHECK #3	
Evaluator's Signature:	Date:

Name _____ **Date** _____ **Score** _____

COMPETENCY ASSESSMENT

Procedure 45-8:   Perform an Inventory of Equipment and Supplies

Task: To develop an inventory of expendable administrative and clinical supplies in a medical office.

Conditions:
- Computer
- Printout of most recent inventory spreadsheet
- Inventory checklist
- Clipboard, pad of reorder forms, pen or pencil

Standards: Perform the Task within 15 minutes with a minimum score of ___ points, as determined by your instructor.

Time began: _____   **Time ended:** _____   **Total time:** _____

No.	Step	Points	Check #1	Check #2	Check #3
1	*Pay attention to detail.* Compare number of items on hand corresponding to each name or code identification number with the printout, and write in the new inventory number on the printout.				
2	If the number of any item is less than the minimum quantity, fill out a reorder form listing completely the name, identification number, and quantity required.				
3	Repeat the previous step for each storage location on the inventory printout sheet.				
4	After completing the inventory, enter the new inventory information, including date of inventory, quantity, and date of reorder request, into the computer database.				
5	Forward the reorder forms to the person responsible for purchasing.				
	Student's Total Points				
	Points Possible				
	Final Score (Student's Total Points/Possible Points)				

Instructor's/Evaluator's Comments and Suggestions:

_____

_____

_____

_____

_____

_____

CHECK #1	
Evaluator's Signature:	Date:

CHECK #2	
Evaluator's Signature:	Date:

CHECK #3	
Evaluator's Signature:	Date:

ABHES Competency: MA.A.1.8.z Maintain inventory equipment and supplies

CAAHEP Competency: V.P.10 Perform an office inventory

Work Documentation Form(s): Inventory Checklist

Inventory Performed By:

Date:

Item	Supply Minimum	Amount on Hand	Reorder?

© Cengage Learning 2014

Name _____ **Date** _____ **Score** _____

COMPETENCY ASSESSMENT

Procedure 45-9:   Perform Routine Maintenance and Calibration of Clinical Equipment

Task: To ensure the operability and calibration of clinical equipment.

Conditions: • Equipment list with maintenance or calibration requirements
               • Clipboard, pen with black ink, maintenance log and service calendar log forms, and deficiency tags
               • Access to operation and service manuals of equipment to be serviced
               • Access to any necessary maintenance tools and supplies

Standards: Perform the Task within 30 minutes with a minimum score of ___ points, as determined by your instructor.

Time began: _____   **Time ended:** _____   **Total time:** _____

No.	Step	Points	Check #1	Check #2	Check #3
1	Locate the number assigned by the clinic manager to identify the equipment being serviced and verify serial number, manufacturer/maker, technical support phone number, warranty information, and last date of service.				
2	*Pay attention to detail by* visually inspecting each piece of equipment associated with the clinical area. • *Practice risk management principles* by checking for any frayed electrical cords, loose connections, or safety issues such as tripping hazards associated with electrical cords. • Clean each item according to manufacturer specifications, and replace light bulbs and batteries if necessary.				
3	Check to ensure the equipment meets operational/calibration standards as defined in the operation and service manual. Recalibrate the equipment following the instructions in the manual if required.				
4	*Follow necessary safety precautions* and tag any equipment not meeting operational standards and report the deficiency.				
5	Fill out and sign the maintenance record sheet if the equipment meets operations standards.				
6	*Pay attention to detail.* Complete documentation form by verifying information for each piece of equipment serviced and/or calibrated. Complete the appropriate information for service using the Service Calendar Log form.				
Student's Total Points					
Points Possible					
Final Score (Student's Total Points/Possible Points)					

Instructor's/Evaluator's Comments and Suggestions:

CHECK #1	
Evaluator's Signature:	Date:

CHECK #2	
Evaluator's Signature:	Date:

CHECK #3	
Evaluator's Signature:	Date:

ABHES Competency: MA.A.1.8.y Perform routine maintenance of administrative and clinical equipment

CAAHEP Competency: V.P.9 Perform routine maintenance of office equipment with documentation

Work Documentation Form(s)

Maintenance Log

Name of Equipment	Serial Number	Mfg/Maker	Technical Support Phone Number	Purchase Date	Service Plan	Last Serviced	Completed By
EKG #8	80462	HP	xxx-xxx-xxxx	1/20/xx	On file	6/12/xx	bql
Centrifuge #3	79031	HP	xxx-xxx-xxxx	7/20/xx	On file	6/12/xx	bql

Service Calendar Log Form

January	February	March	April	May	June	July	August	September	October	November	December

Name _____ **Date** _____ **Score** _____

COMPETENCY ASSESSMENT

Procedure 46-1: Develop and Maintain a Policy Manual

Task: To develop and maintain a comprehensive, up-to-date policy manual of all clinic policies relating to employee practices, benefits, clinic conduct, and so on.

Conditions:
- Computer
- Three-ring binder
- Paper
- Standard policy manual format

Standards: Perform the Task within 20 minutes with a minimum score of ___ points, as determined by your instructor.

Time began: _____   **Time ended:** _____   **Total time:** _____

No.	Step	Points	Check #1	Check #2	Check #3
1	*Paying attention to detail,* develop precise, written clinic policies detailing all necessary information pertaining to the staff and their positions. The information should include benefits, vacation, sick leave, hours, dress codes, evaluations, rules of conduct, and grounds for dismissal.				
2	Identify procedures for reimbursing overtime, preventing discrimination and harassment, creating a safe workplace, and allowing for jury duty.				
3	Include a policy statement related to rules of conduct.				
4	Identify steps to follow should an employee become disabled during employment.				
5	Determine what employee opportunities for continuing education will be reimbursed and include requirements for recertification and licensure.				
6	Provide a copy of the policy manual for each employee.				
7	Review and update the policy manual regularly. Add or delete items as necessary, dating each revised page.				
Student's Total Points					
Points Possible					
Final Score (Student's Total Points/Possible Points)					

Instructor's/Evaluator's Comments and Suggestions:

_____
_____
_____
_____
_____
_____
_____

CHECK #1	
Evaluator's Signature:	Date:

CHECK #2	
Evaluator's Signature:	Date:

CHECK #3	
Evaluator's Signature:	Date:

CAAHEP Competency: IV.P.4 Explain general office policies

Name _____ **Date** _____ **Score** _____

COMPETENCY ASSESSMENT

Procedure 46-2: Prepare a Job Description

Task: To develop a precise definition of the tasks assigned to a job; to determine the expectations and level of competency required; and to specify the experience, training, and education needed to perform the job for purposes of recruiting and performance evaluation.

Conditions: • Computer
• Paper
• Standard job description format

Standards: Perform the Task within 20 minutes with a minimum score of ___ points, as determined by your instructor.

Time began: _____ **Time ended:** _____ **Total time:** _____

No.	Step	Points	Check #1	Check #2	Check #3
1	*Paying attention to detail,* describe each task that creates the job.				
2	List special medical, technical, or clerical skills required.				
3	Determine the level of education, training, and experience required for the position.				
4	Determine where the job fits into the overall structure of the practice.				
5	Specify any unusual working conditions (hours, locations, etc.) that may apply.				
6	Describe career path opportunities.				
7	Review and update the job description regularly. Add or delete items as necessary, dating each revision.				
Student's Total Points					
Points Possible					
Final Score (Student's Total Points/Possible Points)					

Instructor's/Evaluator's Comments and Suggestions:

_____

_____

_____

_____

_____

_____

_____

CHECK #1	
Evaluator's Signature:	Date:

CHECK #2	
Evaluator's Signature:	Date:

CHECK #3	
Evaluator's Signature:	Date:

CAAHEP Competency: IV.P.4 Explain general office policies

Name_____   **Date**_____   **Score**_____

COMPETENCY ASSESSMENT

Procedure 46-3:   Conduct Interviews

Task: To screen applicants for training, experience, and characteristics to select the best candidate to fill the position vacancy.

Conditions: • Interview questions
              • Policy manual (for referencing)
              • Applicant's résumé, application, and cover letter

Standards: Perform the Task within 40 minutes with a minimum score of ___ points, as determined by your instructor.

Time began: _____   **Time ended:** _____   **Total time:** _____

No.	Step	Points	Check #1	Check #2	Check #3
1	*Paying attention to detail,* review résumés and applications received.				
2	Select candidates who most closely match the education and experience being sought.				
3	*Develop a strategic plan* for conducting the interviews by creating an interview worksheet for each candidate listing points to cover.				
4	Select an interview team; this team should always include the HR or clinic manager and the immediate supervisor to whom the candidate will report.				
5	Call personally to schedule interviews.				
6	*Maintain ethical standards* by reminding the interviewers of various legal restrictions concerning questions to be asked.				
7	Conduct interviews in a private, quiet setting.				
8	Put the applicant at ease by beginning with an overview about the practice and staff, briefly describing the job, and answering preliminary questions.				
9	Ask questions about the applicant's work experience and educational background using the résumé and interview worksheet as a guide.				
10	Provide the most promising applicants additional information on benefits and a tour of the clinic, if practical.				
11	Applicant's general salary requirements may be discussed, but avoid discussion of a specific salary until a formal offer is tendered.				
12	Inform the applicants when a decision will be made and thank each for participating in the interview.				

No.	Step	Points	Check #1	Check #2	Check #3
13	Do not make a job offer until all the candidates have been interviewed.				
14	Check references of all prospective employees.				
15	Establish a second interview between the provider–employer(s) and the qualified candidate if necessary.				
16	Confirm accepted job offers in writing, specifying details of the offer and acceptance.				
17	*Show respect* by notifying all unsuccessful applicants by letter when the position has been filled.				
Student's Total Points					
Points Possible					
Final Score (Student's Total Points/Possible Points)					

Instructor's/Evaluator's Comments and Suggestions:

_____

_____

_____

_____

_____

_____

_____

CHECK #1	
Evaluator's Signature:	Date:

CHECK #2	
Evaluator's Signature:	Date:

CHECK #3	
Evaluator's Signature:	Date:

ABHES Competencies: MA.A.1.8.ff Interview effectively; MA.A.1.8.ii Recognize and respond to verbal and non-verbal communication

CAAHEP Competencies: IV.P.2 Report relevant information to others succinctly and accurately; IV.P.4 Explain general office policies

Name _____ **Date** _____ **Score** _____

COMPETENCY ASSESSMENT

Procedure 46-4: Orient Personnel

Task: To acquaint new employees with clinic policies, staff, what the job encompasses, procedures to be performed, and job performance expectations.

Conditions: • Policy manual

Standards: Perform the Task within 30 minutes with a minimum score of ___ points, as determined by your instructor.

Time began: _____   **Time ended:** _____   **Total time:** _____

No.	Step	Points	Check #1	Check #2	Check #3
1	Tour the facilities and introduce the clinic staff.				
2	Complete employee-related documents and explain their purpose. Explain the benefits program.				
3	Present the clinic policy manual and discuss its key elements.				
4	*Review federal and state regulatory precautions for medical facilities.*				
5	Review the job description.				
6	Explain and demonstrate procedures to be performed and the use of procedure manuals supporting these procedures.				
7	Demonstrate the use of any specialized equipment (such as time clocks, key entries, etc.). Medical equipment would be demonstrated by clinical staff.				
8	Assign a mentor from the staff to help with the orientation.				
Student's Total Points					
Points Possible					
Final Score (Student's Total Points/Possible Points)					

Instructor's/Evaluator's Comments and Suggestions:

_____

_____

_____

_____

_____

_____

_____

CHECK #1	
Evaluator's Signature:	Date:

CHECK #2	
Evaluator's Signature:	Date:

CHECK #3	
Evaluator's Signature:	Date:

ABHES Competency: MA.A.1.1.d Have knowledge of the general responsibilities of the medical assistant

CAAHEP Competency: IV.P.4 Explain general office policies